RETINA AND VITREOUS

RETINA *and* VITREOUS

edited by
Rudolph M. Franklin

Proceedings of the Symposium on Retina and Vitreous,
New Orleans, LA, USA, March 12-15, 1992
organized by the
New Orleans Academy of Ophthalmology

Kugler Publications
Amsterdam/New York

Library of Congress Cataloging-in-Publication Data

Symposium on Retina and Vitreous (1992 : New Orleans, La.)
Retina and vitreous : proceedings of the Symposium on Retina and Vitreous, New Orleans, LA, USA, March 12-15. 1992 / organized by the New Orleans Academy of Ophthalmology : edited by Rudolph M. Franklin.
p. cm.
Includes bibliographical references.
ISBN 9062990916 :
1. Retina--Diseases--Congresses. 2. Vitreous body--Diseases--Congresses. 3. Vitreous humor--Diseases--Congresses. 4. Diabetic Retinopathy--therapy--congresses. I. Franklin, Rudolph M. II. New Orleans Academy of Ophthalmology. III. Title.
[DNLM: 1. Retinal Diseases--surgery--congresses. 2. Retinal Diseases--pathology--congresses. 3. Vitreous Body--surgery--congresses. 4. Vitreous Body--physiopathology--congresses. WW 270 S98807r 1992]
RE551.S927 1992
617.7'3--dc20
DNLM/DLC
for Library of Congress 93-12350
CIP

ISBN 90-6299-091-6

Distributor:
Kugler Publications
P.O. Box 11188
1001 GD Amsterdam, The Netherlands
Telefax (+31.20) 638-0524

TABLE OF CONTENTS

Preface

The New Orleans Academy of Ophthalmology provides its members and guests with educational forums throughout the year. The Annual Meeting of the Academy exposes the audience to the views and opinions of national and international experts. Each Annual Meeting reviews an area of ophthalmology in order to update the practicing ophthalmologist with the latest information on diagnosis, therapy, and surgical technique. The 41st Symposium of the New Orleans Academy of Ophthalmology, "Retina and Vitreous", heard a series of presentations from seven world-renowned ophthalmic investigators, teachers, and practitioners.

The Symposium was held in New Orleans on March 12-15, 1992. The lectures were organized in mini-symposia which were followed by round-table discussions by the seven guest speakers or by question and answer periods. The round-table discussions enhanced the symposia, and have been included in this volume. This review of retina and vitreous disorders was well received by all who attended, and should provide a timely update for the reader of this volume.

R.M. Franklin, M.D.
Editor

Acknowledgments

The Program Committee deserves much of the credit for organizing the excellent Symposium.

William F. Rachal, M.D., Chairman
Laurence W. Arend, M.D.
Rudolph M. Franklin, M.D.

The members of the New Orleans Academy of Ophthalmology, especially the Officers and Executive Committee, deserve thanks for the important roles in making this Symposium a success. The leadership of Rodney Kahlil, M.D., then President, with the assistance of Emily Busby, Executive Secretary, assured the success of this 41st Annual Symposium.

Rudolph M. Franklin, M.D., President
New Orleans Academy of Ophthalmology

CONTRIBUTORS

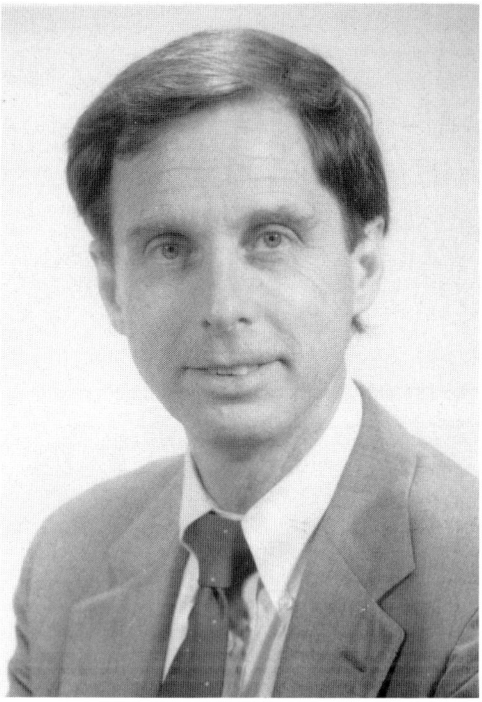

THOMAS M. AABERG, MD, FACS
Department of Ophthalmology
Emory University School of Medicine
Atlanta, Georgia, USA

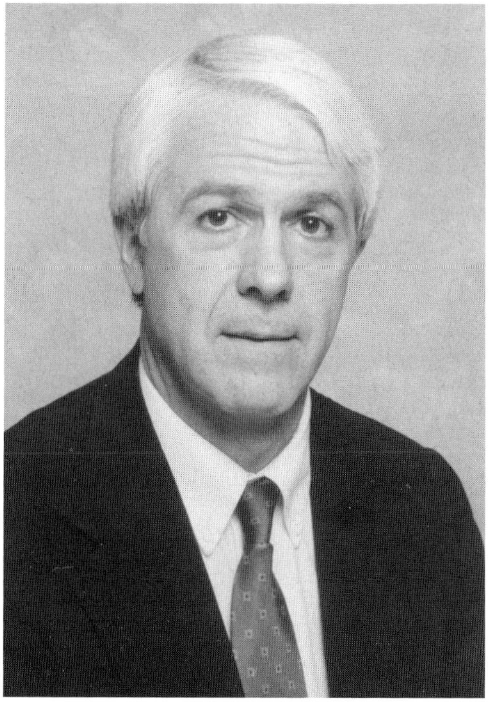

GARY W. ABRAMS, MD
Associated Retinal Consultants
Royal Oak, Michigan, USA

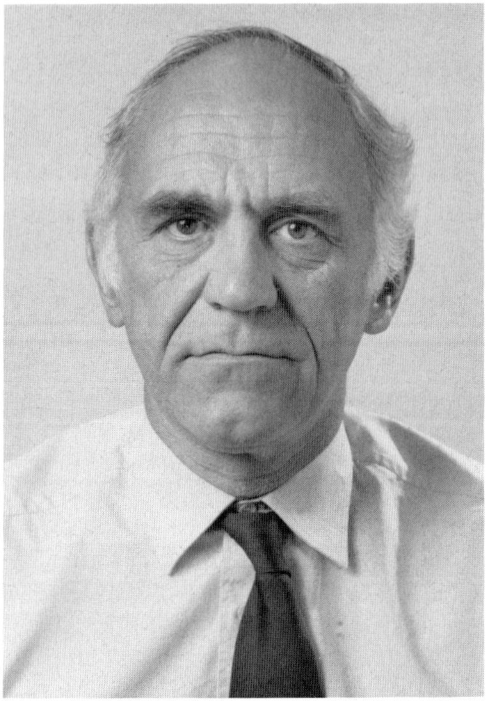

A.C. BIRD, MD
Department of Clinical Ophthalmology
Institute of Ophthalmology
Moorfields Eye Hospital
London, United Kingdom

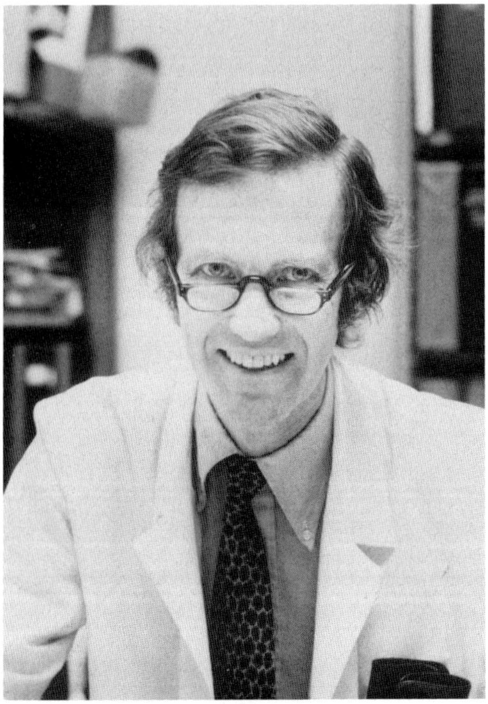

MATTHEW D. DAVIS, MD
Department of Ophthalmology
University of Wisconsin-Madison
Madison, Wisconsin, USA

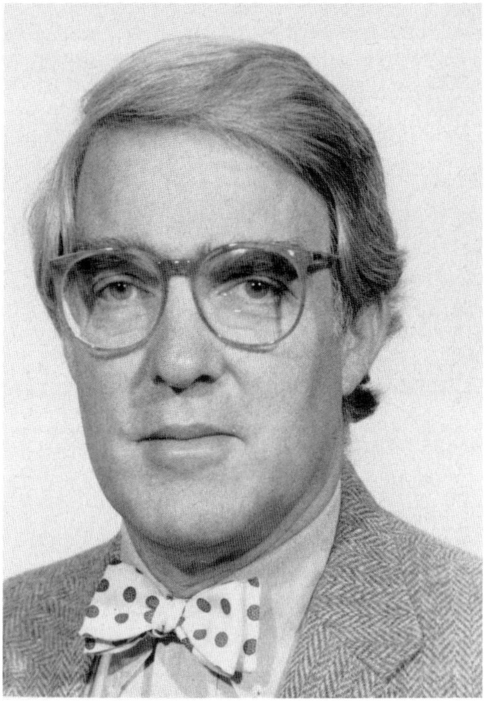

STUART L. FINE, MD
Department of Ophthalmology
Scheie Eye Institute
Philadelphia, Pennsylvania, USA

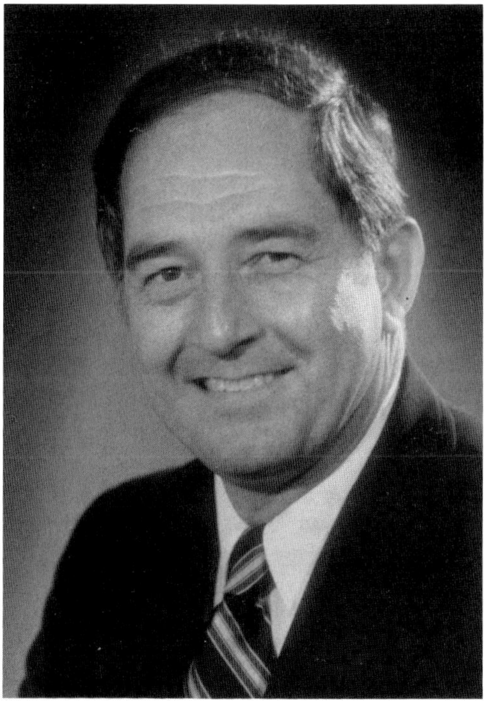

J. DONALD M. GASS, MD
Bascom Palmer Eye Institute
University of Miami School of Medicine
Miami, Florida, USA

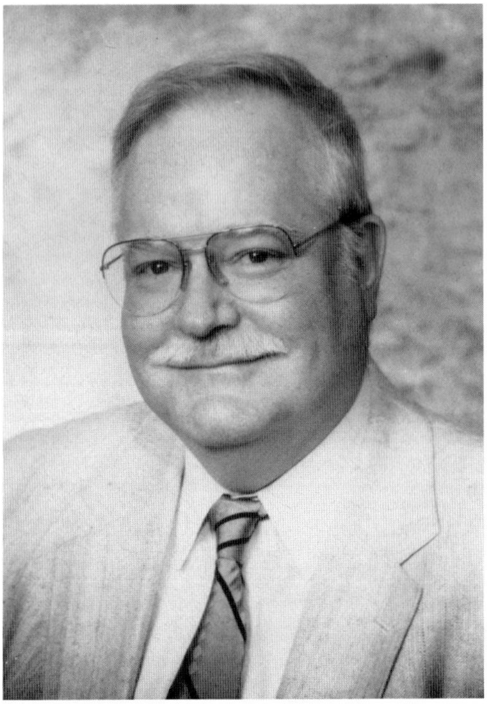

W. RICHARD GREEN, MD
The Eye Pathology Laboratory
Johns Hopkins Hospital
Baltimore, Maryland, USA

I

AGE-RELATED MACULAR DEGENERATION

AGE-RELATED MACULAR DEGENERATION, NATURAL COURSE AND RISK FACTORS

J. Donald M. Gass

Bascom Palmer Eye Institute, University of Miami School of Medicine, Miami, Florida, USA

The appearance of drusen in the macular region of both eyes is the earliest reliable sign of age-related macular degeneration (AMD)[1]. Although they typically appear during the sixth and seventh decades of life, they may be evident in the fourth decade or earlier. Most drusen are sharply circumscribed round mound-shaped elevations of the retinal pigment epithelium (RPE) and vary in size and color depending upon their consistency. In most patients there is a remarkable symmetry in the two eyes as to the number, size, shape and location of the drusen[2]. Although in most patients the drusen are clustered in the central macular areas, in others they may be located eccentrically. Drusen are described by various names depending upon their biomicroscopic appearance that does, in part, relate to their histologic appearance. Nodular or hard drusen are small, usually less than 50 microns in diameter, yellowish lesions. Histologically, they are hyaline deposits beneath the RPE. These small drusen probably have less to do with visual morbidity than the larger so-called soft drusen, which are grey or slightly yellowish, less well defined, and are often confluent[3,4]. Histologically, the sub-RPE material in these larger drusen is more granular and less eosinophilic. They are indistinguishable histopathologically from small serous detachments of the pigment epithelium. The biomicroscopic counterpart of diffuse thickening of the inner layers of Bruch's membrane is more difficult to recognize biomicroscopically. Patients with drusen may remain symptom free for many years. The evolution of drusen is variable. In general, drusen increase in size and number with age. In some cases, however, they disappear. As they increase in number and size, the patient begins to experience visual difficulties related to loss in contrast sensitivity and ability to adapt to change in lighting[5]. They frequently voluntarily stop driving at night even when their acuity is near normal.

Loss of central vision may occur slowly because of geographic atrophy of the RPE that often begins in the area of one or more large drusen and which becomes confluent and gradually enlarges concentrically over a period of many months[6,7]. As an area of eccentric geographic atrophy moves into the center of the macula, the patient may complain of relative rapid drop in acuity. There is a striking tendency for patients who develop geographic atrophy in one eye to do so in the other.

Slow loss of visual acuity may result from the progressive accumulation, enlargement and confluence of soft drusen to form a serous detachment of the RPE, that often has a scalloped border and a pigment figure on its surface[8]. These avascular RPE detachments develop slowly and the patient may maintain good acuity for many months or years. They occasionally flatten spontaneously. This may be accompanied by improvement in

Address for correspondence: J. Donald M. Gass, MD, Bascom Palmer Eye Institute, University of Miami School of Medicine, Miami, FL 33101, USA

Retina and Vitreous, pp. 3-6
Proceedings of the Symposium on Retina and Vitreous,
organized by the New Orleans Academy of Ophthalmology
New Orleans, LA, USA, March 12-15, 1992
edited by Rudolph M. Franklin

visual acuity and lessening of metamorphopsia. In others, however, the vision continues to worsen and geographic atrophy of the RPE appears in the area of RPE detachment.

Another mechanism of slow loss of visual acuity is the development of irregular elevation of the RPE caused by the ingrowth of occult choroidal neovascularization and fibrous tissue beneath the RPE. Because these occult areas of sub-RPE fibrovascular ingrowth may be unaccompanied by any evidence of exudation or hemorrhage and only minimal changes in the appearance of the overlying RPE, they are easily overlooked in patients complaining of mild metamorphopsia and visual loss. They are most easily detected by contact lens examination that permits detection of the often irregular area of RPE elevation. Stereo fluorescein angiography is also helpful in detecting these areas that may not show any, or often only minimal, late punctate staining. Visual loss in patients with occult neovascularization generally occurs at a slower rate than in those with well-defined actively leaking membranes[9].

Rapid loss of visual acuity in patients with AMD is caused by leakage of exudate and blood from choroidal neovascular membranes. In approximately 10 to 15% of cases, the recent dramatic change in acuity is caused by a sharply circumscribed, smooth-surfaced serous detachment of the RPE caused by a plaque or mound-shaped choroidal neovascular complex that, in most cases, lies within a notched area at one edge of the RPE detachment[10]. In some cases the new vessels lie beneath the RPE detachment, and in others, in the center of a donut-shaped area of serous RPE detachment. Stereoangiography is helpful in determining the location of this complex. Spontaneous tears in the RPE at a site away from the new vessels may occur and usually are accompanied by a rapid decline in visual acuity[11]. When this occurs in one eye, there is a great risk of the same complication occurring in the second eye[12,13].

In 80 to 90% of patients rapid loss of central vision is caused by a combination of serous and hemorrhagic detachment of the RPE and retina. In the majority of these patients, angiography will demonstrate that the neovascular complex is either poorly defined or is subfoveal[14]. When the membrane is well defined, the chances of the visual acuity declining to 20/200 or less within one year are approximately 50% for extrafoveal membranes, and 70% for juxtafoveal and subfoveal membranes. Regardless of their location, most of these lesions untreated will progress within months or several years to form a hypertrophic disciform scar with or without chronic serous and hemorrhagic exudative retinal detachment confined to the macula[15]. There is a tendency for symmetry in the appearance of the end-stage disciform scar in the two eyes[16]. In some patients the degree of scarring is less and involution of the new vessels is so complete that they may be difficult or impossible to detect within a large zone of geographic atrophy of the RPE. In probably 5% of eyes, spontaneous involution of the neovascularization may occur prior to spread into the center of the macula, or in spite of spread through the central macula it may not cause major damage to the overlying sensory retina[17]. Although most patients retain central vision in the range of 20/200 to 5/200 after disciform detachment, the disciform exudative and hemorrhagic process may continue to expand over a period of years into the peripheral macular area and beyond. In some, the amount of subretinal yellow exudation may become so massive that the term senile Coat's disease is used. This may be associated with multicentric areas of neovascularization and occasionally bullous exudative retinal detachment. In 5% or less of cases, the initial sub-RPE and subretinal hemorrhage may involve most of the macular area, and within weeks the blood pigment may extend into the vitreous and obscure the fundus for many months. In a few cases, particularly in patients with systemic diseases, hypertension, leukemia or receiving anticoagulants, the initial hemorrhagic event may be so severe that a massive hemorrhagic detachment of the retina and choroid will produce narrowing of the anterior chamber angle and acute glaucoma[18,19].

AMD is one of the four most common causes of blindness in the United States[20]. Its cause is probably multifactorial[21]. The most important risk factors for development of AMD are probably the patient's genetic make-up, race, and age. Other risk factors of possible lesser importance include: cutaneous elastosis, exposure to visible light, sex, hand-grip strength, other medical diseases, mineral deficiency, white blood count, smoking, autoantibodies to retinal astrocytes, and increased scleral rigidity[22-25]. Other suggested factors with little supporting evidence include: alcoholic intake, smoking, refractive error, and height.

Most patients with macular drusen, the earliest sign of AMD, will go through life without becoming legally blind from the disorder. The mean age for patients to lose vision in the first eye caused by disciform detachment is approximately 65 years, and in the second eye is approximately 70 years of age. Risk factors for visual loss in a patient with early signs of AMD include the number, size, and location of drusen. The greater their number, the larger their size, and the more they are concentrated in the central macular area, the greater the risk of visual loss[26,27]. Other factors include patient's age and the presence of focal areas of RPE hyperpigmentation. The risk for severe visual loss in the first eye in a patient presenting with bilateral drusen is approximately 5 to 20% in five years. The risk of visual loss in the second eye is between 4 and 15% each year. The risk of the fellow eye loosing vision is only 10% in five years if it contains only small drusen and no focal areas of RPE hyperpigmentation, compared to a risk of 60% in five years if it has primarily large drusen (>50 μm) and focal RPE hyperpigmentation[27].

In summary, AMD is a prevalent disorder among Caucasians and while a variety of environmental risk factors for its development and progression have been suggested, genetic characteristics, race, and age appear to be its most important determinants.

References

1. Gass JDM: Drusen and disciform macular detachment and degeneration. Arch Ophthalmol 90:206-217, 1973
2. Barondes MJ, Pauleikhoff D, Chisholm IC, Minassian D, Bird AC: Bilaterality of drusen. Br J Ophthalmol 74:180-182, 1990
3. Coffey AJH, Brownstein S: The prevalence of macular drusen in postmortem eyes. Am J Ophthalmol 102:164-171, 1986
4. Sarks SH: Drusen and their relationship to senile macular degeneration. Austral J Ophthalmol 8:117-130, 1980
5. Sunness JS, Massof RW, Johnson MA, Bressler NM, Bressler SB, Fine SL: Diminished foveal sensitivity may predict the development of advanced age-related macular degeneration. Ophthalmology 96:375-380, 1989
6. Maguire P, Vine AK: Geographic atrophy of the retinal pigment epithelium. Am J Ophthalmol 102:621-625, 1986
7. Schatz H, McDonald HR: Atrophic macular degeneration. Ophthalmology 96:1541-1551, 1989
8. Pauleikhoff D, Barondes MJ, Minassian D, Chisholm IH, Bird AC: Drusen as risk factors in age-related macular disease. Am J Ophthalmol 109:38-43, 1990
9. Soubrane G, Coscas G, Francais C, Koenig F: Occult subretinal new vessels in age-related macular degeneration. Ophthalmology 97:649-657, 1990
10. Gass JDM: Serous retinal pigment epithelial detachment with a notch. Retina 4:205-220, 1984
11. Chuang EL, Bird AC: The pathogenesis of tears of the retinal pigment epithelium. Am J Ophthalmol 105:285-290, 1988
12. Chuang EL, Bird AC: Bilaterality of tears of the retinal pigment epithelium. Br J Ophthalmol 72:918-920, 1988
13. Schoeppner G, Chuang EL, Bird AC: The risk of fellow eye visual loss with unilateral retinal pigment epithelial tears. Am J Ophthalmol 108:683-685, 1989
14. Bressler NM, Bressler SB, Gragoudas ES: Clinical characteristics of choroidal neovascular membranes. Arch Ophthalmol 105:209-213, 1987

15. Bressler NM, Frost LA, Bressler SB, Murphy RP, Fine SL: Natural course of poorly defined choroidal neovascularization associated with macular degeneration. Arch Ophthalmol 106:1537-1542, 1988
16. Lavin MJ, Eldem B, Gregor ZJ: Symmetry of disciform scars in bilateral age-related macular degeneration. Br J Ophthalmol 75:133-136, 1991
17. Campochiaro PA, Morgan KM, Conway BP, Stathos J: Spontaneous involution of subfoveal neovascularization. Am J Ophthalmol 109:668-675, 1990
18. El Baba F, Jarrett WH II, Harbin TS, Fine SL, Michaels RG, Schachat AP, Green WR: Massive hemorrhage complicating age-related macular degeneration. Ophthalmology 93:1581-1592, 1986
19. Lewis H, Sloan SH, Foos RY: Massive intraocular hemorrhage associated with anticoagulation and age-related macular degeneration. Graefe's Arch Clin Exp Ophthalmol 226:59-64, 1988
20. Ferris FL III, Fine SL, Hyams L: Age-related macular degeneration and blindness due to neovascular maculopathy. Arch Ophthalmol 102:1640-1642, 1984
21. Tso MO: Pathogenetic factors of aging macular degeneration. Ophthalmology 92:628-635, 1985
22. Blumenkranz MS, Russell SR, Robey MG, Kott-Blumenkranz R, Penneys N: Risk factors in age-related maculopathy complicated by choroidal neovascularization. Ophthalmology 93:552-558, 1986
23. Friedman E, Ivry M, Ebert E, Glynn R, Gragoudas E, Seddon J: Increased scleral rigidity and age-related macular degeneration. Ophthalmology 96:104-107, 1989
24. Jampol LM: Hypertension and visual outcome in the Macular Photocoagulation Study. Arch Ophthalmol 109:789-790, 1991
25. Penfold PL, Provis JM, Furby JH, Gatenby PA, Billson FA: Autoantibodies to retinal astrocytes associated with age-related macular degeneration. Graefe's Arch Clin Exp Ophthalmol 228:270-274, 1990
26. Bressler NM, Bressler SB, Seddon JM, Gragoudas ES, Jacobson LP: Drusen characteristics in patients with exudative versus non-exudative age-related macular degeneration. Retina 8:109-114, 1988
27. Bressler SB, Maguire MG Bressler NM, Fine SL of MPS Group: Relationship of drusen and abnormalities of the retinal pigment epithelium to the prognosis of neovascular macular degeneration. Arch Ophthalmol 108:1442-1446, 1990

AGE-RELATED MACULAR DEGENERATION

W. Richard Green

Eye Pathology Laboratory, The Johns Hopkins Hospital, Baltimore, MD, USA

Ladies and gentleman, I would like to thank the Academy for the privilege of participating in this symposium.

Over the past 25 years or so, I have studied over 500 eyes with age-related macular degeneration and I have come to the conclusion that diffuse deposits under the retinal pigment epithelium (Fig. 1A and B) are the principal morphologic change leading to vision loss in macular degeneration[1-3]. I call this diffuse drusen, but it can also be called basal linear deposits. This material is rich in phospholipids and ultrastructurally consists of vesicular, linear and curvilinear profiles, basement membrane-like material, clusters of widely spaced collagen, electron dense particles and fibrillogranular material (Fig. 2). It is this change that leads to many of the risk factors talked about by Dr. Gass – hypopigmentation and atrophy of the retinal pigment epithelium, pigment clumping, localized areas of detachment (soft drusen), and larger areas of detachment (drusenoid detachments), serous detachments of the retinal pigment epithelium, choroidal neovascularization, and finally, fibrous disciform scarring. This material is deposited between the basement membrane of the retinal pigment epithelium and the remainder of Bruch's membrane. In other words, it is located in the inner collagenous zone of Bruch's membrane. A portion of the thickening as seen by light microscopy may include widely spaced collagen (basal laminar deposits), which are located between the plasma membrane and the basement membrane of the retinal pigment epithelium (Fig. 2). These two deposits are often present in the same eye, but basal laminar deposits in themselves are not as prominent a risk factor for visual loss as are basal linear deposits (diffuse drusen).

Diffuse drusen are detected early only by associated changes in the retinal pigment epithelium. Subtle pigmentary changes are an early feature that can be seen in age-related macular degeneration. These changes are often referred to as pigment modelling in the posterior pole. These changes include RPE attenuation with depigmentation (Fig. 1), RPE atrophy, and pigment clumps with pigmented cells in the subretinal space (Fig. 3) and outer retinal layers. These changes are associated with diffuse drusen and variable photoreceptor cell atrophy. In postmortem eyes there is often artifactitious detachment of the diffuse drusen from the rest of Bruch's membrane. While this is an artefact, it is a meaningful artefact, for there is a tendency for cleavage in the same plane *in vivo* with the formation of soft drusen[2] (Figs. 1C, 4 and 5) and serous detachment of the retinal pigment epithelium.

This is an eye in which we prepared serial sections through the macular area and constricted a two-dimensional drawing of the histopathologic features (Figs. 6 and 7). The solid line represents the area of diffuse drusen and the dotted line is an area of areolar RPE atrophy. An area of hyperpigmentation is present within the area of atrophy. There-

Address for correspondence: W. Richard Green, MD, Eye Pathology Laboratory, The Johns Hopkins Hospital, 600 N. Wolfe Street, Baltimore, MD 21287-9248, USA

Retina and Vitreous, pp. 7-13
Proceedings of the Symposium on Retina and Vitreous,
organized by the New Orleans Academy of Ophthalmology
New Orleans, LA, USA, March 12-15, 1992
edited by Rudolph M. Franklin

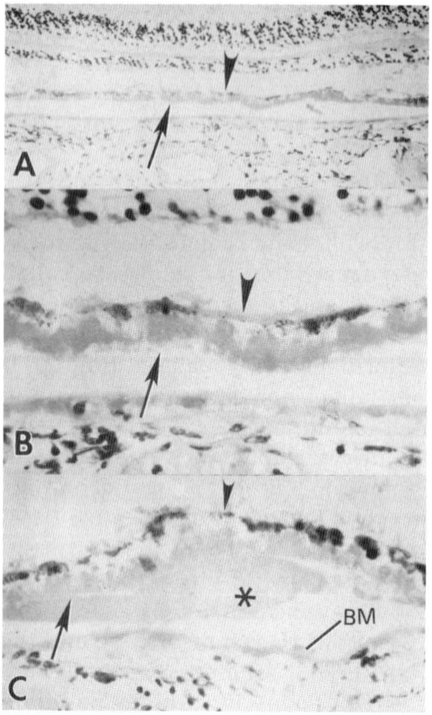

Fig. 1.

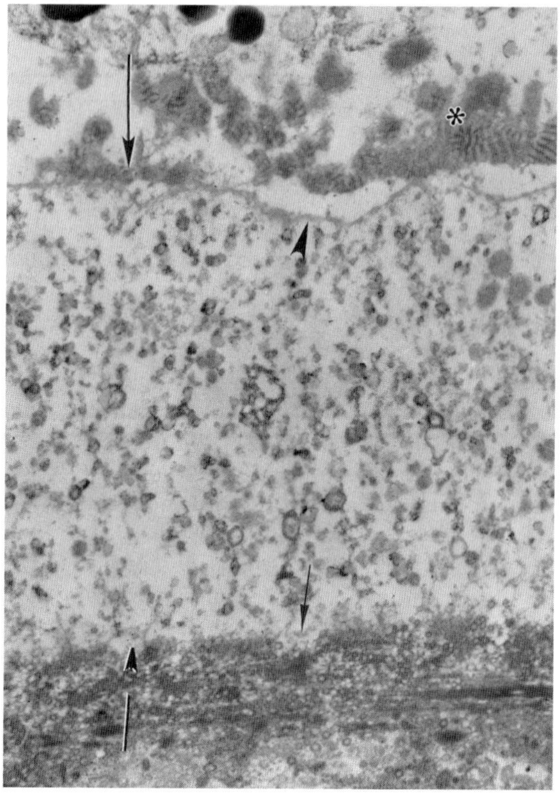

Fig. 2.

Fig. 1. A. Macular area with diffuse thickening of the inner aspect of Bruch's membrane (arrow) (diffuse drusen), which is artifactitiously detached from the remainder of Bruch's membrane. There is marked attenuation of the retinal pigment epithelium (arrowhead) and thinning of the photoreceptor cell layer (hematoxylin and eosin ×340). B. Closer view of diffuse drusen (arrow), attenuated retinal pigment epithelium (arrowhead), atrophy of the outer and inner segments of the photoreceptors, and artifactitious detachment from the remaining portion of Bruch's membrane (hematoxylin and eosin ×544). C. Soft druse. An area where the diffuse drusen (arrow) and the attenuated retinal pigment epithelium (arrowhead) is separated from the remainder of Bruch's membrane (BM) by a proteinaceous material (hematoxylin and eosin ×544).

Fig. 2. Ultrastructural appearance of the diffuse thickening of the inner aspect of Bruch's membrane (diffuse drusen) (basal linear deposits) (between large arrows). The material consists of mainly vesicular material and is located between the basement membrane of the retinal pigment epithelium (arrowhead) and the remainder of Bruch's membrane (small arrow). A layer of wide-spaced collagen (asterisk) (basal laminar deposit) is located between the plasma membrane and basement membrane of the retinal pigment epithelium (×15,000).

fore, areolar atrophy is another component of age-related macular degeneration which is associated with diffuse drusen (Fig. 7B). There was also an area of peripapillary neovascularization where an artery from the choroid extends through a defect in Bruch's membrane and into some fibrous tissue located between the thickened and detached inner aspect of Bruch's membrane along with RPE and the remainder of Bruch's membrane (Fig. 8).

When choroidal neovascularization was first recognized, it was in conditions such as angioid streaks, choroidal ruptures, lacquer cracks, Fuchs' dots in which there were pre-

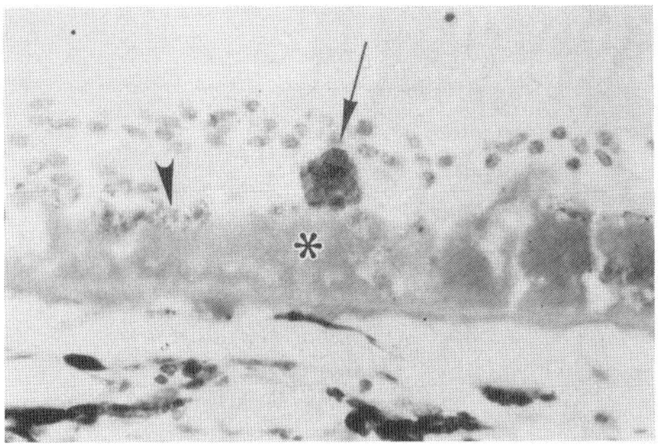

Fig. 3. Area of diffuse drusen (asterisk) with marked attenuation of the retinal pigment epithelium (arrowhead). A large pigmented macrophage is present in the subretinal area (arrow) and there is atrophy of the photoreceptors (periodic acid-Schiff ×1300).

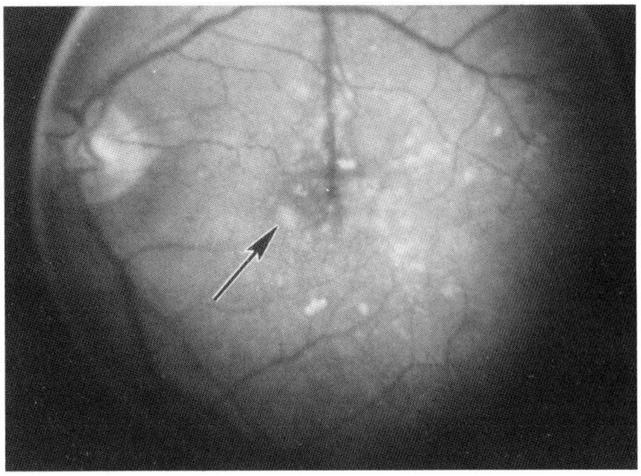

Fig. 4. Clinicopathologic correlation of a soft druse. Ophthalmoscopic appearance of numerous soft drusen, some with calcification. One large soft druse just inferior and nasal to the point of fixation is shown in section in Fig. 5.

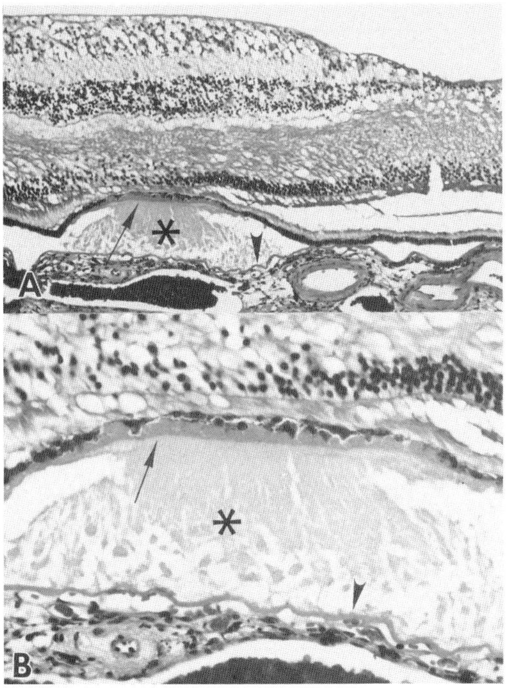

Fig. 5. Area of soft druse noted in Fig. 4 is an area where the thickened inner aspect of Bruch's membrane (diffuse drusen) (basal linear deposits) (arrows) is detached from the remainder of Bruch's membrane (arrowhead) by a proteinaceous material (asterisks) (hematoxylin and eosin: A, ×115; B, × 320). (Figs. 4 and 5 are from: Green WR, McDonnell PJ, Yeo JH: Pathologic features of senile macular degeneration. Ophthalmology 92:615-627, 1985.

existing defects in Bruch's membrane. We now know that cellular breakdown of Bruch's membrane may occur. In, for example, Fig. 9, a little mound of elevation can be seen with a large multinucleated giant cell in a region where Bruch's membrane is absent. Another example is shown in Fig. 10, with a defect in Bruch's membrane, a large multinucleated

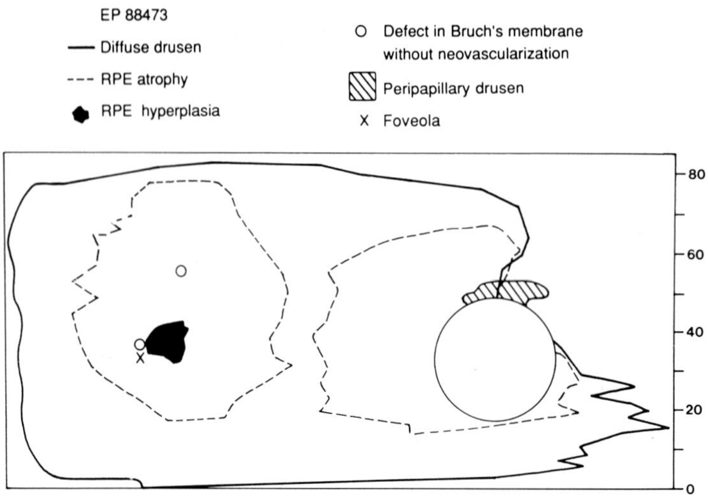

Fig. 6. Two-dimensional map constructed from the study of serial sections discloses the relationships of diffuse drusen area of retinal pigment epithelial atrophy and focal area of retinal pigment epithelium hyperplasia.

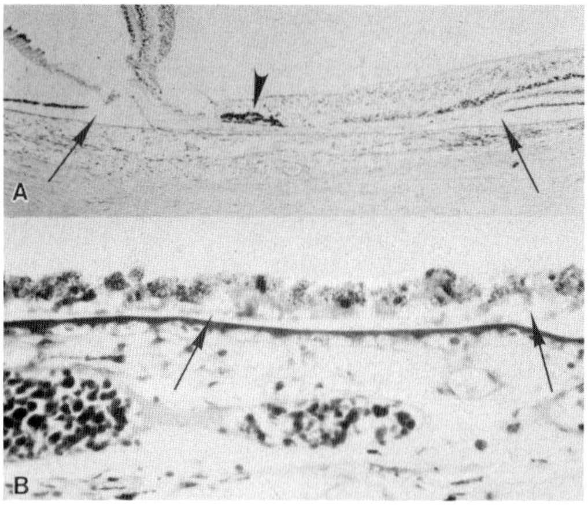

Fig. 7. A. View of level of macula with retinal pigment epithelial and photoreceptor cell atrophy (between arrows) and localized area of retinal pigment epithelial hyperplasia (arrowhead) (hematoxylin and eosin ×13.6). B. Area adjacent to the area of atrophy where retinal pigment is intact over diffuse drusen (arrows) (hematoxylin and eosin ×544).

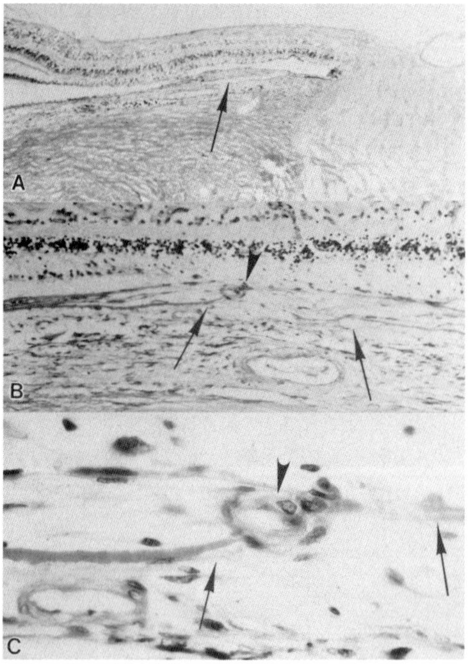

Fig. 8. Peripapillary choroidal neovascularization. A. Thin subretinal pigment epithelial scar (arrow) in temporal peripapillary area is associated with marked atrophy of the photoreceptor cells (Van de Grift ×13.6). B and C. A small choroidal vessel (arrowheads) extends through a defect in Bruch's membrane (between arrows) and into a fibrocellular tissue located under the attenuated retinal pigment epithelium (periodic acid-Schiff: B, ×340; C, ×544).

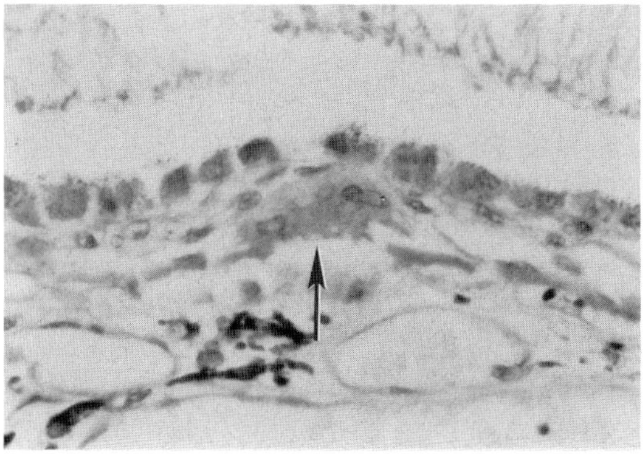

Fig. 9. Area where a large foreign body giant cell (arrow) is located in a defect of Bruch's membrane (hematoxylin and eosin ×544).

giant cell and early neovascularization. A small capillary-like vessel is located between the thickened inner aspect of Bruch's membrane and the remainder of Bruch's membrane.

The eye illustrated in Figs. 11 and 12 has neovascularization associated with diffuse drusen. Three defects in Bruch's membrane had a capillary-like vessel going from the choroid and into the subretinal pigment epithelial area. There is some hypopigmentation of the retinal pigment epithelium and marked loss of the photoreceptor cell layer. In some instances we have observed subretinal pigment epithelium neovascularization with intact retinal pigment epithelium and photoreceptor cells (Fig. 13). As Dr. Gass points out, such cases may not be detected clinically.

We have 23 eyes which were studied by serial sections through the macula. Of these 23 eyes, 14 (61%) had two or more defects in Bruch's membrane with neovascularization. Undetected points of neovascularization may be a factor in the high incidence of persist-

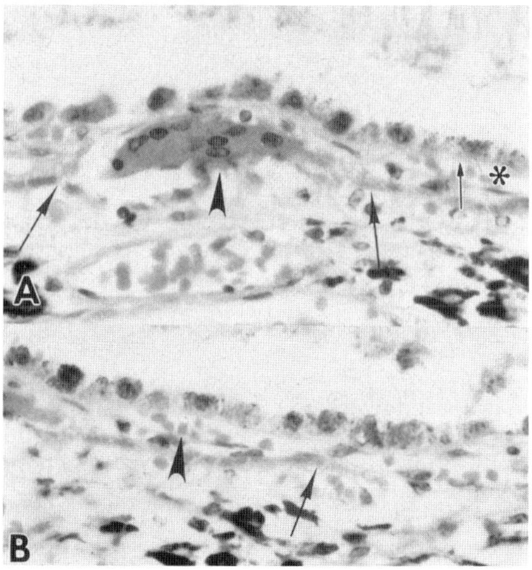

Fig. 10. Early choroidal neovascularization. A. A large multi-nucleated giant cell (arrowhead) is present in an area where Bruch's membrane is discontinuous (between large arrows). Capillary-like vessels (asterisk) extend between the slightly thickened inner and outer portions of Bruch's membrane (small arrow) (periodic acid-Schiff ×544). B. New vessels (arrowhead) extend in the same plane for a short distance beyond one margin of the defect in Bruch's membrane (arrow) (periodic acid-Schiff ×544).

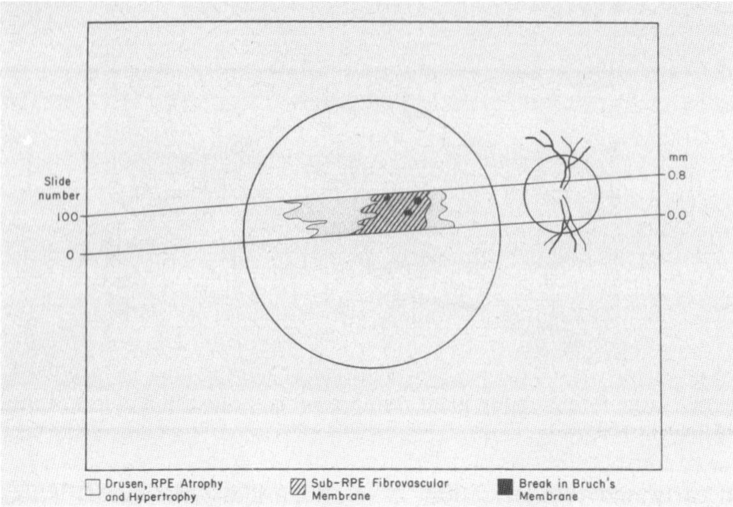

Fig. 11. Two-dimensional reconstruction depicts the areas of diffuse drusen, sub-RPE neovascularization and three defects in the outer layer of Bruch's membrane.

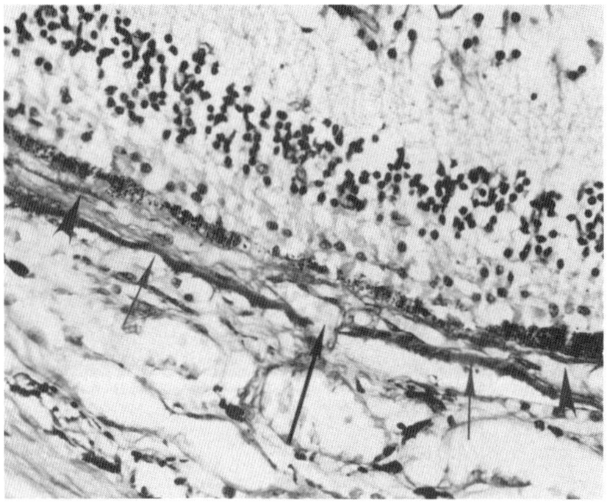

Fig. 12. Area discloses one of the three areas of neovascularization depicted in Fig. 14. Here a capillary (large arrow) extends through a minute defect in the outer layer of Bruch's membrane and extends to both sides, where the fibrovascular membrane is located between the thickened inner portion of Bruch's membrane (arrowheads) and the remainder of Bruch's membrane (small arrows) (periodic acid-Schiff ×370). (Figs. 11 and 12 are from: Green WR, Key SN III: Senile macular degeneration: A histopathologic study. Trans Am Ophthalmol Soc 75:180-254, 1977. Permission courtesy of the American Ophthalmological Society.)

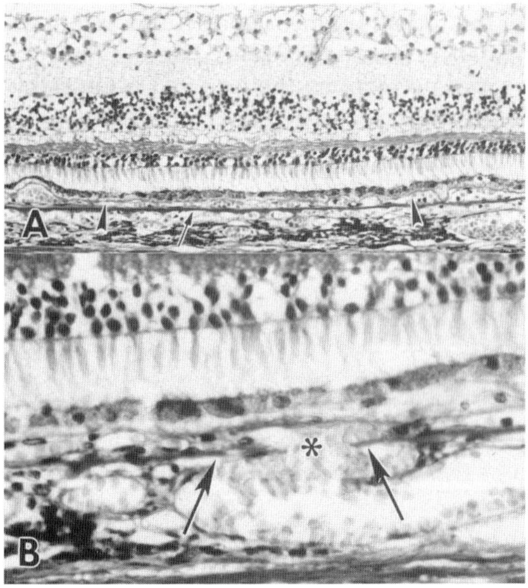

Fig. 13. A. The thin vascular membrane is located between the slightly thickened inner (arrowheads) and outer (arrow) portions of Bruch's membrane. The adjacent retinal pigment epithelium and photoreceptors are intact (Verhoeff van Giesen ×185). B. Area of defect in the outer portion of Bruch's membrane (between arrows) where a capillary-like vessel extends in an intra-Bruch's membrane plane (Verhoeff van Giesen ×500). (From: Green WR, Key SN III: Senile macular degeneration: A histopathologic study. Trans Am Ophthalmol Soc 75:180-254, 1977. Permission courtesy of the American Ophthalmological Society.)

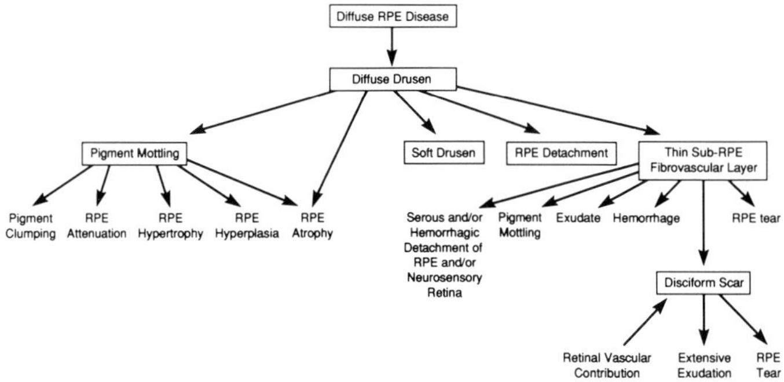

Fig. 14. Flow diagram illustrates the relationships of the various morphologic features of age-related macular degeneration.

ence or recurrence of neovascularization after laser treatment.

We have examined 12 eyes with neovascular lesions which received laser treatment and we found that nine of the 12 or 75% of the lesions had persistent neovascularization or had developed an additional source of neovascularization[4].

We believe that diffuse thickening of the inner aspect of Bruch's membrane (diffuse drusen) is the principal change that leads to the various morphologic features and visual loss in age-related macular degeneration (Fig. 14). Effects on the retinal pigment epithelium lead to the appearance of pigment mottling with small pigment clumps and retinal pigment epithelium attenuation, hypertrophy, hyperplasia and atrophy. Separation of the thickened layer leads to small focal areas of detachment (soft drusen), and large areas of detachment (retinal pigment epithelium detachment). Diffuse drusen predispose to choroidal neovascularization and the new vessel membrane is located between the thickened inner aspect and the remainder of Bruch's membrane. The early thin fibrovascular tissue may have a variety of effects including pigment mottling, exudate, hemorrhage and contribute to retinal pigment epithelium tears and stimulate fibrocellular proliferation with the formation of a disciform scar.

References

1. Green WR, Schwartz DM: Aspects Histopathologiques. In: Coscas G (ed) Dégénérescences Maculaires Acquises Liées à l'Age et Néovaisseaux Sous-Rétiniens, pp 90-119. Paris: Masson 1991
2. Green WR, McDonnell PJ, Yeo JH: Pathologic features of senile macular degeneration. Ophthalmology 92:615-627, 1985
3. Green WR, Key SN III: Senile macular degeneration: A histopathologic study. Trans Am Ophthalmol Soc 75:180-254, 1977
4. Green WR: Clinicopathologic studies of treated choroidal neovascular membranes: a review and report of two cases. Retina 11:328-356, 1991

PATHOPHYSIOLOGY OF AGE-RELATED MACULAR DISEASE

A.C. Bird

Department of Clinical Ophthalmology, Institute of Ophthalmology, Moorfields Eye Hospital, London, UK

Despite early hopes[1-3], it has become evident that laser treatment will not have a major impact on blindness from age-related macular disease[-6]. This requires that our knowledge of the behavior and etiology of age-related macular disease be re-examined, and alternative approaches to therapy sought. There is still incomplete information on the natural history and epidemiology of the disease. Those factors which determine the nature of the eye disease and magnitude of risk of visual loss have not been identified. As a result of recent clinical observation and laboratory research, new pathogenetic concepts have been formulated, and it is hoped that these will form a rational basis for future studies and provide novel therapeutic approaches to this disorder.

The lesions identified as causing loss of central vision are subretinal neovascularization, detachment of the retinal pigment epithelium and geographic atrophy. These are widely believed to occur in response to deposition of abnormal material within Bruch's membrane[7,8] which is a progressive phenomenon with age. Accumulation of debris may be detected by microscopy as early as ten years, and is seen consistently by the age of 60 years[9-12]. There is now increasing circumstantial evidence that the chemical composition as well as the quantity and distribution of the deposits in Bruch's membrane determine the effect of retinal function. The functional consequences, and the reactions provoked by the accumulated material are important to the outcome of disease.

In the normal state it is likely that the inward growth of choroidal blood vessels is suppressed by the metabolic environment of Bruch's membrane. This may be due to the intrinsic composition of Bruch's membrane or to the presence of diffusible agents produced by the retinal pigment epithelium. Changes induced by the accumulation of abnormal material within Bruch's membrane, and the presence of macrophages appear to be important in the induction of new vessel growth[13].

The pathogenesis of retinal pigment epithelial detachments has been re-examined recently. In the early discussion it was suggested that the detachment was induced by passage of fluid through Bruch's membrane from the choriocapillaris, the physical attachment of pigment epithelium to Bruch's membrane having been disturbed by progressive accumulation of debris on the inner surface of Bruch's membrane[7]. The assumption that fluid was derived from choroid is understandable since the fluorescein which fills the subpigment epithelial space during fluorescein angiography is derived from the choroid rather than the retina. This concept presumes high hydrostatic pressure in choroid, although experimental evidence implies that it is unlikely that the hydrostatic pressure in

These studies were supported in part by MRC and The Wellcome Trust

Address for correspondence: A.C. Bird, MD, FRCS, FCOphth, Department of Clinical Ophthalmology, Institute of Ophthalm- ology, Moorfields Eye Hospital, City Road, London EC1V 2PD, UK

Retina and Vitreous, pp. 15-27
Proceedings of the Symposium on Retina and Vitreous,
organized by the New Orleans Academy of Ophthalmology
New Orleans, LA, USA, March 12-15, 1992
edited by Rudolph M. Franklin

the choroid is greater than the pressure within the retina[14]. Indeed the little evidence that exists suggests that it may be somewhat lower. As an alternative mechanism fluid might be drawn into the subpigment epithelial space from the choroid by high osmotic pressure within this cavity, although the little that is known concerning the constituents of the subpigment epithelial space does not imply that this is the case. The acceptance that choroidal blood vessels may grow through Bruch's membrane and proliferate on the outer surface of flat pigment epithelium as a primary response to age-related Bruch's membrane disease, has led to the proposal that exudation from such a new vessel complex may be an alternative source of fluid causing pigment epithelium to detach[15]. However, neovascularization is not universal in pigment epithelial detachments[16,17]. It is undeniable that such blood vessels may modify the outcome of pigment epithelial detachments, but it is unlikely that this represents the initiating event in the pathogenesis of the lesion.

One major weakness of these concepts is that none explains certain clinical behavior characteristics of pigment epithelial detachments. It is hard to conceive how scattered photocoagulation over the surface of the pigment epithelial detachment would induce the pigment epithelium to flatten[4]. In addition it is difficult to explain the drop in vision which appears to be a common, if not invariable, association of spontaneous flattening of the pigment epithelium at least in the elderly[18]. Finally, any hypothesis concerning the pathogenesis of these lesions would need to account for the phenomenon of tearing of the pigment epithelium[19].

In 1986 a new concept was proposed in which it was suggested that the subpigment epithelial fluid is derived from the retinal pigment epithelial rather than from the choroid[20]. It is widely accepted that fluid is pumped from the retina to Bruch's membrane due to active movement of ions by the pigment epithelial cells. If Bruch's membrane became hydrophobic a significant resistance to water flow may be generated at this level causing fluid to collect between the pigment epithelium and Bruch's membrane. Such a mechanism demands that there be progressive accumulation of lipid in Bruch's membrane, and that this would vary from one patient to another. The observed entry of fluorescein from the choroid into the subpigment epithelial space would be explained by movement down a concentration gradient rather than the movement following fluid flow. This alternative explanation for the pathogenesis of retinal pigment epithelial detachments had the attraction over previous concepts in that it was compatible with the three observed behavioral characteristics of pigment epithelial detachments which were unexplained at that time:

1. The destruction of pigment epithelial cells, and therefore some of the pump, by photocoagulation would cause reduction in the volume of fluid being moved into the subpigment epithelial space, and predictably would be followed by flattening of the pigment epithelium.
2. This concept explains the observation that flattening of pigment epithelial detachments is accompanied by loss of vision. Tissue failure as manifest by visual loss might be associated with reduction of fluid pumped into the subpigment epithelial space which would itself be accompanied by flattening of the pigment epithelium onto Bruch's membrane.
3. The pigment epithelial pump might be powerful enough to produce tangential stress in the detached tissues sufficient to cause tearing of the pigment epithelium since it resists the influence of trans-cellular hydraulic pressure differences[21]. The observed slow flow of fluorescein into the subpigment epithelial space in patients at risk of suffering a pigment epithelial tear would be in accord with the proposal that in these patients the hydrophobicity in Bruch's membrane would be high.

Therefore, this alternative hypothesis concerning the pathogenesis of retinal pigment epithelial detachments has many attractions for the clinician. It does not exclude new vessels growing within the inner portion of Bruch's membrane as a contributor to the detachment. It is evident that decreased hydraulic conductivity of Bruch's membrane would be an essential prerequisite for these vessels to cause accumulation of fluid in the sub-pigment epithelial space.

Some support for this concept is derived from both histopathological and biophysical observations. There is evidence that the hydraulic conductivity of Bruch's membrane becomes progressively less with age[22]. Clefts seen by histopathology in Bruch's membrane with linear deposits have been interpreted as water clefts consequent upon hydrophobicity of Bruch's membrane[23].

During the last four years a series of laboratory and clinical studies have been undertaken which were stimulated by these considerations.

Laboratory studies

Evidence has been sought to support the proposal that there is progressive accumulation of lipids in Bruch's membrane with age. Increase of basophilia and PAS staining of Bruch's membrane has been long recognized by pathologists[24-26] and was thought to reflect progressive lipid deposition. However, because routine histological procedures removes most lipids from the specimen, no systematic analysis of lipid content of the debris had been reported until recently. A study of frozen tissue has been undertaken using histochemical staining techniques on human eyes with an age range between one and 95 years[27]. The composition and ultrastructure of Bruch's membrane were recorded by electron microscopy on the same specimens. The results analyzed in three age groups, 0-30 years, 30-59 years and older than 60 years, showed progressive accumulation of lipids in Bruch's membrane with age. Differences were found in the specific types of lipids present. Some eyes stained for neutral lipids alone, some stained predominantly for phospholipids, and others stained equally for both neutral lipids and phospholipids. The deposits were associated with the progressive destruction of the native architecture of Bruch's membrane but no correlation was identified between specific inclusions in Bruch's membrane with a particular lipid.

To confirm these conclusions, material extracted by lipid solvents from tissue of eye-bank fresh eyes has been analyzed by thin layer and subsequently gas chromatography[28]. After separation, the chemical species were identified by mass spectroscopy. This study confirmed the conclusion that the quantity of lipid in Bruch's membrane increases with age. Eyes from donors over the age of 60 years showed wide variation of total lipid extracted from donors of similar age that the ratios of phospholipids to neutral fats was different from one specimen to another.

In order to investigate further the potential determinants of fluorescence of drusen and Bruch's membrane and the correlation of fluorescence with biophysical properties of the tissue, a series of macular specimens from human donors older than 60 years of age were examined[29]. *In vitro* fluorescein binding was recorded microscopically and the presence of fibronectin was sought by immunohistochemistry. The results were correlated with the proportions of phospholipids to neutral fats as shown by histochemical and biochemical studies. It was found that high content of neutral fats was associated with lack of both fluorescein binding and fibronectin, and conversely in those specimens with high proportions of phospholipids fluorescein binding was strong and fibronectin was present. Fibronectin is found in plasma and in tissue which is diffusion continuity with blood. Thus, the presence or absence of fibronectin indicates that the tissue is hydrophilic or hydrophobic. These observations support the central hypothesis concerning biophysical changes in Bruch's membrane with age.

Therefore, evidence from laboratory studies give support to the proposal in that lipids accumulate in Bruch's membrane with age, and that the nature and quantity of the lipids varies widely between patients of a similar age. This is compatible with the proposal that the hydrophobicity of Bruch's membrane increases with age, and that there is considerable variation from one subject to another.

Clinical studies

Microscopic studies show that thickening of Bruch's membrane may be in the form of discrete deposits on its inner surface, or diffuse (linear) accumulation which is seen as a continuous layer in the inner or outer portion of Bruch's membrane. This thickening may be compounded by secretion of material by pigment epithelium between its basal plasma membrane and basement membrane[10]. There is associated reduction of the cross-sectional area of the choriocapillaris[30,31], and the normal pattern of sinusoidal capillaries may be replaced by a tubular system[32,33].

Clinical studies have been directed towards the analysis of discrete deposits on the inner surface of Bruch's membrane which can be recognised clinically as drusen. However, they have largely ignored the potential importance of diffuse Bruch's membrane thickening, due to the lack of any recognised clinical manifestations of linear change. Logically, the diffuse deposits would be expected to play a major role in determining the outcome of disease. It is fortunate that the chemical composition of two forms of deposit appear to be similar[27], such that studies based upon drusen characteristics may indicate also the influence of diffuse change.

Drusen

The hypotheses concerning the pathogenesis of sight-threatening lesions in age-related maculopathy can be tested by studying the behavior of disease, and seeking correlation of outcome with the clinical characteristics of Bruch's membrane change. It would be predicted that the highest resistance to water flow in Bruch's membrane would be found in eyes destined to suffer tears of the detached retinal pigment epithelium in which the concept implies that sufficient tangential stress is induced in the detached tissues to cause them to rupture. The determination that a tear in one eye implied high risk of a similar event occurring in the fellow eye[34] provided the opportunity to test the concept. A comparison was made of the drusen in the fellow eye of one with a tear with those of a fellow eye of one with visual loss due to subretinal neovascularization. It was shown in two studies that the drusen were larger, more confluent, and less fluorescent in the former group than in the latter[35,36].

There is doubt as to the determinants of fluorescence of drusen, and therefore the significance of this finding to disease. Fluorescence may be dependent upon the quantity of pigment in the overlying pigment epithelium, but perhaps more important is the presence or absence of fluorescein within the drusen material itself. It has been hypothesized that drusen that are hyperfluorescent must be hydrophilic allowing free diffusion of water soluble sodium fluorescein into the abnormal deposit; there may also be binding of sodium fluorescein to polar molecules[20,29]. By contrast, the hypofluorescence of other drusen would imply that they are hydrophobic and lack polar compounds. It was suggested that the former are rich in protein and phospholipids, while the latter are rich in neutral fats. If these conclusions are correct, they would indicate high hydrophobicity of Bruch's membrane in an eye at risk of having a tear of the retinal pigment epithelium, and support the concept that the subpigment epithelial fluid is derived from the pigment epithelium.

The observations that the form of drusen correlate with the type lesion consequent upon Bruch's membrane change, and that there is some symmetry of behavior of the two eyes in an individual[37] imply that drusen are symmetrical in their characteristics. This is a concept which dates from the last century[38], and several newer observations support the proposal[8,39]. Nevertheless, symmetry had not been tested in a formal way until recently. A study of the drusen characteristics in patients with bilateral age-related changes at the level of Bruch's membrane and good vision has shown that very close symmetry exists between the two eyes[39]. The greatest symmetry was of fluorescence, both early and late in the fluorescein angiogram, indicating that the chemical composition, and therefore the biophysical properties, of the deposits in Bruch's membrane vary from one patient to another but are similar in the two eyes of a single individual.

Another possible implication of these observations is that the form of drusen may determine not only the type of lesions which may cause visual loss but also the magnitude of risk of such an event. This was tested in patients with unilateral visual loss due to tears of the retinal pigment epithelium[37]. This study showed that the annual risk of fellow eye visual loss was between 35% and 50%, 80% losing second eye vision within the first three years of review. This is considerably higher than the accepted figure of about 12% per year in all age-related macular disease[8,41,42]. This study also confirmed the symmetry of sight-threatening lesion in that 31 of the 36 losing vision in the second eye did so as a consequence of a retinal pigment epithelial detachment.

Diffuse Bruch's membrane change

As a result of studies on Sorsby's fundus dystrophy[43-45], it was suggested that a prolonged choroidal filling phase on fluorescein angiography may be a clinical sign of diffuse thickening of Bruch's membrane. In this autosomal dominant condition a continuous layer of abnormal material of up to 30 microns in thickness is deposited between the inner collagenous layer of Bruch's membrane and the basement membrane of the retinal pigment epithelium[46]. In contrast with the normal rapid filling, a contiguous area of prolonged, patchy choroidal fluorescence is seen during the transit phase of the angiogram[43-45]. Major choroidal blood vessels are seen prior to filling of the choriocapillaris so that obscuration of choroidal fluorescence by pigment could not explain the angiographic sign. The dye appears initially in the inner choroid as small points of fluorescence which gradually enlarge and coalesce with one another over several frames of the angiogram. Continuous fluorescence indistinguishable from the surrounding normal fundus is not apparent until the venous phase of the retinal circulation. This pattern of choroidal filling is characteristically seen in patients with known choroidal hypoperfusion as part of general vascular disease[47-49].

Fluorescein angiography transit photographs were analyzed in eyes of consecutive patients with age-related changes at the level of Bruch's membrane[50]. Of these, 26% had evidence of a prolonged choroidal filling phase during the initial dye transit. This angiographic sign could represent the clinical correlate of changes in the choriocapillaris as identified by microscopy[30-33].

In order to establish the potential significance of this clinical sign, visual sensitivity was measured in eight eyes with this angiographic finding, and in six eyes with similar amount of drusen but normal choroidal filling[51]. Scotopic threshold was measured using the Humphrey automated perimeter and fine matrix mapping. In eyes without delayed choroidal perfusion, no discrete area of increased threshold was found when compared with the background sensitivity. By contrast, in seven of the eight eyes with fluorescein angiographic evidence of prolonged choroidal filling, discrete areas of scotopic threshold elevation of up to 3.4 log units were recorded which corresponded closely to regions of choroidal perfusion abnormality.

The visual acuity and the fundus appearance were identical in patients with and without abnormal choroidal perfusion such that neither clinical attribute segregates these two populations. Although no simple clinical clues exist to identify those patients with loss of scotopic sensitivity and abnormal choroidal perfusion, functional correlates were evident to the patients. They report the need for increased light intensity for reading, fading vision after a few minutes in bright light, and easy fatiguability when doing close work.

Dark adapted threshold elevation in the macular area in eyes with age-related macular disease had been documented by others[52,53]. However, no correlation between the sensitivity and the number of drusen was found, and the threshold elevation over drusen and non-drusen areas was similar. On the basis of these findings, it was concluded that more diffuse pigment epithelial or retinal dysfunction must be present other than that caused by drusen.

No established pathogenetic concepts are readily available to explain either the changes in choroidal fluorescence or the functional loss. Diminution of the choroidal capillary bed with age has been shown by structural studies[30-33], but the absence of change in the arteries makes it unlikely that it is due to arterial obstruction or systemic hypertension[54-56]. It is doubtful whether capillary changes are due to physical displacement by the debris since the same angiographic phenomenon occurs in Sorsby's fundus dystrophy[44,45] in which the deposits are internal to the inner collagenous layer of Bruch's membrane[46]. Furthermore, observations on acute and chronic choroidal ischemia make it unlikely that there would be significant retinal dysfunction as a consequence of the observed perfusion abnormality[48,49,57].

A unifying mechanism has been proposed by which these changes may be generated. It has been suggested that a continuous layer of debris in Bruch's membrane may act as a barrier to metabolic exchange between the retinal pigment epithelium and the choroidal capillaries. If this is the case it could explain both the psychophysical and angiographic findings observed in this and other studies. Normal photoreceptor function is dependent on the free diffusion through Bruch's membrane of large molecule complexes as they pass from the choriocapillaris to the pigment epithelium[58]. Predictably such molecules would not pass freely through a continuous layer of debris. This has been suggested with respect to alteration of proteoglycans in the inter-fiber matrix of Bruch's membrane[59]. However, the debris deposited into Bruch's membrane by the retinal pigment epithelium is likely to be a more important determinant of conductivity. The magnitude of change would depend upon the thickness and chemical composition of the material within Bruch's membrane; the disturbance would be particularly marked in the presence of a large quantity of neutral fats[27,28].

There is circumstantial evidence that the behavior characteristics of the choriocapillaris are determined by the retinal pigment epithelium[60,61], and it has been proposed that the diffusible agents from the pigment epithelium modulate the choroidal vasculature[62]. Based on these hypotheses, it has been proposed that a barrier to diffusion at the level of Bruch's membrane would result in changes in choroidal capillaries[45,46]. If the normal characteristics of the choroidal capillaries are dependent upon the diffusible agent, failure of this agent to reach the choroid would result in the vessels reverting to the more common tubular arrangement of capillary beds.

It cannot be assumed that angiographic appearance implies perfusion deficit alone, since it may also be modified directly by the accumulated material in Bruch's membrane. Although the initial choroidal fluorescence is likely to be derived from the dye in the choroidal blood vessels and extracellular space of the choroid, the subsequent distribution of fluorescein has not been well defined particularly in disease. Fluorescence microscopy shows the dye to be in Bruch's membrane and some drusen rather than in the extracellular space of the choroid soon after injection[20]. It is probable that the dye is bound to extracellular polar molecules. If this is the case, choroidal fluorescence would be modified by changes in the speed of effusion of dye from the choroidal capillaries, the diffusion characteristics of the tissues, and the binding properties of Bruch's membrane as well as by the speed of blood flow. The influence of neutral fats upon fluorescence characteristics may be complex, and by modifying several of these functions would serve to modify the appearance of dye during angiography.

Consequences of Bruch's membrane change

It is evident that there is correlation between the number, density, confluence and fluorescence angiographic characteristics of drusen on the one hand, and the subsequent outcome of disease on the other.

The mechanisms by which the deposits cause the sight-threatening complications have not been clearly identified, but these finding allow some speculation as to the relevant pathogenetic mechanisms. The major lesions causing visual loss are the growth of new blood vessels from the choroid through Bruch's membrane towards the retina, detachment of the retinal pigment epithelium, and atrophy of the outer retina and choriocapillaris[7]. Some correlation exists between the type of drusen and the form of lesion causing visual loss.

Drusen which are hyperfluorescent, and therefore presumed to be hydrophilic, appear to predispose to sub-retinal neovascularization[35,36]. Over the last decade some determinants of blood vessel growth have been identified, although the precise mechanisms leading to neovascularization in various clinical situations have not been defined. The chemical nature of the inter-fiber matrix of Bruch's membrane, change in the pigment epithelial influence upon blood vessel growth, and the presence of macrophages[13] which stimulate neovascularization, may all be relevant. In particular, polar molecules may stimulate invasion of Bruch's membrane by macrophages or neutral fats may suppress blood vessel growth.

Patients with large confluent drusen in the central area which are hypofluorescent have a predisposition towards pigment epithelial detachments with or without subretinal neovascularization[35,36]. It has been proposed that these presumed lipid-rich deposits reduce hydraulic conductivity of Bruch's membrane, so that water which is pumped from the retina towards the choroid by the retinal pigment epithelium or fluid leaking from blood vessels growing in the inner surface of Bruch's membrane accumulates in the sub-pigment epithelial space. In its extreme form the pigment epithelial detachment becomes progressively larger, generating sufficient tangential stress in the detached tissues to cause a tear[19,35].

Loss of photoreceptors in the outer neuro-retina is a constant association with age[63]. Areas of well-defined geographic atrophy supervene, a process which has been well documented histologically[31]. Atrophy may follow spontaneous resolution of retinal pigment detachments[18], although this probably accounts for a small proportion of such lesions. To what extent a diffusion barrier is responsible for geographic atrophy is unknown. It is easy to conceive that movement of molecules between the choroidal capillaries and the pigment epithelium would be impeded by the interposition of a layer of debris particularly if it was composed largely of neutral fats rather than polar molecules. Just as the diffusion across Bruch's membrane of water and growth factors produced by the retinal pigment epithelium would be hampered, complexes containing molecules essential for photoreceptor function would not pass freely from the choroid to the retinal pigment epithelium. Consequent functional deficit might be expected, and that major sensitivity loss has been identified in those with the angiographic sign of slow choroidal perfusion, and therefore presumed diffuse disease despite good visual acuity lends support to these concepts[51].

The symmetry of drusen in terms of quantity, distribution and chemical composition, and the hypothesis that the form of Bruch's membrane deposits determine the nature and magnitude of risk to vision, together suggest that the two eyes of a patient should behave in a similar manner, and that there would be differential risk from one patient to another. Several observations are compatible with this concept. In patients with unilateral visual loss, there is the good correlation between the form of drusen in one eye and the type of lesion in the other. It has also been shown in patients with a retinal pigment epithelial tear in one eye that there is a very high risk of a similar event occurring in the other[34,40].

These clinical observations give circumstantial support to the original concept that there may be change in hydraulic conductivity of Bruch's membrane with age and that the effect differs from one subject to another. The functional deficits imply that it is not just water movement that is affected but that there may be global reduction of metabolic exchange between the retinal pigment epithelium and choriocapillaris.

Pathogenesis of Bruch's membrane change

The question arises as to whether or not these conclusions of selective deposition of material into Bruch's membrane are compatible with the current concepts of the pathogenesis of Bruch's membrane disease with age. It is widely believed that the material within the abnormal deposits is derived from the pigment epithelium[12,63-66]. The distribution of phospholipids implies that the lipids are of cellular origin rather than being from blood. Shedding of the photoreceptor cell outer segment tip occurs daily; the cell fragments are phagocytosed by the retinal pigment epithelium, and degraded by various lysosomal enzymes which are specific to their substrate[67-75]. There is good evidence that the retinal pigment epithelium discharges cytoplasmic material throughout life into the inner portion of Bruch's membrane[76,78] which subsequently diffuses through Bruch's membrane to be cleared by the choroidal capillaries. By this mechanism it is believed that the pigment epithelium voids the products of phagosomal degradation. Thus it was believed that the material discharged into Bruch's membrane consisted of degradation products photoreceptor outer segment material.

However, it has not been proven that the photoreceptors represent the original source of abnormal material or that it derived from phagosomes. Neither rhodopsin sequences nor phagosomal enzyme activity have been shown in Bruch's membrane deposits using monoclonal antibodies[79]. A major alternative source of material results from retinal pigment epithelial autophagy, a phenomenon common to all long-lived cells with high metabolic activity by which cytoplasmic renewal takes place[78,80]. It is now believed by many that the debris discharged into Bruch's membrane is a product of retinal pigment epithelial metabolic activity in general rather than being directly derived from outer segment material. This is not to deny that a relationship may exist between the state of the photoreceptors and the volume of material produced, since retinal pigment epithelial activity is likely to reflect the quantity outer segment membrane renewal.

Accumulation in Bruch's membrane is thought to result from failure to clear the debris deposited into this region. It is possible that the material discharged into Bruch's membrane is abnormal as a consequence of incomplete phago-lysosomal degradation, and in particular may contain large molecules and membrane complexes, such that free outward diffusion does not occur. Both lipids and proteins are contained within the phagosomes. Failure of those enzymes responsible for degrading or modifying the lipids, might results in the accumulation of fats within Bruch's membrane, and conversely defective protease activity might cause protein accumulation. In addition to the contents of phagosomes and cytoplasmic material discharged into Bruch's membrane, the membranes surrounding the vesicles and any plasma membrane shed would add to the load.

Finally, there is formation of an additional layer of material internal to the retinal pigment epithelial basement membrane which has been called basal linear deposit[10]. This is believed to be a product of retinal pigment epithelium. It is not known if this process is central to age-related macular disease or simply a reaction of an abnormal cell. The observation that this linear thickening is not seen before the changes are well established implies that it does not initiate the disease. Once thickening of Bruch's membrane is established, the deposits would be expected to aggravate the situation by changing the diffusion characteristics of Bruch's membrane, and further hamper outward diffusion.

Increasing work is being undertaken in order to identify the possible importance of the retinal pigment epithelial cell dysfunction in the pathogenesis of aging changes. There is net reduction of the number of retinal pigment epithelial cells with age[63,81] implying that each cell will have greater metabolic load since it relates to a larger number of photoreceptors. There is also a reduction in the melanin content of the cells[82], and the spectral properties of the melanin changes[83]. Perhaps of greater significance is the accumulation of lipofuscin within the pigment epithelial cells. Lipofuscin granules are yellow-brown autofluorescent lipid aggregates. They are thought to result from fusion of long-term phagolysosomes containing the end products of phagocytosis of photoreceptor outer segments and cytoplasmic constituents[84-87]. Lipofuscin appears to increase in the first two decades of life, and then remains stable until middle life rising thereafter[88]. The density of lipofuscin increases from the peripheral retina to the macula with a drop at the fovea[89], a distribution which corresponds to the density of rods[63]. At the age of 40 years, lipofuscin occupies about 8% of the cytoplasmic volume and by the age of 80 this figure has risen to 19%[85]. With increasing age the lipofuscin granules and melanin granules fuse to form large complex structures called melanolysosomes[84]. The effect of this accumulation upon cell function is not clear. For example, it is not known whether the displacement of cytoplasm interferes with cell activity.

It is possible that the accumulation of melanolysosomes may be due to an absolute deficiency of lysosomal enzymes such that there is defective degradation of phagosomal material. However, the evidence concerning the absolute level of activity is mixed, some workers finding the levels to be raised[70], while others have reported it to be reduced[71]. The first would accord with the observation that the residual bodies are all acidified (K. Dorey, personal communication), an indication that lysosomal vesicles are constantly fusing with the long-term phagosomes. In addition, there is experimental evidence that increasing phagosomal load in cultured retinal pigment epithelial cells results in a rise in degradative enzyme activity, although the levels achieved did not reach those seen in the elderly[90,91]. These findings suggest the possibility that there may competition from the newly produced vesicles containing lysosomal enzymes such that they may be not be freely available to new phagosomes. Thus, even if there is an increased total enzyme activity, there may still be defective breakdown of newly ingested photoreceptor outer segment material within the pigment epithelium.

A final consideration concerns the possibility that the phagocytosed material has been altered. The high oxygen tension and light levels in the retina, and the presence of long-chain unsaturated fatty acids imply high risk of free radical damage to outer segment membrane lipids. Should there be peroxidation of these lipids, large complexes would form such that may not be degraded efficiently by lysosomal enzymes. Some protection against this event would be expected from the presence in neuroretina and pigment epithelium of enzymes such as superoxide dismutase, catalase and glutathione peroxidase which protect from free radical damage[93-95]. Comparison of the lipid content of the new basal discs and old apical discs shows that there is no evidence of diminution of docoso-hexanoic acid (24:6), a change that might have been expected if there was significant peroxidation of lipids in the photoreceptor outer segment[96].

Conclusions

From the evidence available to date, it is possible to formulate hypotheses as to the origin of the abnormal material in Bruch's membrane, and the mechanisms by which this material is generated. That it is derived from the pigment epithelium is not questioned, although the nature of the metabolic defects and their cause are poorly understood. Nevertheless, however uncertain we are as to the basic pathogenetic defects, it is evident that the current concepts are compatible with the proposal that there may be selective deposition of protein or lipid into Bruch's membrane, and that the form of lipid may be different from one subject to another.

The lesions which cause visual loss represent reactions to the abnormal material which may be determined by the nature of the material, and the evidence now supports this proposal. Many clinically identifiable clues exist which allow the variants of disease to be defined and which provide a basis upon which the determinants of disease may be defined. Both laboratory and clinical observations lend circumstantial support to the concept that reduced hydraulic conductivity of Bruch's membrane gives rise to retinal pigment epithelial detachments. In addition, the functional deficits so common in the elderly can be explained by alteration of the diffusion characteristics of Bruch's membrane. The corollary is that subretinal neovascularization as the initiating event in age-related macular degeneration occurs as a result of changes that are different from those which give rise to pigment epithelial detachments.

An additional factor may be the variable response of the individual to the deposits. It is widely believed that prevalence of visual loss as a consequence of age-related macular disease is much less in some races when compared with others. However, it has not been shown that this represents the influence of genetic or environmental factors. If either of these is important, they may cause differences in either the genesis of the abnormal material, or the mechanism by which it accumulates, or in the modulation of the response it evokes.

References

1. Macular Photocoagulation Group: Argon laser photocoagulation for senile macular degeneration: results of a randomized clinical trial. Arch Ophthalmol 100:1347-1357, 1982
2. Coscas G, Soubranne G: Photocoagulation des neovaisaux souretiens dans le dégenerescence maculaire sénile par laser à argon: résultats d'une étude randomisée de 60 cas. Bull Mem Soc Fr Ophtalmol 94:149-154, 1982
3. Moorfields Macular Study Group: Treatment of senile macular degeneration: a single blind randomised trial by argon laser photocoagulation. Br J Ophthalmol 66:745-753, 1982
4. Moorfields Macular Study Group: Retinal pigment epithelial detachments in the elderly: a controlled trial of argon laser photocoagulation. Br J Ophthalmol 66:1-16, 1982
5. Chisholm IH: The recurrence of neovascularization and late failure in senile disciform lesions. Trans Ophthalmol Soc UK 103:354-359, 1983
6. Macular Photocoagulation Group: Argon laser photocoagulation for neovascular maculopathy: three year results for randomized clinical trials. Arch Ophthalmol 224:493-501, 1986
7. Gass JDM: Pathogenesis of disciform detachment of the neuro-epithelium. 3. Senile disciform macular degeneration. Am J Ophthalmol 63:617-644, 1967
8. Gass JDM: Drusen and disciform macular detachment and degeneration. Arch Ophthalmol 90:206-217, 1973
9. Hogan MJ, Alvarado J: Studies on the human macula. IV. Aging changes in Bruch's membrane. Arch Ophthalmol 77:410-420, 1967
10. Sarks SH: Ageing and degeneration in the macular region: A clinico-pathological study. Br J Ophthalmol 60:324-341, 1976
11. Green WR, Key SN: Senile macular degeneration: a histopathological study. Trans Am Ophthalmol Soc 75:180-250, 1977

12. Feeney-Burns L, Ellersieck M: Age-related changes in the ultrastructure of Bruch's membrane. Am J Ophthalmol 100:686-697, 1985
13. Penfold PL, Killingsworth MC, Sarks SH: Senile macular degeneration: The involvement of giant cells in atrophy of the retinal pigment epithelium. Invest Ophthalmol Vis Sci 27:364-371, 1986
14. Foulds WS: Clinical significance of trans-scleral fluid transfer. Trans Ophthalmol Soc UK 96:290-308, 1976
15. Gass JDM: Pathogenesis of tears of the retinal pigment epithelium. Br J Ophthalmol 68:513-519, 1984
16. Barondes MJ, Pagliarini S, Chisholm IH, Hamilton AM, Bird AC: Controlled trial of laser photocoagulation of pigment epithelial detachments in the elderly: a four year review. Br J Ophthalmol 76:5-7, 1992
17. Pagliarini S, Barondes MJ, Chisholm IH, Hamilton AM, Bird AC: Detection of subpigment epithelial neovascularization in cases of retinal pigment epithelial detachments: a review of the Moorfields treatment trial. Br J Ophthalmol 76:8-10, 1992
18. Casswell AG, Kohen D, Bird AC: Retinal pigment epithelial detachments in the elderly: classification and outcome. Br J Ophthalmol 69:397-403, 1985
19. Hoskin A, Bird AC, Sehmi KS: Tears of detached retinal pigment epithelium. Br J Ophthalmol 65:417-422, 1981
20. Bird AC, Marshall J: Retinal pigment epithelial detachments in the elderly. Trans Ophthalmol Soc UK 105:674-682, 1986
21. Tsuboi S: Measurement of the volume flow and hydraulic conductivity across the isolated dog retinal pigment epithelium. Invest Ophthalmol Vis Sci 28:1776-1782, 1987
22. Fisher RF: The influence of age on some ocular basement membranes. Eye 1:184-189, 1987
23. Loffler KU, Lee WR: Basal linear deposits in the human macula. Graefe's Arch Clin Exp Ophthalmol 224:493-501, 1986
24. Spencer WH: Symposium: Macular diseases, pathogenesis: light microscopy. Trans Am Acad Ophthalmol 69:662-667, 1965
25. Hogan MJ: Symposium: macular diseases, pathogenesis: electron microscopy of Bruch's membrane. Trans Am Acad Ophthalmol 69:683-690, 1965
26. Farkas T, Sylvester V, Archer D, Altona M: The Histochemistry of drusen. Am J Ophthalmol 71:1206-1215, 1971
27. Pauleikhoff D, Harper CA, Marshall J, Bird AC: Aging changes in Bruch's membrane: a histochemical and morphological study. Ophthalmology 97:171-178, 1990
28. Sheraidah G, Steinmetz R, Maguire J, Pauleikhoff D, Marshall J, Bird AC: Analysis of lipids extracted from Bruch's membrane in age related macular disease. Ophthalmology 100:47-51, 1993
29. Pauleikhoff D, Zuels S, Sheraidah G, Marshall J, Wessing A, Bird AC: Determinants for the fluorescence of drusen in Bruch's membrane. Ophthalmology 99:1548-1553, 1992
30. Sarks SH: Changes in the region of the choriocapillaris in aging and degeneration. 23rd Concilium Ophthalmol, Kyoto 228-238, 1978
31. Sarks SH, Sarks J, Killingsworth C: Evolution of geographic atrophy of the retinal pigment epithelium. Eye 2:552-577, 1988
32. Tso MOM: Pathogenetic factors of aging macular degeneration. Ophthalmology 92:628-635, 1985
33. Olver J, Pauleikhoff D, Bird AC: Morphometric analysis of age changes in the choriocapillaris. Invest Ophthalmol Vis Sci (Suppl) 31:47, 1990
34. Chuang EL, Bird AC: Bilaterality of tears of the retinal pigment epithelium. Br J Ophthalmol 72:918-920, 1988
35. Chuang EL, Bird AC: The pathogenesis of tears of the retinal pigment epithelium. Am J Ophthalmol 105:185-190, 1988
36. Pauleikhoff D, Barondes MJ, Minassian D, Chisholm IH, Bird AC: Drusen as a risk factor in age related macular disease. Am J Ophthalmol 109:38-43, 1990
37. Schoeppner G, Chuang EL, Bird AC: Retinal pigment epithelial tears: risk to the second eye. Am J Ophthalmol 108:683-685, 1989
38. Hutchinson J, Tay W: Symmetrical central chorio-retinal disease occurring in senile persons. Roy Lond Ophthalmol Hosp Rep 83:275-285, 1875
39. Coffrey AJH, Brownstein S: The prevalence of macular drusen in postmortem eyes. Am J Ophthalmol 102:164-171, 1986
40. Barondes M, Pauleikhoff D, Chisholm IH, Minassian D, Bird AC. Bilaterality of drusen: Br J Ophthalmol 74:180-182, 1990
41. Gregor Z, Bird AC, Chisholm IH: Senile disciform macular degeneration in the second eye. Br J Ophthalmol 61:141-147, 1977

42. Bressler SB, Bressler NM, Fine SL, Hillis A, Murphy RP, Olk BJ, Patz A: Natural course of choroidal neovascular membranes with the foveal avascular zone in senile macular degeneration. Am J Ophthalmol 93:157-163, 1983
43. Hoskin A, Sehmi K, Bird AC: Sorsby's pseudo-inflammatory macular dystrophy. Br J Ophthalmol 65:859-865, 1981
44. Capon MRC, Polkinghorne PJ, Bird AC: Sorsby's pseudo-inflammatory dystrophy: Sorsby's fundus dystrophy. Eye 2:114-122, 1988
45. Polkinghorne PJ, Capon MRC, Berninger TA, Lyness AL, Sehmi K, Bird AC: Sorsby's fundus dystrophy: a clinical study. Ophthalmology 96:1763-1768, 1989
46. Capon MRC, Marshall J, Kraft JI, Alexander RA, Hiscott PS, Bird AC: Sorsby's fundus dystrophy: a light and electron microscopic study. Ophthalmology 96:1769-1777, 1989
47. Foulds WS, Lee WR, Taylor WOG: Clinical and pathological aspects of choroidal ischaemia. Trans Ophthalmol Soc UK 91:325-341, 1971
48. Van Buskirk EM, Lessell S, Friedman E: Pigment epitheliopathy and erythema nodosum. Arch Ophthalmol 85:369-372, 1971
49. Gaudric A, Coscas G, Bird AC: Choroidal ischemia. Am J Ophthalmol 94:489-498, 1982
50. Pauleikhoff D, Chen JC, Chisholm IH, Bird AC: Choroidal perfusion abnormalities in age related macular disease. Am J Ophthalmol 109:211-217, 1990
51. Chen JC, Fitzke FW, Pauleikhoff D, Bird AC: Poor choroidal perfusion is a cause of visual morbidity in age-related macular degeneration. Invest Ophthalmol Vis Sci 33:334-340, 1992
52. Sunness JS, Massof RW, Johnson MA, Finkelstein D, Fine SL: Peripheral retinal function in age-related macular degeneration. Arch Ophthalmol 103:811-816, 1985
53. Sunness JS, Johnson MA, Massof RW, Marcus S: Retinal sensitivity over drusen and nondrusen areas: a study using fundus perimetry. Arch Ophthalmol 106:1081-1084, 1988
54. Meves H: Die pathologisch-anatomischen Gefassveränderungen des Auges bei der beningen und malingen Nephrosklerose. Graefes Arch Ophthalmol 168:287, 1948
55. Friedman E, Smith TR, Kuwabara T: Senile choroidal vascular patterns and drusen. Arch Ophthalmol 69:220-230, 1963
56. Friedman E, Smith TR, Kuwabara T, Beyer CK: Choroidal vascular patterns in hypertension. Arch Ophthalmol 71:842-850, 1964
57. Tso MOM, Bettman JW: Occlusion of the choriocapillaris in primary nonfamilial amyloidosis. Arch Ophthalmol 86:281-286, 1971
58. Bok D: Retinal photoreceptor-pigment epithelium interactions. Invest Ophthalmol Vis Sci 26:1659-1694, 1985
59. Hewitt TA, Nakazawa, K, Newsome DA: Analysis of newly synthesized Bruch's membrane proteoglycans. Invest Ophthalmol Vis Sci 30:478-486, 1989
60. Korte GE, Repucci V, Henkind P: RPE destruction causes choriocapillary atrophy. Invest Ophthalmol Vis Sci 25:1135-1145, 1984
61. Andracchi S, Korte GE: Expression of plasma membrane alkaline phosphatase in normal and regenerating choriocapillaris of the rabbit. Invest Ophthalmol Vis Sci (Suppl) 32:1081, 1991
62. Glaser BM, Campochiaro PA, Davies JL, Sato M: Retinal pigment epithelial cells release an inhibitor of neovascularization. Arch Ophthalmol 103:1870-1875, 1985
63. Marshall J: The ageing retina: physiology or pathology. Eye 1:282-295, 1987
64. Farkas T, Sylvester V, Archer D: The ultrastructure of drusen. Am J Ophthalmol 71:1196-1205, 1971
65. Hogan MJ: Role of the retinal pigment epithelium in macular disease. Trans Am Acad Otolaryngol Ophthalmol 76:64-80, 1972
66. Grindle CFJ, Marshall J: Aging changes in Bruch's membrane and their functional implications. Trans Ophthalmol Soc UK 98:172-175, 1978
67. Shichi H: Microsomal electron transfer system in bovine retinal pigment epithelium. Exp Eye Res 8:60-68, 1969
68. Shichi H, Atlas SA, Nebert DW: Genetically regulated aryl hydroxylase induction in the eye: possible significance of drug-metabolizing enzyme system in the retinal pigment epithelium-choroid. Exp Eye Res 21:557-567, 1976
69. Hayasaki S, Hara S, Mizuno K: Distribution and some properties of cathepsin D in the retinal pigment epithelium. Exp Eye Res 24:307, 1975
70. Hayasaki S, Hara S, Mizuno K: Distribution of acid lipase in the bovine retinal pigment epithelium. Exp Eye Res 24:1, 1977
71. Hayasaki S, Shiono T, Hara S, Mizuno K: Regional distribution of lysosomal enzymes in the retina and choroid of human eyes. Graefe's Arch Clin Exp Ophthalmol 216:269-273, 1981

72. Stramm LE, Desnick RJ, Hoskins ME, Agguire GD: Aryl sulphatase B activity in cat retinal pigment epithelium: regional studies in feline mucopolysaccharidosis VI. Invest Ophthalmol Vis Sci 27:1050-1057, 1986
73. Cabral L, Unger W, Boulton M, Lightfoot R, McKechnie N, Grierson I, Marshall J: Regional distribution of lysosomal enzymes in the canine retinal pigment epithelium. Invest Ophthalmol Vis Sci 31:670-676, 1990
74. Wilcox D: Extracellular release of acid hydrolases from cultured retinal pigment epithelium. Invest Ophthalmol Vis Sci 28:6-11, 1987
75. Yamada T, Hara S, Tamai M: Immunohistochemical localization of Cathepsin D in ocular tissue. Invest Ophthalmol Vis Sci 31:1217-1223, 1990
76. Burns RP, Feeney-Burns L: Clinico-morphological correlations of drusen and Bruch's membrane. Trans Am Ophthalmol Soc 78:206-225, 1980
77. Ishibashi T, Sorgente N, Patterson R, Ryan SJ: Pathogenesis of drusen in the primate. Invest Ophthalmol Vis Sci 27:184-193, 1986
78. Rungger-Branche E, Englert U, Leuenberger PM: Exocytic clearing of degraded membrane material from pigment epithelial cells in frog retina. Invest Ophthalmol Vis Sci 28:2026-2037, 1988
79. Feeney-Burns L, Gao Chun Lan, Tidwell M: Lysosomal enzyme cytochemistry of human RPE, Bruch's membrane and drusen. Invest Ophthalmol Vis Sci 28:1138-1147, 1987
80. Reme C: Autophagy in visual cells and pigment epithelium. Invest Ophthalmol Vis Sci 16:807-814, 1977
81. Dorey CK, Wu G, Ebenstein D, Garsd A, Weiter JJ: Cell loss in the ageing retina: relationship to lipofuscin accumulation and macular degeneration. Invest Ophthalmol Vis Sci 30:1691-1699, 1989
82. Feeney-Burns L, Hilderbrand ES, Eldred S: Aging human RPE: morphometric analysis of macular, equatorial and peripheral cells. Invest Ophthalmol Vis Sci 25:195-200, 1983
83. Boulton ME, Docchio F, Dayhaw-Braker P, Ramponi R, Cubeddu R: Age related changes in the morphology, absorption and fluorescence of melanosomes and lipofuscin granules of the retinal pigment epithelium. Vis Res 30:1291-1303, 1990
84. Feeney L: Lipofuscin and melanin of human retinal pigment epithelium: fluorescence, enzyme cytochemical and ultrastructural studies. Invest Ophthalmol Vis Sci 17:583-600, 1978
85. Feeney-Burns L, Eldred GE: The fate of the phagosome: conversion to "age-pigment" and impact in human retinal pigment epithelium. Trans Ophthalmol Soc UK 103:416-421, 1984
86. Katz ML, Drea C, Robinson WG: Relationship between retinol and lipofuscin in the retinal pigment epithelium. Mech Ageing Dev 35:291-305, 1986
87. Boulton ME, McKechnie NM, Breda J, Bayly M, Marshall J: The formation of autofluorescent granules in cultured human RPE. Invest Ophthalmol Vis Sci 30:83-89, 1989
88. Weale RA: Do years or quanta age the retina? Photochem Photobiol 50:249-538, 1989
89. Wing GL, Blanchard GC, Weiter JI: The topographical and age relationship of lipofuscin concentration in the retinal pigment epithelium. Invest Ophthalmol Vis Sci 17:601-607, 1978
90. Boulton M: Aging of the retinal pigment epithelium. In: Osborne NN, Chader GJ (eds) Progress in Retinal Research, Vol 11, Ch. 6, pp 125-152. Oxford: Pergamon Press
91. Wyszynski RE, Brunar WE, Cano DB, Morgan KM, Davis CB, Sternberg P: A donor age-dependent change in the activity of alpha-mannosidase in human cultured RPE cells. Invest Ophthalmol Vis Sci 30:2341-2347, 1989
92. Boulton M. Moriarty P, Unger W, Bishop P: Modulation of lysosomal enzyme content in cultured human RPE. Invest Ophthalmol Vis Sci (Suppl) 32:1056, 1991
93. Akeo K, Curren S, Dorey CK: Superoxide dismutase activity and growth of retinal pigment epithelial cells are suppressed by 20% oxygen. Curr Eye Res 7:961-967, 1988
94. Bouma E, Unger W, Boulton M, Marshall J: Catalase activity in cultured human RPE during phagocytosis. Invest Ophthalmol Vis Sci (Suppl) 29:441, 1988
95. Penn JS, Naash MI, Anderson RE: Effect of light history on retinal antioxidants and light damage susceptibility in the rat. Exp Eye Res 44:779-788, 1987
96. Haldeman M, Boesze-Battaglia K, Albert AA: Lipid distribution in bovine disc membranes as a function of age. Invest Ophthalmol Vis Sci (Suppl) 32:1009, 1991

THE CASE FOR TREATING SUBFOVEAL NEOVASCULARIZATION IN PATIENTS WITH AGE-RELATED MACULAR DEGENERATION

Stuart L. Fine

Department of Ophthalmology, Scheie Eye Institute, Philadelphia, Pennsylvania, USA

The idea of deliberately obliterating the fovea with laser photocoagulation is egregious to most ophthalmologists.

Consequently it may be difficult to accept the recommendations from a multicentered clinical trial, supported by the National Eye Institute, which actually recommended foveal photocoagulation as a treatment for certain patients with age-related macular degeneration (AMD) and subfoveal neovascularization. In fact, in a series of three papers published in the September 1991 *Archives of Ophthalmology*, the Macular Photocoagulation Study (MPS) Group reported that laser treatment for subfoveal new vessels was the appropriate management for patients with AMD who met the entrance criteria for the Foveal Photocoagulation Study (FPS)[1-3].

The decision to make this recommendation, or even to assess laser treatment for subfoveal new vessels, was not undertaken lightly. Initially, the MPS evaluated laser treatment for AMD patients with new vessels not involving the center of the fovea. In studies conducted between 1979 and 1988, the MPS group found that laser treatment was preferable to observation in reducing the risk of severe vision loss in neovascularization that did not extend through the foveal center[4,5]. During the mid 1980's, a natural history study concluded that approximately 70% of AMD patients with subfoveal new vessels progressed to severe vision loss within two years[6]. Next, a pilot trial of laser treatment, conducted at two MPS centers, showed promising results in that laser treated eyes lost vision less often than untreated eyes. Accordingly, the MPS group, with continuing support from the National Eye Institute, agreed to conduct a prospective randomized trial of laser treatment for subfoveal new vessels.

In general, ophthalmologic treatment actually makes patients better. Whether prescribing glasses for a myopia, using cycloplegic and steroid drops to reduce the discomfort of anterior uveitis, or removing a cataract to promote better vision, ophthalmologic treatment makes patients better. In the case of treating subfoveal new vessels with laser, the treatment is more like removing a gangrenous digit to prevent extension. We are performing a destructive treatment in an effort to contain the ultimate damage. Consequently, the MPS group reports that laser treatment is preferable to no treatment, it means that the likelihood of severe vision loss is reduced by the laser treatment in a way that is both statistically significant and clinically meaningful.

Nevertheless, it may be difficult for some ophthalmologists to explain to a patient and a family that the recommended treatment not only will not improve the vision but actually will make the vision worse, both immediately and irrevocably. That is precisely

Address for correspondence: Stuart L. Fine, M.D., Department of Ophthalmology, Scheie Eye Institute, Myrin Circle, 51 North 39th Street, Philadelphia, PA 19104, USA

Retina and Vitreous, pp. 29-30
Proceedings of the Symposium on Retina and Vitreous,
organized by the New Orleans Academy of Ophthalmology
New Orleans, LA, USA, March 12-15, 1992
edited by Rudolph M. Franklin

what we must tell the patient, however. In the same breath, we must explain that according to data from many patients with a similar appearance, the likelihood of severe vision loss is less in treated eyes than in non-treated eyes.

In reviewing the data published in September 1991, I find it particularly helpful to have available those graphs and tables which depict how particular subgroups of eyes fare with and without treatment. Specifically, I find it helpful to talk to patients about the visual outcome, with or without laser treatment, as a function of the size of the neovascular lesion and as function of the visual acuity at the time that treatment is being considered. In general, eyes with smaller membranes and poorer baseline acuity will have the better outcomes after laser treatment whereas eyes with larger membranes and better acuity at baseline will have the worse visual outcomes, comparing treated *vs.* non-treated eyes[2]. Recently MPS investigators have analyzed outcomes for treated eyes and non-treated eyes which consider baseline visual acuity and neovascular lesion size together[7].

In summary, it is important for ophthalmologists to be convinced beyond any reasonable doubt that, based on the best available data in 1993, eyes with subfoveal neovascular lesions that meet FPS eligibility criteria have a better prognosis with laser treatment than with observation alone. Treatment surely is not a panacea; however, successful laser treatment can limit the damage and reduce the likelihood of severe visual acuity loss in the future for eyes with new and recurrent subfoveal neovascular lesions that meet FPS eligibility criteria.

References

1. MPS Group: Laser photocoagulation of subfoveal neovascular lesions in age-related macular degeneration. Results of a randomized clinical trial. Arch Ophthalmol 109:1219-1231, 1991
2. MPS Group: Laser photocoagulation of subfoveal recurrent neovascular lesions in age-related macular degeneration. Results of a randomized clinical trial. Arch Ophthalmol 109:1232-1241, 1991
3. MPS Group: Subfoveal neovascular lesions in age-related macular degeneration. Guidelines for evaluation and treatment in the Macular Photocoagulation Study. Arch Ophthalmol 109:1242-1257, 1991
4. MPS Group: Argon laser photocoagulation for neovascular maculopathy after five years: Results from randomized clinical trials. Arch Ophthalmol 109/8:1109-1114, 1991
5. MPS Group: Krypton laser photocoagulation for choroidal neovascularization: Five year results from randomized clinical trials. Arch Ophthalmol. Submitted for publication March 31, 1993
6. Guyer DR, Fine SL, Maguire MG et al: Subfoveal choroidal neovascularization membranes in age-related macular degeneration: visual prognosis in eyes with relatively good visual acuity. Arch Ophthalmol 104:702-705, 1986
7. MPS Group: The influence of initial lesion size and initial visual acuity on the effects of laser photocoagulation for subfoveal choroidal neovascularization. Arch Ophthalmol. Submitted for publication May 1993

SURGICAL EXCISION OF SUBFOVEAL NEOVASCULAR MEMBRANES

H. Michael Lambert and Thomas M. Aaberg, Sr.

Department of Ophthalmology, Emory University School of Medicine, Atlanta, Georgia, USA

Age-related macular degeneration (AMD) is the number one cause of blindness in persons over the age of 50 in the United States[1,2]. The disease has two specific presentations, non-exudative or "dry" macular degeneration and exudative or "wet" macular degeneration. Eighty percent of patients with AMD have the non-exudative type, consisting of atrophy and migration of the retinal pigment epithelium and drusen. Only 20% of AMD patients have the exudative type which consists of the "dry" findings plus retinal pigment epithelial detachments and/or subretinal neovascular membrane formation. Although the wet form accounts for the minority of patients with AMD, it can lead to serous retinal detachment and subretinal hemorrhage which, in turn, are the cause of 80% of legal blindness in AMD.

The subretinal neovascular membrane formation that is responsible for the marked visual loss in AMD also occurs in many other conditions, most notably in the presumed ocular histoplasmosis syndrome (POHS), myopia, associated with angioid streaks in various conditions, and as an idiopathic entity. For the last 15 years the Macular Photocoagulation Study (MPS) has addressed the treatment of subretinal neovascular membranes in these diseases with long-term multi-centered clinical trials[3-6]. The efficacy of extrafoveal and juxtafoveal membrane photocoagulation treatment was proven, and recently the results of the subfoveal portion of the study were released[7,8]. The MPS subfoveal study criteria included patients with 20/40 to 20/320 vision and a subfoveal membrane of less that 3.5 disc areas. Results showed that laser treatment was definitely preferable over observation, however, the treated patients suffered an immediate three line visual loss (on average) following treatment. At two years following treatment, laser treated patients had an average visual acuity of 20/250 compared with 20/320 average vision for non-treatment patients. Contrast sensitivity also proved to be better in the photocoagulation treated patients.

Although the MPS showed the above benefits in treating subfoveal membranes, photocoagulation really only limited the loss of vision in these patients and vision is initially worsened with treatment. Patients had little hope of improving vision with subfoveal photocoagulation. With these results in mind and the knowledge that vitreoretinal techniques have improved greatly in recent years with instruments now precise enough for subretinal work, we undertook the study of the surgical removal of subfoveal membranes. Questions we wished to answer in this ongoing study include:

1. can subfoveal membranes be removed safely; and
2. can visual function be restored or improved with surgery? We elected to choose patients with the poorest prognosis for visual recovery, but with a clearly identifiable subfoveal neovascular membrane for ease of surgical approach.

Address for correspondence: H. Michael Lambert, MD, Department of Ophthalmology, Emory University School of Medicine, 1327 Clifton Road, NE, Atlanta, GA 30322, USA

Retina and Vitreous, pp. 31-34
Proceedings of the Symposium on Retina and Vitreous,
organized by the New Orleans Academy of Ophthalmology
New Orleans, LA, USA, March 12-15, 1992
edited by Rudolph M. Franklin

Our criteria include:
1. 20/200 or worse vision;
2. a clearly identifiable subfoveal membrane occupying the entire foveal avascular zone; and
3. an overlying serous retinal detachment.

Our technique has evolved over the course of our ongoing study. Initially we performed the surgery similarly to Thomas and Kaplan[10] who reported the results of vitrectomy and subfoveal membrane removal in two patients with POHS. We have since modified the technique considerably. We start with a routine pars plana vitrectomy with careful peripheral vitreous removal. The posterior hyaloid is then addressed with complete dissection in all patients. At this point the balanced saline solution (BSS) infusion bottle is raised to increase intraocular pressure to just below arterial closure to minimize hemorrhage. A small retinotomy is performed with a microvitreoretinal knife, BSS is used to form a bleb at the retinotomy site, and the retinotomy is extended with vertical vitreoretinal scissors. No cauterization of the retina is performed and minimal bleeding occurs. The retinotomy site is chosen:
1. to avoid larger vessels;
2. to minimize manipulation under the fovea;
3. to maximize the approach to the membrane; and
4. to minimize the damage to the nerve fiber layer.

Using a 30-gauge bent disposable cannula (chosen for its very smooth surface) BSS is injected very slowly and carefully between the membrane and retina and the membrane and retinal pigment epithelium to attempt to hydrodissect the subretinal neovascular membrane from surrounding structures. Great care is taken to avoid the extrusion of BSS through the retina. Mechanical dissection to insure complete separation is then performed with the cannula tip. Vertical membrane forceps are then used to "tease" the membrane without actually grasping it. The membrane will usually contract and thicken with manipulation simplifying removal. The membrane is then grasped and gently rocked free from surrounding structures. Constant traction is applied and the membrane is slowly removed to the vitreous cavity. A small bubble of perfluoro-N-octane is then injected through the infusion light pipe (no instrument is removed from the eye to allow constant hemostasis) to tamponade the macula. A full five minutes is allowed to pass before removal of the membrane from the eye. The perfluoro-N-octane is then removed followed by a total air-fluid exchange. The retinotomy site is not treated.

In performing this surgery, we have learned several interesting facts. The vitreous is attached to the retina in the vast majority of cases (37 of the first 42 cases). In this age group (particularly the AMD patients) one would expect a much higher incidence of posterior vitreous detachment. This finding leads to the speculation that traction from the posteriorly attached vitreous on the macular region may play a role in subretinal neovascular membrane formation. Additionally, the subretinal neovascular membranes have uniformly proven to be much larger than indicated by fluorescein angiography. A thin ring of tissue surrounds each membrane. Perhaps this is, in part, the reason for the high failure/recurrence rate (50+%) of photocoagulation in the Macular Photocoagulation Study. Histopathology of the membranes reveals tissue and cells including endothelial lined vascular channels, new collagen, fibrocytes, retinal pigment epithelium, erythrocytes, and myofibroblasts as well as chronic inflammatory cells (macrophages, lymphocytes, and plasma cells), basal laminar deposits and diffuse drusen, photoreceptors, Bruch's membrane, and fibrin[11]. These all suggest that subretinal neovascular membrane formation is nothing more than the ingrowth of granulation tissue attempting to heal the diseased macular area.

The results of this surgical approach have been encouraging to date. In the first ten AMD patients 60% showed visual improvement by three months and 70% showed improvement by six months (Table 1)[12]. Although these patients were improved over the preoperative levels, none returned to driving levels, probably reflecting the low prognosis patients chosen in our study. The results in POHS and idiopathic membrane patients have been even more encouraging (Table 2). At the one month postoperative point, five of eight were 20/100 or better, by three months five of five patients were 20/100 or better, and at six months the one idiopathic membrane patient had improved to 20/80 from her 20/400 preoperative level and the one POHS patient had improved from counting fingers at two feet preoperatively to 20/20-.

Complications are those expected from performing vitreous surgery and removing vascular structures, but have been less than expected. Hemorrhage has been minimal and controllable. In the first ten patients, five had minimal hemorrhage from the choroid with subretinal membrane removal removed at surgery. Elevation of the balanced salt solution bottle and the use of perfluoro-N-octane have greatly reduced this problem. Several patients have suffered subretinal hemorrhages postoperatively. All but one cleared

Table 1. Characteristics of 10 AMD patients with subfoveal membranes

Patient	*Age*	*Sex*	*Preoperative visual acuity**	*Postoperative visual acuity*		
				1 Month	*3 Months*	*6 Months*
1	68	F	CF 3′	20/80	20/60	20/100
2	71	F	CF 1′	20/400	20/400	20/400
3	70	F	20/200	20/400	20/200	20/100
4	75	F	20/400	20/400	20/400	20/400
5	91	M	20/400	20/300	20/300	20/300
6	70	F	CF 1′	20/300	20/300	20/400
7	83	M	CF 3′	20/400	20/400	20/400
8	73	M	20/200	CF 3′	CF 3′	CF 3′**
9	91	F	CF 5′	20/300	20/400	20/400
10	76	F	20/200	20/200	20/200	20/200

*Standard visual acuity chart (20/20-20/400) used for acuity measurements. Counts fingers vision obtained when patient unable to recognize Snellen letters at any distance. Best corrected visions via standard refraction techniques were measured upon initial evaluation, confirmed one day preoperatively, and at each visit by ophthalmic technologists masked to the study. **Patient suffered central retinal vein occlusion three weeks postoperatively

Table 2. Characteristics of eight idiopathic and POHS patients with subfoveal membranes

Patient	*Age*	*Dx**	*Preoperative visual acuity***	*Postoperative visual acuity*		
				1 Month	*3 Months*	*6 Months*
1	36	I	20/400	20/100	20/80	20/80
2	49	I	20/400	20/40		
3	33	P	CF 2′	20/40	20/40	20/20-
4	19	P	20/200	20/100	20/100	
5	18	P	20/300	20/30-	20/30+	
6	43	P	20/400	20/400	20/100	
7	48	P	20/200	20/400***		
8	29	P	20/200	20/200		

*I: idiopathic; P: presumed ocular histoplasmosis syndrome. **Standard visual acuity chart (20/20-20/400) used for acuity measurements. Counts fingers vision obtained when patient unable to recognize Snellen letters at any distance. Best corrected visions via standard refraction techniques were measured upon initial evaluation, confirmed one day preoperatively, and at each visit by ophthalmic technologists masked to the study. ***Recurrent subfoveal membrane without sequelae. One patient suffered a massive subretinal hemorrhage one week postoperatively which broke into the vitreous cavity causing a hemorrhagic glaucoma (cleared with treatment). Hydrodissection leads to macular hole formation in several early patients, however, this problem has been eliminated by more careful control of the hydrodissection infusate. Retinal detachment which occurred in three of the first 12 patients (all repaired successfully without sequelae) has not, however, occurred in any of the following 30 patients. The high incidence of retinal detachment in the first 12 patients is thought to be secondary to manipulation at the sclerotomy sites and contraction of the newly detached posterior vitreous along with pressure on this area by the air bubble. Careful dissection of the vitreous base and external cryopexy of the sclerotomy sites in selected cases have reduced this complication. Endophthalmitis has not occurred in any patient to date. Subretinal membranes have recurred in three of the 42 patients to date.

The surgical excision of subfoveal neovascular membranes in patients with 20/200 or worse vision has been shown in our studies to be a safe and beneficial procedure in the short term. Complications have been limited and controllable. We feel that this technique may be a definite alternative to the laser photocoagulation of these membranes. However, long-term study is necessary to prove the efficacy of this technique. Both techniques should be compared in a multi-centered prospective double-blind trial to determine the relative benefits of each.

References

1. Leibowitz HM, Krueger DE, Maunder LR, Milton RC, Kini MM, Kahn HA, Nickerson RJ, Pool J, Colton TL, Ganley JP, Lowenstein JI, Dawber TR: The Framingham Eye Study monograph: an ophthalmological and epidemiological study of cataract, glaucoma, diabetic retinopathy, macular degeneration, and visual acuity in a general population of 2631 adults, 1973-1975. Surv Ophthalmol 24:335, 1980
2. Ferris FL: Age-related macular degeneration and blindness due to neovascular maculopathy. Arch Ophthalmol 102:1640, 1984
3. Macular Photocoagulation Study Group: Argon laser photocoagulation for senile macular degeneration: results of a randomized clinical trial. Arch Ophthalmol 100:912, 1982
4. Macular Photocoagulation Study Group: Argon laser photocoagulation for neovascular maculopathy: three-year results from randomized clinical trials. Arch Ophthalmol 104:694, 1986
5. Macular Photocoagulation Study Group: Recurrent choroidal neovascularization after argon laser photocoagulation for neovascular maculopathy. Arch Ophthalmol 104:503, 1986
6. Macular Photocoagulation Study Group: Krypton laser photocoagulation for neovascular lesions of age-related macular degeneration: results of a randomized clinical trial. Arch Ophthalmol 108:816, 1990
7. Macular Photocoagulation Study Group: Laser photocoagulation of subfoveal neovascular lesions in age-related macular degeneration: results of a randomized clinical trial. Arch Ophthalmol 109:1220, 1991
8. Macular Photocoagulation Study Group: Laser photocoagulation of subfoveal recurrent neovascular lesions in age-related macular degeneration: results of a randomized clinical trial. Arch Ophthalmol 109:1232, 1991
9. Hanscom TA, Diddie KR: Early surgical drainage of macular subretinal hemorrhage. Arch Ophthalmol 105:1722, 1987
10. Thomas MA, Kaplan HJ: Surgical removal of subfoveal neovascularization in the presumed ocular histoplasmosis syndrome. Am J Ophthalmol 111:1, 1991
11. Lopez PF, Grossniklaus HE, Lambert HM, Aaberg TM, Capone A, Sternberg P Jr, L'Hernault N: Pathologic features of surgically-excised subretinal neovascular membranes in age-related macular degeneration. Am J Ophthalmol 112:647, 1991
12. Lambert HM, Capone A Jr, Aaberg TM, Sternberg P Jr, Mandell BA, Lopez PF: Surgical excision of subfoveal neovascular membranes in age-related macular degeneration. Am J Ophthalmol 113:30, 1992

ROUND TABLE: ARMD: TREATMENT WITH VITAMINS AND MINERALS OR IS THERE A ROLE FOR VITAMINS AND MINERAL TREATMENT?

J. Donald Gass, moderator

J. Donald Gass: It is evident from the information presented earlier that we certainly do not have good treatment for age-related macular degeneration. I think it is appropriate that they set aside some time to discuss some therapeutic possibilities during the pre-disciform, or the pre-neovascular phase of this disease. Although this round table is entitled "Vitamins and minerals", I think there are some other questions that are more pressing at the moment. One concerns interferon. Another is the feasibility of vitreous surgery for excision of subretinal neovascular membrane. Another, should surgical removal of large areas of subretinal pigment epithelial and subretinal blood be considered? Perhaps other panel members have other suggested subjects for discussion. I hope we will leave some time for comments concerning where to go from here; because none of the topics I have mentioned previously offer a great deal of promise. Let us begin with the subject of vitamins and minerals. As all of you are aware, I think it was in 1988 that Dr. Newsome and his co-workers reported the results of a randomized study in which they gave 200 mg of zinc sulfate to a group of patients – it was a randomized controlled trial – and they felt that the information they derived from this study showed some possible benefit. They cautioned that it was premature to use this approach in a widespread fashion because of the potential risk of side effects, and because the findings were inconclusive. First of all, I wish to ask the panelists, do you recommend the use of these vitamins, selenium, vitamin E, and zinc? Tom?

Thomas M. Aaberg, Sr.: I think ophthalmologists right now are in a real bind when it comes to the patient coming into the office, that if you do not at least discuss that aspect with the patient you may end up discussing it with the patient's lawyer at some time in the future. It is proper for all of us to present the data, as it has just been presented by Don, indicating that this evidence has been in the literature. One needs then to color it with your own philosophy. My philosophy is that it is preliminary, that it does not at all indicate that this will hold up under further scrutiny, and that if the patient wishes to take that course, then he or she may do so. As long as they have some caution that they do not say, well, if one is better, four pills are better yet, and get into toxicity problems, I am content to approach it that way.

Gass: Dr. Fine, do you have any comment?

Stuart L. Fine: If patients ask whether they should take it, I tell them I do not think so. If they ask should they stop, I say yes, I think you should. The article that was published did show a difference between the two groups, but in the realm of science and medicine, it is important for there to be verification in order to establish validity. Those studies have not been repeated. While it was a randomized trial, it was carried out on a

Retina and Vitreous, pp. 35-40
Proceedings of the Symposium on Retina and Vitreous,
organized by the New Orleans Academy of Ophthalmology
New Orleans, LA, USA, March 12-15, 1992
edited by Rudolph M. Franklin

relatively small group of patients. They were representing a few families in Utah. The studies were carried out carefully, but in the field, and although visual acuity was the outcome of interest, the visual acuity measurements were not made in the same rigid, standardized way that they were done in the Diabetic Retinopathy Study, and the Early Treatment Diabetic Retinopathy Study, and a lot of the other large randomized trials. Perhaps more important is whether or not it is possible to generalize about the whole population from that study on a relatively small group of patients, and I think not. Another interesting question is whether those results are going to hold up over time. What you would like to see, if you had a prophylactic treatment that reduced the likelihood of a bad outcome, is that as time progressed the differences between treated eyes and untreated eyes actually increased over time. And if you look at even the data which were published, the differences at 24 months, as I recall, were less than the differences at 12 months. One might legitimately ask the question that if there had been follow-up for 36 months, would the differences have been obliterated? And is it possible that at 48 months treated eyes would have been doing worse than untreated eyes! Another thing which made me raise my eyebrows was that if one looks at the actual loss of visual acuity, there is a lot of information in the literature about how quickly eyes with drusen and good visual acuity or with mild geographic atrophy lose vision. The published rate is about the same rate of vision loss that was reported in the patients who were treated with zinc. The patients who were in the control group had a much worse rate of visual acuity loss, which suggests that there might be something peculiar about that group of patients. This makes me conclude that perhaps we ought not to be generalizing about the entire population from that small study group. In other words, it would have been more credible if the patients who had been given the placebo had had about the same rate of vision loss as any other group of untreated patients with macular degeneration, and the group of patients treated with zinc had had a lower rate of vision loss, but that was not the case. So the facts are that the study comprised a small population of related individuals, that the studies were conducted in the field without rigorous visual acuity measurements, and that the differences between groups were small, and they tended to disappear over time. The study nevertheless was interesting and probably should have been reported. As Alan Bird says, we have not cured this disease with photocoagulation, and we are certainly not going to cure it with submacular surgery. We ought to have access to lots of new ideas and information, but I do not think that this study establishes the value of zinc in the treatment of macular degeneration. Moreover, I do not think it is incumbent upon ophthalmologists to feel as though they must treat AMD patients with zinc. There are lots of questions involved about the interpretation of the study data. Furthermore, Dr. Rick Ferris, who is the director of the biometry branch of the National Eye Institute, wrote an editorial in the *Archives* about a year ago pointing out some of the deficiencies in the zinc study and applying a slightly different interpretation, some of which I have just highlighted. So, I do not think there needs to be any concern about the medical-legal aspects of not treating patients with AMD.

Gass: Stuart, I understand there is a trial being organized at the National Institutes of Health. Does that involve zinc?

Fine: Well, that is the Age-Related Eye Disease Study, and it may be that Dr. Matthew Davis can comment on that because he is involved in that study.

Davis: No, I can not say very much, except that the study is still being designed. It is almost completely designed, and will start in July of this year. Patients will be randomized to zinc and high dose vitamins, as anti-oxidants. We will also be studying cataract. I am sure there will be editorial or other notification of the study probably this summer when it gets started.

Gass: Thank you, Matt. Anyone else, Alan? Tell us about zinc in the United Kingdom.

Alan C. Bird: The concept that an abnormality of zinc metabolism may be relevant to age-related macular disease and that zinc supplementation may be helpful in management is attractive in some ways. There are very high quantities of zinc at the level of the pigment epithelium, and there are zinc-dependent enzymes in the pigment epithelium. If pigment epithelial cell dysfunction is important in the genesis of age-related macular disease and that this was due to a deficiency in zinc levels, it would be reasonable to advocate zinc as an appropriate treatment. I am unaware of any laboratory investigation demonstrating reduced levels of zinc in the pigment epithelium in the elderly. It appears, therefore, that treatment with zinc is not correcting a deficiency, although it could be argued that more zinc is required in the elderly than in the young since there may be a large metabolic demand for zinc-dependent enzymes with age. It is evident to all that the paper in question does not present convincing evidence of a therapeutic effect and this was freely admitted by the authors. At present, in England, it is not a practice to recommend that people take zinc routinely for age-related macular disease.

Gass: Well, I think we can summarize that very briefly by saying that no-one on the panel, at least, is very enthusiastic about recommending zinc to the patients. Now, I think we ought to go on. Yes, Dick, I am sorry.

W.R. Green: I think, though, we have to keep in mind that light is toxic to the retina, and that the active metabolism that takes place between the photoreceptors and the pigment epithelium does generate toxic oxygen radicals. Drugs that will combine and remove toxic oxygen provide a distinct rationale for their use. But, at this date that rationale has not been established by clinical trials.

Gass: Well, let us move on to the topic of interferon. Within the past year – I do not remember the date – Dr. Fung wrote a letter to the editor, and described his results, I believe in the treatment of seven patients with juxtafoveal membranes – possibly some subfoveal membranes. He thought the results he observed following the interferon treatment were better than he would have expected. Since that time, there has just been an unbelievable flood of phone calls and people inquiring about interferon. If one reads that letter, the only thing surprising to me is how it ever got into the literature. But, anyway, it is there, we are stuck with it, and I would like to open this subject up for discussion. Anyone wish to start? First of all, what is the rationale for it, Dr. Fine?

Fine: I think the rationale is that interferon-alpha 2A inhibits neovascularization in certain biologic systems Dr. Judah Folkman in Boston has shown that in some childhood cancers, including pulmonary hemangiomatosis and hairy cell leukemia, there can be rather dramatic effects. Apparently the capillary bed behaves differently in different parts of the body. Therefore, although there has been a dramatic response in those two situations, I am not aware that the results are applicable to the treatment of choroidal neovascularization. I must say that I was flabbergasted when I realized how often interferon was being used to treat patients with AMD. Just like zinc, we have to accept the possibility that it might be helpful. However, I am aware of absolutely no tangible evidence that there have been any patients actually helped by interferon. Along with several colleagues, I am conducting an informal survey and have some information now on about 175 patients who have been given interferon. We have not heard of a single patient in whom neovascularization has regressed and the vision improved in response to that drug. Dr. Folkman, who has been a pioneer in using interferon-alpha in children with cancer, has indicated that the dose which most ophthalmologists are giving is just a fraction of what is actually required on a mg/kg basis, to get a biologic response. Also, he has suggested, according to colleagues, that it may not have been given long enough, and so he is not surprised that there have not been good responses. But he is not advocating interferon treatment either. We are now surveying retina specialists by mail to learn whether there have been any good results. The most encouraging thing I have heard was about a patient with new vessels under the right fovea, who was placed on interferon and in the opposite eye, which had been about 20/800 for the last two or three years, some of the fluid dried up a little and the vision improved from 20/800 to 20/600 in the fellow eye, and the patient said he was better. That is about the most encouraging thing! Now, I do not deny the possibility that interferon could promote resolution of fluid in disciform scars, but if that is going to turn out to be the main effect of the drug, I do not think it is going to be very helpful! I do not use interferon. I am astonished that patients actually would agree to take it. But in the 1980s people with cancer went to Mexico to get Laetrile. I cannot imagine what I could tell a patient to convince him/her to take that drug as a treatment for AMD!

Gass: Any comments, Dick?

Green: Stuart, you do not think that there is enough evidence even to warrant a clinical trial at this point?

Fine: No, I have been asked that, and you know I am a very strong proponent of clinical trials, but I think that before one conducts a clinical trial, there has to be some reasonable evidence that the treatment to be tested does something positive. For example, if there is a new vessel membrane, one can see it and see that it leaks fluid, and that it causes exudation. One then can apply photocoagulation and can see an anatomic effect. When you can produce an anatomical effect, and you know what the natural course is, then you can think about doing a clinical trial. I am trying to find a patient who has had some anatomical response to the use of interferon, and so far, I have not found one.

Bird: Can I ask if the treatment is innocuous?

Fine: The treatment is not innocuous. If the treatment were innocuous and cheap, then one could say to a patient, "well, it may not help, but at least it will not hurt". But, in fact, there are many adverse effects. Since I have not used it I would not want to describe those; maybe there are people in the audience who would like to, but flu-like symptoms and liver toxicity are among the toxic effects. Also, it is quite expensive. The treatment can cost anywhere from, I think, $1000 to $4000 dollars and it is an out-of-pocket expense since it is generally not covered by third party payers. I have heard of patients who had withdrawn their life savings from the bank, as I guess any of us would do if we thought that this treatment might be something which would restore our vision. So, it is not innocuous by any means, neither economically nor medically.

Gass: Any other comment?

Aaberg: Don, it would seem to me that this is one area that could justifiably be evaluated in the laboratory, because it is certainly possible to grow retinovascular capillary endothelial cells, and one should be able to then investigate whether interferon indeed stops the growth of these cells. I would think that that should be the way to proceed rather than to be injecting it into human beings at this point in time.

Gass: I did not attend any of the recent vitreoretinal meetings or the Macula Society meeting. I would be interested from those who attended, has there been a shift away from the types of patients in whom interferon was originally suggested as beneficial? Dr. Fung's first seven patients all had early neovascularization that was threatening the macula. Now I understand that in one part of the country interferon is recommended for very large neovascular membranes which are beyond treating with the laser. This would seem to make absolutely no sense at all. Stuart, you mentioned that the only success you had heard of from those using interferon is one patient whose vision in the first affected eye had improved after treatment instituted because of involvement of the second eye.

Green: Well, with regard to that point, Wayne Fung noted improvement in a handful of cases in the fellow eye which already had a disciform scar. Is that not right Stuart?

Fine: Yes.

Gass: Well, anyway, I think we can summarize the situation on interferon as follows: First of all, we need at least another feasibility trial or two. And I would urge that if any of you in the audience have a series of 20 or so patients treated with interferon which met Dr. Fung's criteria, you write a letter to the editor and get your findings into print. I am afraid that a lot of elderly people are taking significant risks with this treatment that has not been adequately investigated. Any other comments?

Davis: In defense of Dr. Fung, I believe he is planning a trial, a randomized controlled trial. Now whether that will happen or not I do not know, but I spoke with him after the meeting, the Macular Society meeting, and I think it is incumbent upon him to do that. Maybe none of the rest of us feel it is reasonable, but I think it is incumbent upon him to do it, and I think he is planning it.

Gass: Well, I think it is good that he is planning it. I just think that it is premature to do a controlled clinical trial. I do not believe it is appropriate to ask a patient to be randomized to a treatment that is risky and is unproven. So, we really do not have an adequate feasibility study.

Davis: One more comment. I think it is more ethical to do it as a trial than to do it uncontrolled.

Gass: That is true! You cannot argue with that statement.

Davis: (in the audience) Half of the people will be randomized to not getting it.

Gass: But my point is that I am not sure there is a need for a further clinical study. Stuart has already collected 170 patients and he has only found one who might have had a favorable response, then that information should be published, which should do much to stifle widespread use of interferon until more laboratory investigation can be done to test the rationale for its use.

Bird: You cannot be sure that the recorded change was a response to treatment. It is possible that this may have occurred spontaneously at a time when the treatment was given, such that there is no proof that functional improvement and the treatment were causally related.

Gass: Well, I think our time is up. Is that correct? And so we will adjourn for lunch.

II

DIABETIC RETINOPATHY

DIABETIC RETINOPATHY: NATURAL COURSE, PREVALENCE, CLASSIFICATION AND RISK FACTORS FOR PROGRESSION

Matthew D. Davis

Department of Ophthalmology, University of Wisconsin-Madison, Madison, Wisconsin, USA

Natural course of diabetic retinopathy

The natural course of diabetic retinopathy is best understood in relation to five fundamental pathologic processes[1-7]:

1. formation of retinal capillary microaneurysms;
2. excessive vascular permeability;
3. vascular occlusion;
4. proliferation of new blood vessels and accompanying fibrous tissue on the surface of the retina and optic disc; and
5. contraction of these fibrovascular proliferations and the vitreous.

Microaneurysms

The retinal capillary microaneurysm is the hallmark of diabetic retinopathy and its earliest reliable clinical sign. Early in their evolution microaneurysms are seen with direct ophthalmoscopy as tiny dots of the same deep red color as the retinal veins. At this stage the wall of the microaneurysm is completely transparent and only the blood within its lumen is visible, as is the case for normal retinal vessels. Ophthalmoscopically visible microaneurysms commonly vary in diameter from about 15-60 μm, *i.e.*, from one-eighth to one-half the diameter of a normal retinal vein at the disc margin, but occasionally may be larger (the dimensions used here are based on the common clinical convention that considers the diameter of the average optic disc to be 1500 μm, although 1800-1900 μm may be a better estimate)[8,9]. It is often difficult to determine ophthalmoscopically whether a given red spot is a microaneurysm or a punctate hemorrhage. Most round red dots with smooth edges fill during fluorescein angiography, proving that they are microaneurysms; some that do not fill can be shown to be microaneurysms packed with red blood cells by clinico-histopathologic correlation[10].

Microaneurysms may show little change over periods of several years or may disappear leaving no trace. Alternatively, their walls may become thickened, sometimes sufficiently to occlude their lumens[10]. As the wall of a microaneurysm thickens it becomes less transparent and its color changes from the bluish-red of venous blood through shades of orange offering little contrast with the fundus background to the yellowish-white color of hard exudate. During the reddish-orange stage the wall of the microaneurysm, seen on edge, may be visible as a white ring surrounding the blood in its lumen (Fig. 1).

Address for correspondence: Matthew D. Davis, MD, Department of Ophthalmology, University of Wisconsin-Madison, 610 N. Walnut Street, P.O. Box 5240, Madison, WI 53705, USA

Retina and Vitreous, pp. 43-61
Proceedings of the Symposium on Retina and Vitreous,
organized by the New Orleans Academy of Ophthalmology
New Orleans, LA, USA, March 12-15, 1992
edited by Rudolph M. Franklin

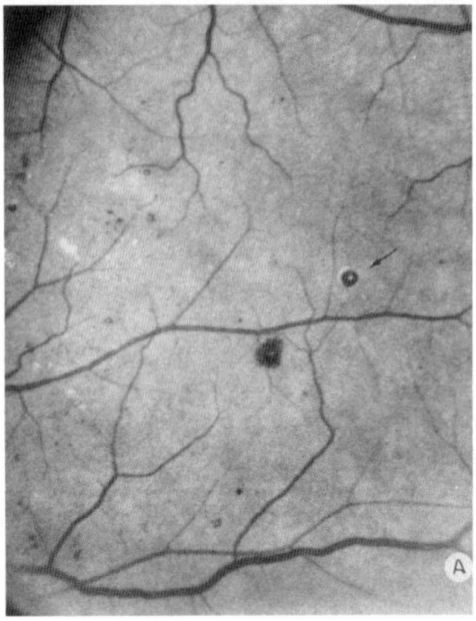

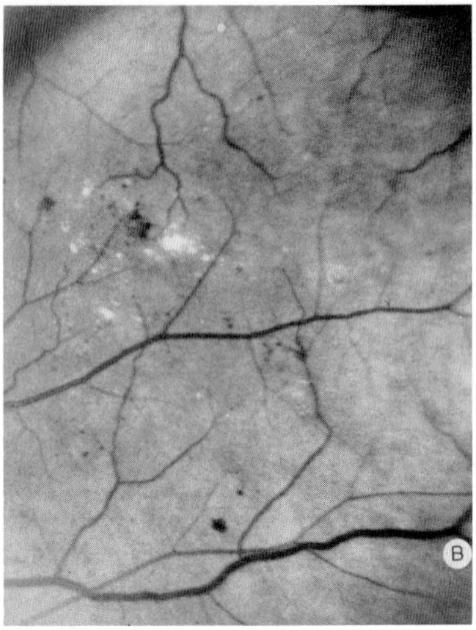

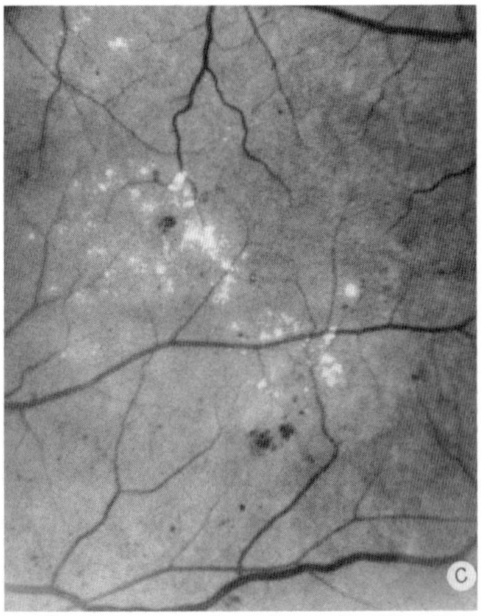

Fig. 1. Evolution of a very large microaneurysm in the left eye of a patient with type II diabetes. *A.* The microaneurysm (arrow) has a central light reflex and its wall is mostly invisible (except from 9 to 12 o'clock) and does not obscure the blood in its lumen. *B.* Fifteen months later the wall of the microaneurysm is apparent as a ring around its lumen and the blood in the lumen is obscured by the wall. *C.* Two years later the microaneurysm is an opaque white spot, its lumen presumably closed. Partial hard exudate rings surround groups of smaller microaneurysms below the large microaneurysm and at the left side of the figure. (Courtesy of Fundus Photograph Reading Center, University of Wisconsin-Madison.)

Excessive vascular permeability

An early and easily detected clinical sign of increased vascular permeability is the accumulation of white or yellowish-white deposits in the deeper layers of the retina ("hard exudates"). Hard exudates are made up mainly of lipid, most of which has presumably leaked from the plasma across excessively permeable capillary walls, particularly those of microaneurysms. Hard exudates may be sprinkled across the fundus in no particular pattern, but more often are arranged in partial or complete rings, each ring marking the circumference of a roughly circular zone of thickened (edematous) retina that surrounds one or more microaneurysms (Fig. 2). The lipid apparently remains dispersed within the retina in the edematous zones and becomes deposited at their edges as water and other small molecules are resorbed across the walls of surrounding more normal capillaries. Thickened retina usually maintains normal or near-normal transparency, and retinal edema was largely overlooked as a characteristic feature of diabetic retinopathy until binocular ophthalmoscopy became widely available. In advanced stages of retinopathy, larger retinal vessels may also demonstrate excessive permeability. Newly formed preretinal vessels are characteristically very permeable, as demonstrated dramatically by fluorescein angiography.

Vaso-obliteration

In the earliest stages of diabetic retinopathy individual acellular (non-perfused) capillaries can be seen histologically, but not ophthalmoscopically. Somewhat later dropout of individual capillaries can often be demonstrated angiographically within one disc diameter of the center of the macula, where choroidal fluorescence is less visible and individual retinal capillaries are normally more clearly seen. As retinopathy becomes more severe

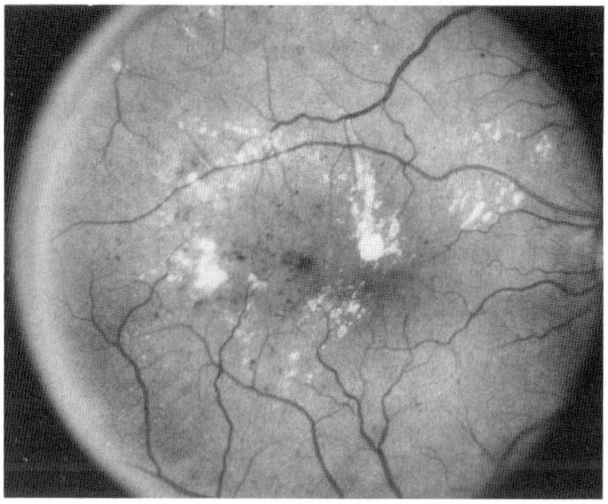

Fig. 2. A hard exudate ring about 1.5 disc diameters in diameter is centered about 1.0 disc diameter superotemporal to the center of the macula in this right eye. Part of the ring is a plaque of hard exudate just above the center of the macula. Within the ring there are many large microaneurysms, some with visible walls. They are slightly out of focus because the retina here is thickened (edematous) and the camera is focused on the surrounding retina. The thickened retina maintains near-normal transparency. With stereoscopic viewing retinal thickening was obvious and could be seen to extend into the center of the macula. (Courtesy of the Early Treatment Diabetic Retinopathy Study (ETDRS) Research Group.)

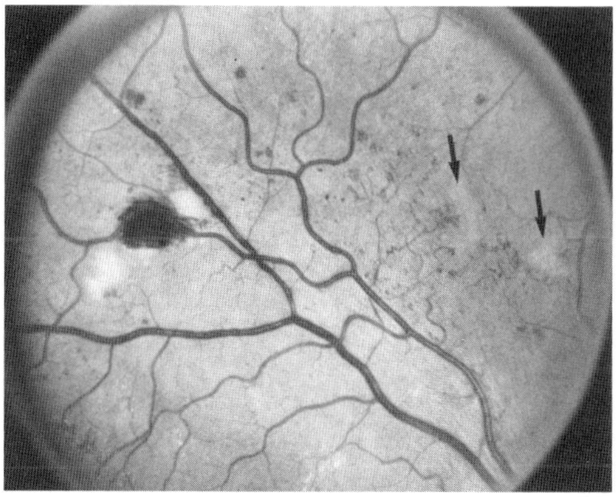

Fig. 3. Severe NPDR. On the left side of the figure there are two prominent soft exudates with a large blot hemorrhage between them. Venous beading is prominent where the superior branch of the superior temporal vein passes by the upper exudate. On the right side of the figure there are two faint soft exudates (arrows) and many prominent IRMA. (Courtesy of the ETDRS Research Group.)

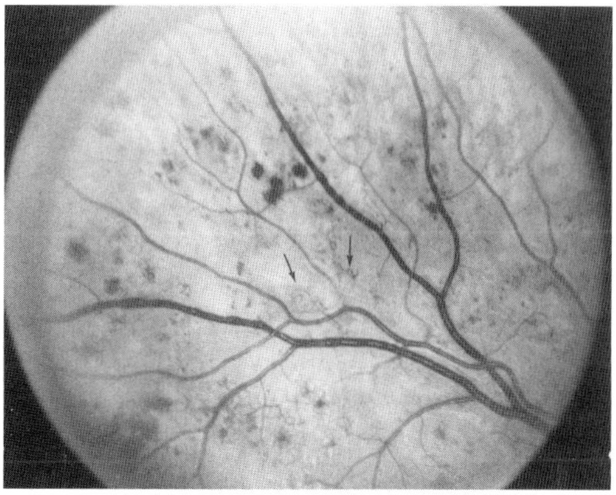

Fig. 4. Transition from severe NPDR to PDR. There are extensive retinal hemorrhages, venous beading, and several large faint soft exudates (just to the left of the center of the figure). Arrows indicate tortuous small vessels that could be either IRMA or early new vessels on the surface of the retina. (Courtesy of the ETDRS Research Group.)

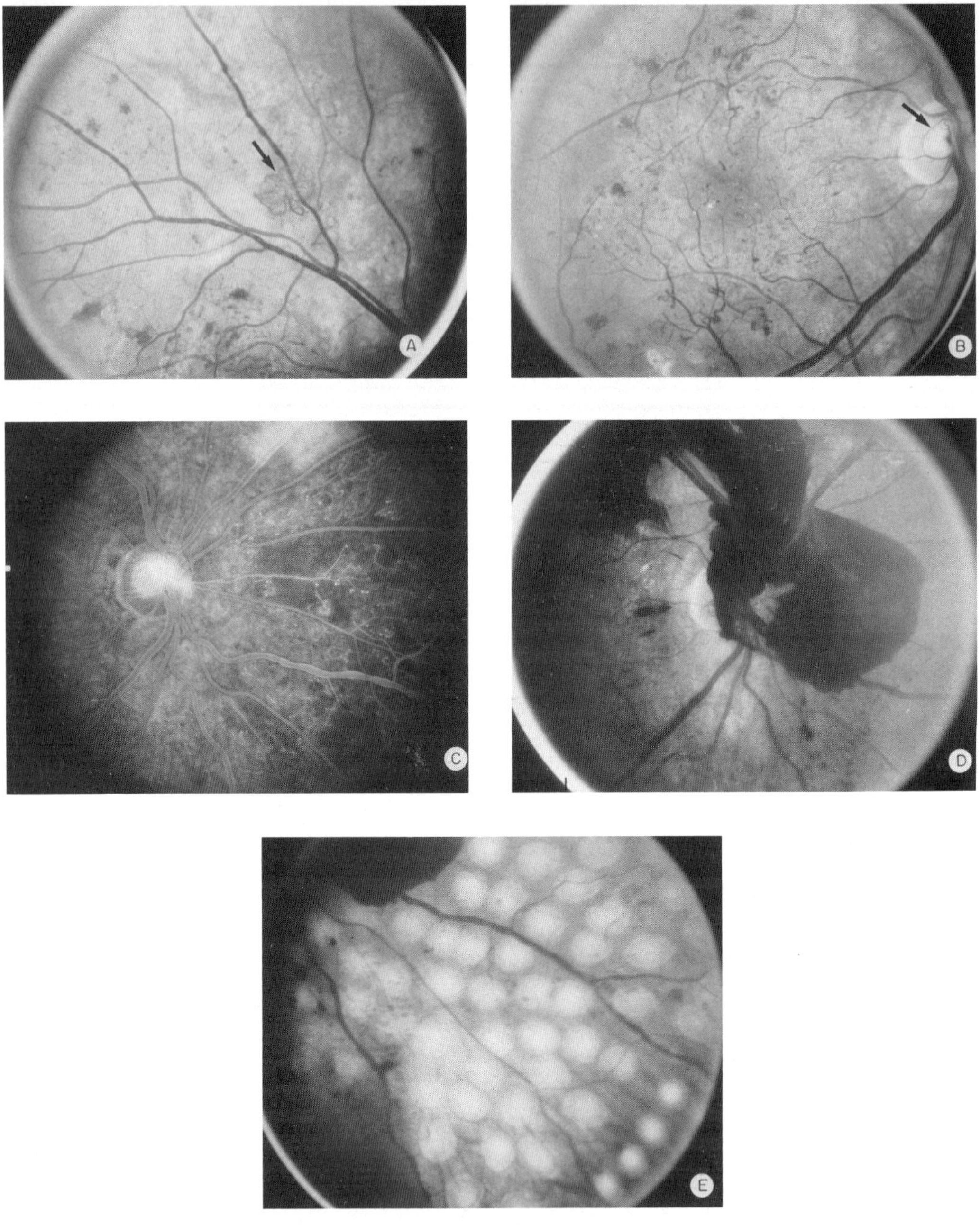

Fig. 5A. New vessels forming a wheel-like network (arrow) in the superior temporal quadrant of an eye with venous beading, soft exudates, IRMA and blot hemorrhages. *B.* Posterior pole of the same eye showing IRMA and retinal hemorrhages centrally and featureless retina near the left edge of the figure. With stereoscopic examination the vascular loop on the disc (arrow) could be seen to bridge the physiologic cup and was clearly a new vessel. *C.* In the late-stage angiogram the position of new vessels on the disc is marked by fluorescein leakage. Fluorescein leakage along the superior nasal vein at the upper edge of the figure is from new vessels here. There is an obvious area of capillary dropout beginning one disc diameter nasal to the disc. *D.* Ten months later, preretinal and vitreous hemorrhage occurred from the new vessels. *E.* Lower nasal quadrant showing fresh burns of the first episode of scatter photocoagulation, carried out on the same day. After repeated photocoagulation almost all the new vessels regressed and good vision was maintained. (Courtesy of the ETDRS Research Group.)

larger patches of capillary closure appear, each typically supplied by an occluded terminal arteriole. Such patches are often marked initially by overlying cotton-wool spots (soft exudates), which tend to fade over periods of many months (Figs. 3 and 4). Adjacent to patches of capillary closure microaneurysms and tiny tortuous vessels are frequently seen. It is difficult to determine whether these vessels are dilated pre-existing capillaries or intraretinal new vessels, and the term "intraretinal microvascular abnormalities" (IRMA) is used to include both possibilities (Figs. 3 and 4)[11]. Histologically, these vessels are hypercellular and most observers agree that the stimulus for them, and for new vessels on the surface of the retina, is probably partial ischemia of the inner retinal layers caused by capillary closure. As capillary closure becomes more extensive dark red blot hemorrhages often appear (Fig. 4), as does segmental dilation of retinal veins (venous beading, Figs. 3, 4 and 5A). When these lesions are prominent, non-proliferative retinopathy (NPDR) is considered severe (preproliferative). When capillary closure becomes very extensive, these intraretinal lesions tend to disappear, leading to a featureless appearance (Fig 5B).

Proliferation of new vessels and fibrous tissue

Although proliferation of endothelial cells is taking place within the retina as a part of IRMA and venous beading, only when new vessels appear on the surface of the retina or optic disc is diabetic retinopathy said to have entered the proliferative stage (PDR). New vessels begin typically as fine loops or networks lying on the surface of the retina or the optic disc, or bridging across the physiologic cup (Fig. 5B). Early new vessels are easily overlooked and may be difficult to distinguish from IRMA (Fig. 4). As they become larger, new vessels are easily identified, either by their tendency to form networks or by their course across both arterial and venous branches of the underlying retinal vessels, a pattern never occurring in the normal vasculature. The most striking networks are roughly circular patches resembling carriage wheels, with vessels radiating like spokes from the center of the patch to a circumferential vessel bounding its periphery (Figs. 5A and 6B and C). The centers of such patches often lie over retinal veins, into which the vessels appear to drain. Eyes with new vessels on the disc are at greater risk of visual loss, and new vessels here (on or within one disc diameter of the disc, or in the vitreous cavity anterior to this area) are commonly designated NVD and considered separately from new vessels elsewhere (NVE)[12-17]. On fluorescein angiography new vessels usually leak profusely (Fig. 5C).

The rate of growth of new vessels is extremely variable. In some patients a patch of vessels may remain essentially unchanged for many months, while in others a definite increase may be seen in as little as a week or two. New vessels characteristically follow a cycle of proliferation and regression[3,4]. Early in their evolution new vessels appear bare, but later translucent fibrous tissue often appears adjacent to them and becomes increasingly opaque as regression of the new vessels occurs (Fig. 6D). Usually regression is incomplete, but occasionally blood-filled new vessels may disappear altogether, being replaced by tufts of white tissue or networks of white lines, or occasionally leaving no trace at all. These fibrovascular proliferations characteristically become adherent to the vitreous framework and such adhesions remain even after the new vessels regress. So long as neither vitreous hemorrhage nor contraction of the vitreous and/or fibrovascular proliferations occurs, the new vessels remain asymptomatic.

Contraction of vitreous and fibrovascular proliferations

Posterior vitreous detachment tends to occur at an earlier age in patients with PDR. In areas free of fibrovascular proliferations the posterior vitreous surface usually pulls away

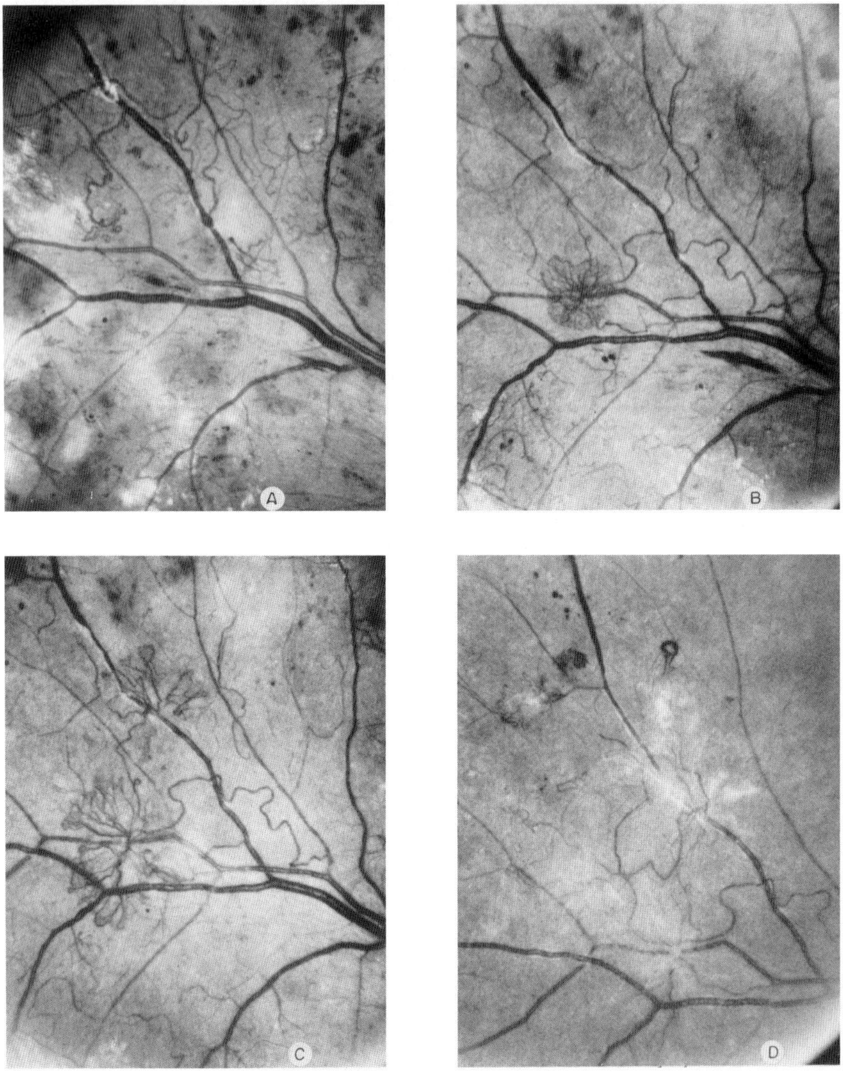

Fig. 6A. Severe NPDR in a patient with newly diagnosed type II diabetes (superior temporal quadrant of the right eye). There are many microaneurysms, hemorrhages and hard exudates, as well as extensive retinal edema and venous beading. Most of the tortuous small vessels appeared to be within the retina (large IRMA), but some may have been on its surface (NVE). *B.* Eight months later there had been marked improvement in the intraretinal abnormalities, but a wheel-like network of new vessels had appeared on the surface of the retina. *C.* Three months later the new vessel patch had enlarged and a second patch had developed above it. During the next two years the new vessels continued to grow slowly at the edges of the patches, while regressing at their centers. *D.* Three years after they had appeared, most of the new vessels had regressed, although there was still one dilated loop at the upper edge of the upper patch. No contraction of fibrous proliferations or vitreous had occurred, there had been no vitreous hemorrhage, and vision remained good. (Courtesy of Fundus Photograph Reading Center, University of Wisconsin-Madison.)

easily from the retina. Where proliferations are present, they are pulled forward, and with them the retina from which they arise, often producing localized areas of tractional retinal detachment (Fig. 7). The fibrovascular proliferations themselves also play an important part in the contraction process, particularly when they are extensive. In addition to pro-

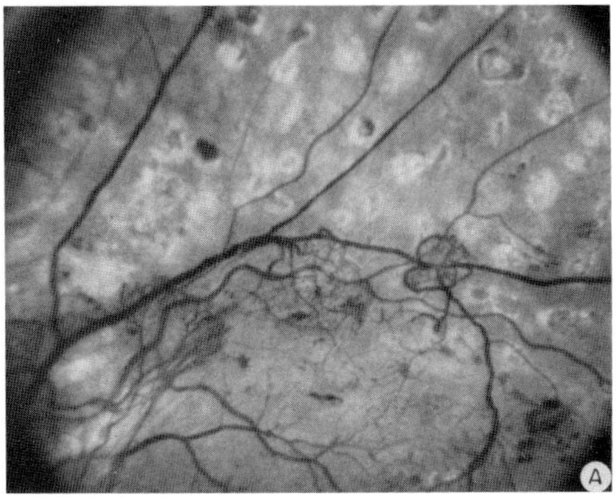

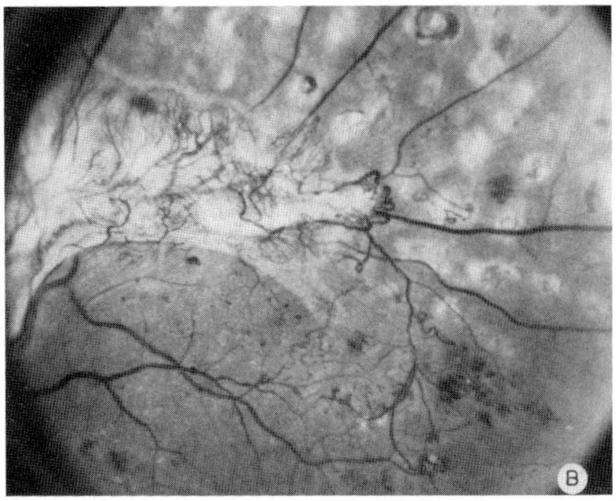

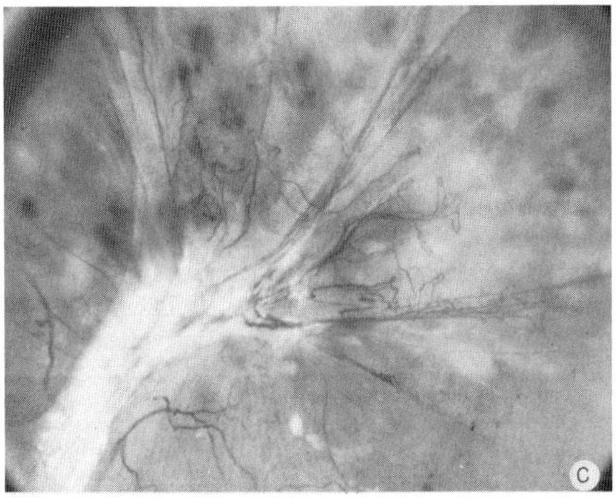

Fig. 7A. Networks of new vessels extend over the surface of the retina along the superior temporal vein. Scars are typical of initial scatter photocoagulation, with ample room for additional treatment (in retrospect, this probably would have been advisable). *B.* Four months later, new vessels had increased and dense fibrous tissue had appeared. *C.* Seven months later, fibrous proliferations had contracted. Broad adhesions prevented them from pulling away from the retina; instead, the retina has been pulled forward (detached) throughout the area included in the figure. The photocoagulation scars are blurred by the overlying detached retina (and are also out of focus). (Courtesy of the Diabetic Retinopathy Vitrectomy Study (DRVS) Research Group.)

ducing a vector of force that tends to pull the retina forward away from the retinal pigment epithelium and choroid, contraction of a sheet of fibrous tissue also tends to pull the surrounding retina towards the center of the sheet (tangential traction). Since fibrovascular membranes are usually centered on or near the optic disc, tangential traction often leads to displacement ("dragging") of the macula nasally toward the disc (Fig. 8).[18].

As contraction begins, traction is exerted upon the new vessels[4,5]. Preretinal and/or vitreous hemorrhage often occurs concomitantly, probably in part because of the traction (Fig. 5D). The severity of visual symptoms varies with the extent of the hemorrhage, from a few floating specks lasting only an hour or two (until the blood disperses or settles inferiorly) to loss of all but hand movement or light perception vision. It is unusual for the first vitreous hemorrhage that occurs in an eye to be massive, but a large hemorrhage often follows an initial small one within a few days or weeks. The rate at which hemorrhages clear is highly variable, from a few weeks when they are small to months, years, or never when they are large. Hemorrhages tend to recur periodically, usually without any obvious precipitating event and often during sleep[19,20].

Prevalence of diabetic retinopathy

PDR has generally been considered to be a more important problem in type I (insulin-dependent) diabetes and macular edema more important in type II (non-insulin-dependent). Accurate comparisons have been difficult, because of uncertainties in the clinical

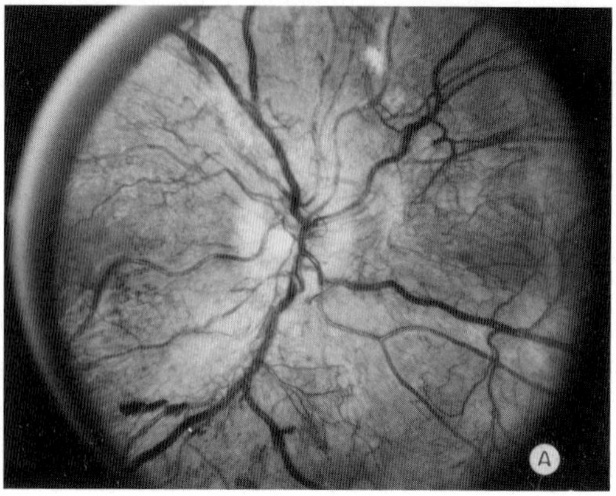

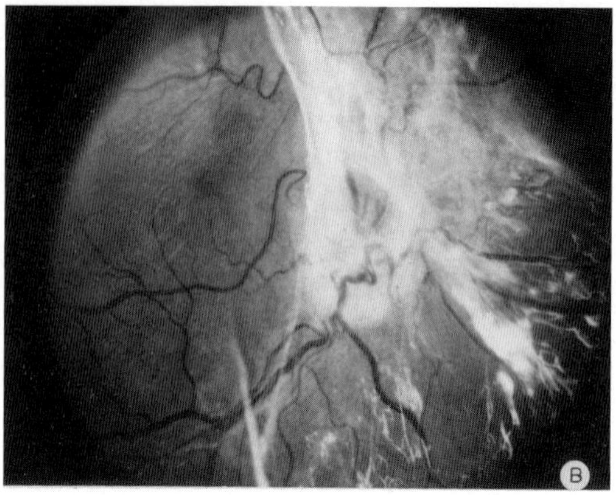

Fig. 8A. There are extensive new vessels on the surface of the disc and retina in this right eye as well as many dilated intraretinal vessels (IRMA). There is a soft exudate about 1 disc diameter superonasally to the disc and several small preretinal hemorrhages near the bottom of the figure to the left. The macula is in its normal position, centered at or just temporal to the left edge of the figure. Fibrous tissue accompanying the new vessels is visible adjacent to the temporal vascular arcades and in a small area 0.5 disc diameter superonasal to the disc. Fibrous proliferations were actually much more extensive, but were transparent and difficult to detect. Visual acuity was 20/20. Contraction of the fibrous proliferations occurred within the next several months, dragging the retina nasally and superiorly, and new vessels regressed. *B.* Four years later, the center of the macula was about 1.5 disc diameters superotemporal to the disc margin. The first major bifurcation of the inferior temporal vein had been pulled upward to the disc margin from its previous position. New vessels had regressed completely, some of them now appearing as networks of fine white lines. Visual acuity was 20/30. (Courtesy of the DRVS Research Group.)

assessment of diabetes type and the paucity of population-based studies. Figs. 9 and 10 from a study by Klein and co-workers summarize the prevalence of any degree of retinopathy and of PDR, respectively, in a population-based sample of diabetic individuals in southwestern Wisconsin[21]. Retinopathy severity was assessed in stereoscopic color fundus photographs graded according to the Modified Airlie House classification[16,17]. In the younger-onset group, which was made up of individuals whose age at diagnosis of

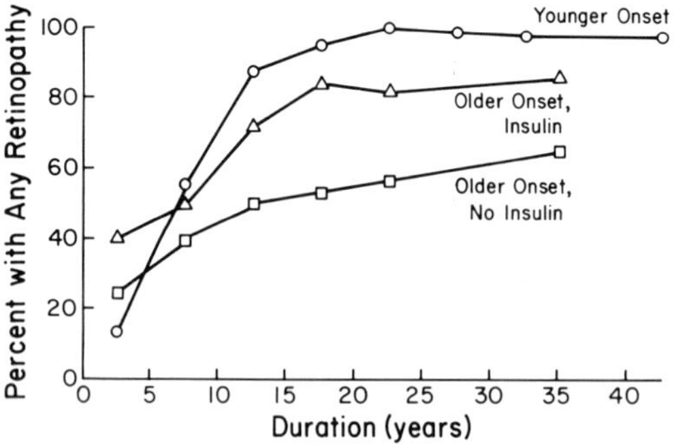

Fig. 9. Percentage of persons with diabetic retinopathy by duration of diabetes in each of three groups classified by age at diagnosis and insulin use. The number of persons in each duration interval in each group was at least 70, with the following exceptions – younger-onset group: interval 30-34 years, 43, interval 35 years and over, 44; non-insulin-taking group: interval 20-24 years, 41, interval 25 years and over, 15.

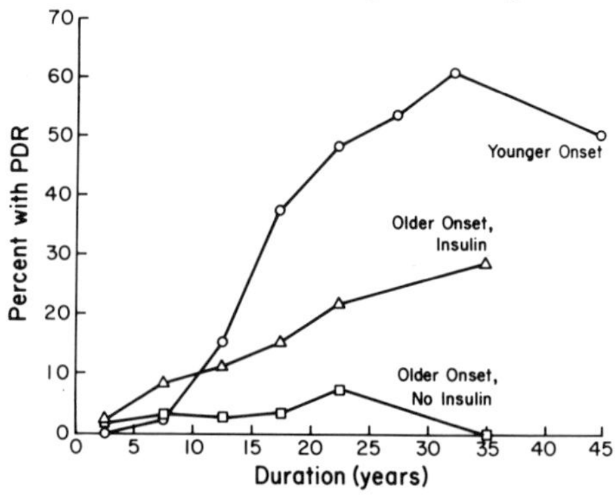

Fig. 10. Percentage of persons with PDR by duration of diabetes in each of the three groups.

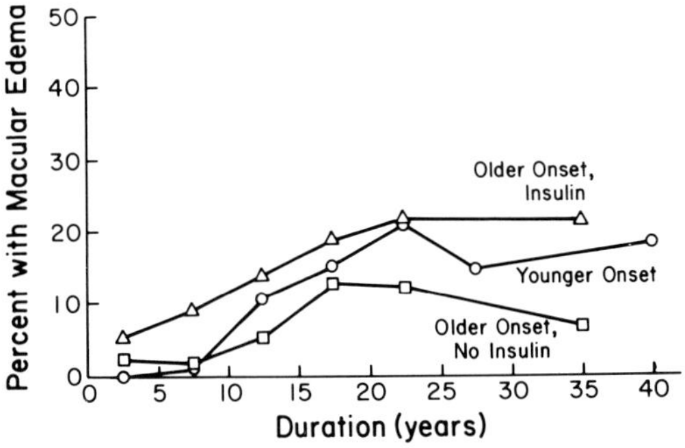

Fig. 11. Percentage of persons with macular edema by duration of diabetes in each of the three groups. (*Figs. 9-11* from: Klein R, Davis MD, Moss SE, Klein BEK, DeMets DL: The Wisconsin Epidemiologic Study of Diabetic Retinopathy: a comparison of retinopathy in younger and older onset diabetic persons. In: Vranic M, Hollenberg C, Steiner G (eds) Comparison of Type I and Type II Diabetes, pp 321-325. New York: Plenum Publishing Corp 1985.)

Table 1. ETDRS Retinopathy Severity Scale (clinical approximation)

Descriptive designation	*Level*	*Definition*
No retinopathy	10	No Ma or other lesions
Very mild (Ma only)	20	Ma, but no other lesions
Mild NPDR	35	Ma plus RH, HE, and/or SE
Moderate NPDR	43	Ma plus H/Ma severe in 1 quadrant *or* IRMA mild in 1-3 quadrants
	47	*Both* Level 43 definitions and/or *one* of the following: - H/Ma severe in 2-3 quadrants - IRMA mild in 4 quadrants - VB mild in 1 quadrant
Severe NPDR	53 A-D	Ma plus ≥ 2 Level 47 definitions and/or *one* of the following: - H/Ma severe in 4 quadrants - VB present in ≥ 2 quadrants - IRMA ≥ moderate in ≥ 1 quadrant
Very severe NPDR	53 E	Ma plus 2 or 3 of above
Mild PRD	61	NVE < 1/2 disc area, or FP only
Moderate PDR	65	NVE ≥ 1/2 disc area and/or NVD < Standard Photograph 10A (about 1/4-1/3 disc area)
High-risk PDR	71, 72	NVD ≥ Standard Photograph 10A and/or VH or PRH present and new vessels visible or assumed to be obscured by VH/PRH
Advanced PDR	81, 85	Fundus obscured by VH or PRH so that new vessels cannot be graded, or retinal detachment involving center of macula

Ma: microaneurysms; NPDR: non-proliferative diabetic retinopathy; RH: retinal hemorrhage; HE: hard exudates; SE: soft exudates; H/Ma: hemorrhages/microaneurysms; IRMA: intraretinal microvascular abnormalities; VB: venous beading; PDR: proliferative diabetic retinopathy; NVE: new vessels elsewhere (≥ 1 DD from disc); FP: fibrous proliferations; NVD: new vessels of the disc (within 1 DD of disc margin); VH: vitreous hemorrhage; PRH: preretinal hemorrhage. (Modified from: Early Treatment Diabetic Retinopathy Study Research Group: Fundus photographic risk factors for progression of diabetic retinopathy. ETDRS Study Report No 12. Ophthalmology 98:823-833, 1991. Courtesy of the ETDRS Research Group.)

diabetes was less than 30 years and who were taking insulin at the time of examination (nearly all presumably had type I diabetes), prevalence of retinopathy (Fig. 9) rose steeply from about 13% in persons with less than five years of diabetes to 90% in those with ten to 15 years. Retinopathy was more common in the older-onset individuals with diabetes of less than five years' known duration and prevalence rose less rapidly with increasing duration, both in the group taking insulin (a mixture of type I and type II diabetes) and in the non-insulin-taking (type II) group.

Prevalence of PDR (Fig. 10) in the younger-onset group was zero when duration of diabetes was less than five years, 2% in the five to ten year duration interval, and then rose rapidly to about 50% or more in persons with 20 or more years of diabetes. In the older-onset insulin-taking group, prevalence rose fairly steadily from 2% in persons with less than five years of diabetes to more than 20% in those with 20 years or more. In the non-insulin-taking group, prevalence remained about 2-5% regardless of duration. Among individuals with PDR, its severity did not appear to differ between the younger-onset and the combined older-onset groups; in each case in the worse eye about 25% of individuals had Diabetic Retinopathy Study (DRS) high-risk PDR and 15% had advanced PDR (see Table 1 for definitions).

Prevalence of macular edema did not vary as widely by diabetes type (Fig. 11), but PDR was significantly more common in younger-onset individuals with macular edema (65% *versus* 36% and 19%, respectively, in the older-onset insulin-taking and non-insulin-taking groups) and moderately extensive hard exudate was significantly less common (2%, 9%, and 18%, in the three groups, respectively).

Because diabetes with onset after age 30 years is more common than the younger-onset type, however, in the population from which Klein and co-workers drew their sample these older-onset individuals comprised a majority of the total number with either macular edema or PDR. Of all persons with macular edema, 20% were estimated to belong to the younger-onset group, 59% to the older-onset insulin-taking group, and 21% to the non-insulin-taking group. Of all persons with PDR, 43% belonged to the younger-onset group, 42% to the older-onset insulin-taking group, and 15% to the non-insulin-taking group[21]. Among patients with PDR entering the DRS or attending the Eye Unit of the Joslin Clinic, the percentage belonging to the younger-onset group appeared to be somewhat higher, in the range of 50-65%[22,23].

Classification of diabetic retinopathy

The Early Treatment Diabetic Retinopathy Study (ETDRS), a randomized clinical trial sponsored by the National Eye Institute, investigated the use of photocoagulation and aspirin in patients with mild to severe NPDR or mild to moderate PDR, with or without macular edema. Patients were randomly assigned to aspirin 650 mg per day or placebo. One eye of each patient was randomly assigned to early photocoagulation, the other to deferral of photocoagulation, *i.e.*, follow-up visits at frequent intervals and prompt initiation of photocoagulation if high-risk PDR developed[24]. Gradings of stereoscopic fundus photographs of eyes assigned to deferral (aspirin and placebo groups combined) were used to refine a retinopathy severity scale developed in earlier studies[25]. A clinical approximation of this ETDRS scale is shown in Table 1. The "severe" category for hemorrhages/microaneurysms and the "moderate" category for IRMA referred to in Table 1 are defined by the Standard Photographs shown in Figs. 12 and 13; Standard Photograph 10A is shown in Fig 14.

Fig. 15 presents cumulative rates of development of high-risk PDR in ETDRS eyes assigned to deferral of photocoagulation, by severity of retinopathy at baseline[24]. Eyes with mild NPDR (Level 35) were at low risk of progression to high-risk PDR, only about 15%

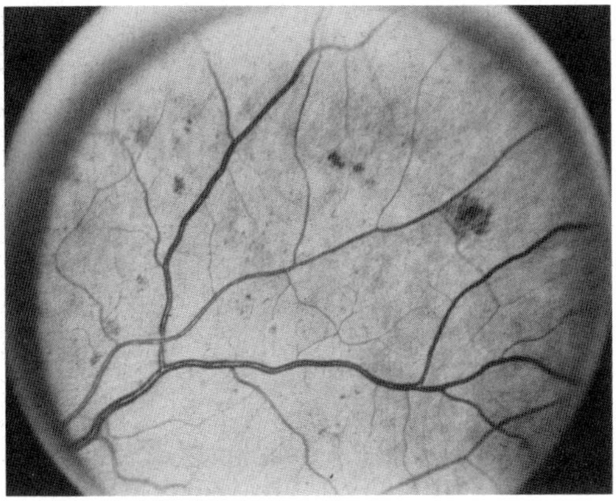

Fig. 12. Standard Photograph 2A of the Modified Airlie House Classification, defining the lower margin of the severe category for retinal hemorrhages/microaneurysms.

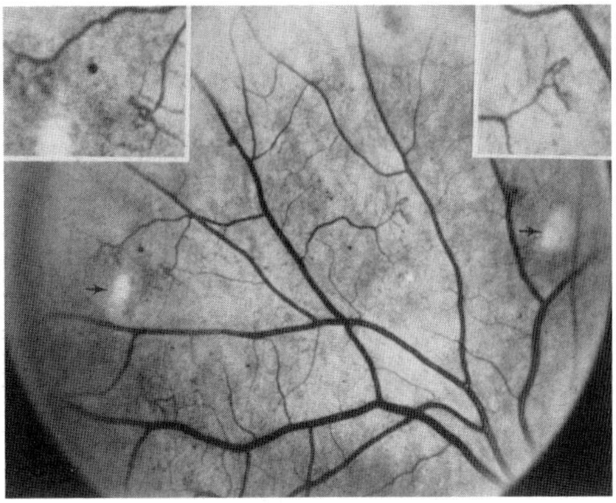

Fig. 13. Standard Photograph 8A of the Modified Airlie House Classification, defining the lower margin of the moderate category for IRMA. Insets show two of several areas of IRMA. Arrows indicated soft exudates.

(*Figs. 12* and *13* from: Early Treatment Diabetic Retinopathy Study Research Group: Grading diabetic retinopathy from stereoscopic color fundus photographs: an extension of the modified Airlie House classification. ETDRS Study Report No 10. Ophthalmology 98:786-806, 1991. Courtesy of the ETDRS Research Group.)

after five years. Eyes with very severe NPDR (Level 53E) or moderate PDR (Level 65) were at much higher risk, about 50% after a little more than a year. This analysis documents the validity of the severity scale and supports the use of progression along the scale as an outcome measure. Table 2 presents the percentages of ETDRS deferral-group eyes with progression of two or more steps along the scale between baseline and the one-, three-, and five-year visits. One-year progression rates were quite similar across baseline levels, but three- and five-year rates increased somewhat with increasing level. The ETDRS used progression along this scale by two or more steps as an outcome measure to

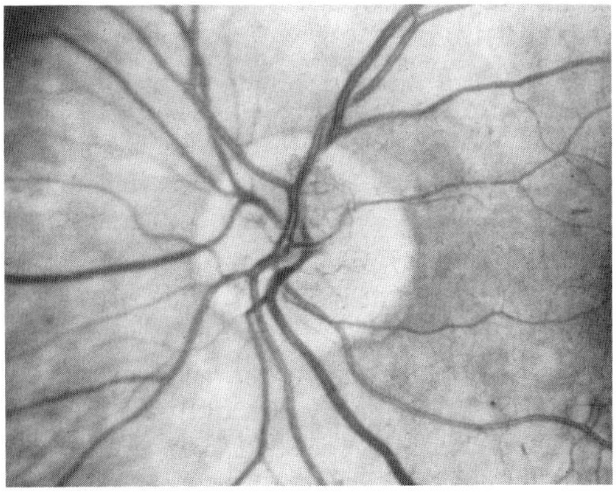

Fig. 14. Standard Photograph 10A of the Modified Airlie House Classification. New vessels cover about 1/4 the area of this disc, which is a little larger than average. New vessels equalling or exceeding those in this photograph are sufficient to place an eye in the high-risk PDR category (without regard to the size of the disc). (Courtesy of the Diabetic Retinopathy Study Research Group.)

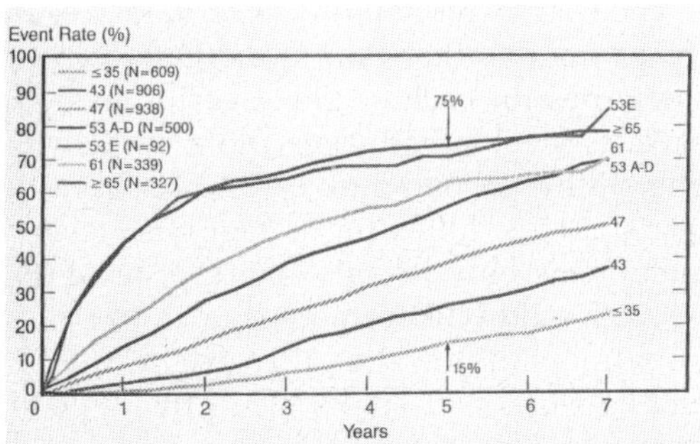

Fig. 15. Cumulative rates of high-risk proliferative retinopathy in ETDRS deferral group eyes, by baseline retinopathy severity level. See Table 1 for definitions of levels. (From: Early Treatment Diabetic Retinopathy Study Research Group: Early photocoagulation for diabetic retinopathy. ETDRS Study Report No 9. Ophthalmology 98:766-785, 1991. Courtesy of the ETDRS Research Group.)

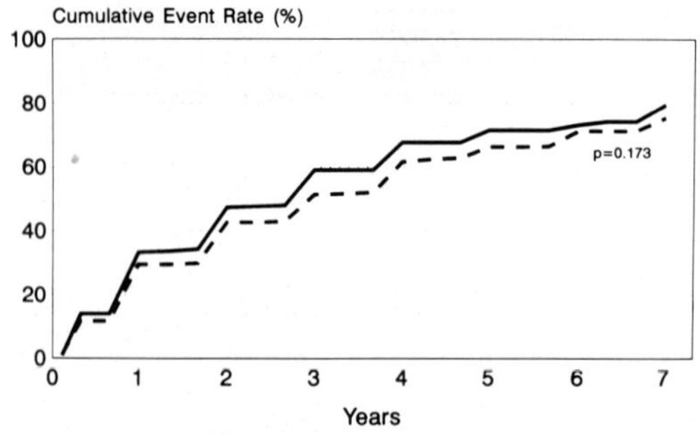

Fig. 16. Cumulative rates of worsening of retinopathy by two or more steps on the scale shown in Table 1, for eyes with severity Level 35 at baseline assigned to deferral of photocoagulation, by patient drug treatment assignment (- - - aspirin, —— placebo). (From: Early Treatment Diabetic Retinopathy Study Research Group: Effects of aspirin treatment on diabetic retinopathy. ETDRS Study Report No 8. Ophthalmology 98:757-765, 1991. Courtesy of the ETDRS Research Group.)

Table 2. Percentage of eyes with retinopathy progression of two or more levels at one-, three-, and five-year visits, by baseline retinopathy severity level

Baseline retinopathy level	*One-year follow-up*		*Three-year follow-up*		*Five-year follow-up*	
	Percent	*No.**	*Percent*	*No.**	*Percent*	*No.**
Level 35	26.2	569	35.7	524	40.0	290
Level 43	22.0	840	37.5	758	50.3	457
Level 47	26.3	864	47.5	793	66.3	472
Level 53	32.4	522	58.1	468	68.1	301
Level 61	21.5	311	52.8	282	62.8	183

*Number at risk (From: Early Treatment Diabetic Retinopathy Study Research Group: Fundus photographic risk factors for progression of diabetic retinopathy. ETDRS Study Report No 12. Ophthalmology 98:823-833, 1991. Courtesy of the ETDRS Research Group.)

assess the effect of aspirin in eyes with mild NPDR (Fig. 16). Aspirin was not found to influence progression even in this mildest subgroup, nor to influence progression to high-risk PDR when all patients were considered. Aspirin also did not increase the risk of vitreous hemorrhage in eyes that had new vessels at baseline[26].

The ETDRS retinopathy severity scale, and others similar to it, can also be used to classify patients, rather than eyes. One convenient way to do this is to provide two patient categories for each ocular severity level, a more severe one for patients with that ocular severity level in both eyes and a milder one for patients with a lesser ocular severity category in the second eye[27]. This has been called the "worse eye emphasized" method and leads to the following categories: level 10/10: no retinopathy; level 20/<20: microaneurysms only in only one eye; level 20/20: microaneurysms only in both eyes; level 35/<35: mild NPDR in one eye and any lesser level (in this case microaneurysms only or no retinopathy) in the other eye; level 35/35: mild NPDR in both eyes; and so on. Klein and co-workers used a scale of this type to study risk factors for retinopathy progression over a four-year period[28,29].

Risk factors for retinopathy progression

Table 3 provides four-year incidence rates of PDR and of progression by two or more steps on a "worse eye emphasized" scale in patients classified by diabetes type and baseline retinopathy severity. Rates of two-or-more step progression ranged from 18 to 57%,

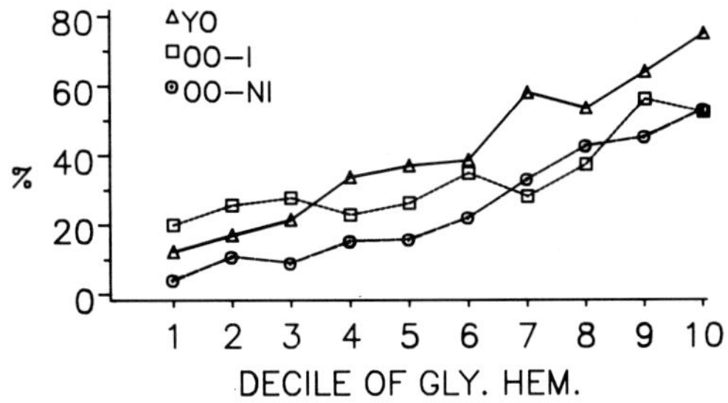

Fig. 17. Percentage of patients with NPDR at baseline showing progression of retinopathy by two or more levels (see text) four years later, by decile of glycosylated hemoglobin at baseline. YO: younger-onset patients; OO-I: older-onset patients taking insulin; OO-NI: older-onset patients not taking insulin. (Courtesy of R. Klein and co-workers.)

with a tendency to be somewhat lower in the older-onset groups but with no systematic difference between baseline retinopathy severity levels. As expected, the rate of progression to PDR increased with increasing baseline retinopathy severity. The high rates of progression by two or more steps on the scale and the relative stability of these rates between baseline retinopathy severity levels make this outcome a useful one in risk factor analyses. Fig. 17 presents such an analysis, in which risk of progression was strongly related to baseline level of glycosylated hemoglobin[30]. There appeared to be a similar, dose-response relationship in each patient group. Comparing the highest to the lowest quartile of glycosylated hemoglobin, the relative risk of progression was four in the younger-onset group, two in the older-onset insulin-taking group and six in the older-onset non-insulin-taking group. In multivariate analyses, baseline glycosylated hemoglobin remained a strong predictor of progression, independent of age, diabetes duration, baseline retinopathy severity, and blood pressure[30,31]. Moreover, none of these other factors was an independent predictor of progression in the younger-onset group (diastolic blood pressure was of borderline significance). In the older-onset groups younger age, longer diabetes duration, and lesser retinopathy severity were risk factors for progression, but the associations were weaker than that for glycosylated hemoglobin.

Table 3. Four-year rates of retinopathy progression by baseline retinopathy severity and diabetes type (after Klein *et al.*[28,29])

Baseline retinopathy level	*YO-I*			*OO-I*			*OO-NI*		
	No. at risk	*% with progression*		*No. at risk*	*% with progression*		*No. at risk*	*% with progression*	
		≥ 2 Steps	*PDR*		*≥ 2 Steps*	*PDR*		*≥ 2 Steps*	*PDR*
10/10	271	36.5	0.4	154	33.1	0	320	20.3	0.6
21/<21	66	36.4	3.0	49	51.0	0	65	36.9	1.5
21/21	105	51.4	4.8	23	56.5	0	24	29.2	0
31/<31	58	46.6	10.3	37	35.1	8.1	27	33.3	0
31/31	74	54.1	20.3	49	18.4	2.0	19	42.1	10.5
41/<41	60	20.0	18.3	43	25.6	16.3	16	18.8	6.2
41/41	59	47.5	42.4	36	19.4	19.4	4	25.0	25.0
51/<51 or 51/51	20	50.0	50.0	27	48.1	48.1	11	36.4	36.4

YO-I: younger-onset taking insulin; OO-I: older-onset taking insulin; OO-NI: older-onset not taking insulin. In this scale Levels 10 and 21 correspond exactly to Levels 10 and 20, respectively, in Table 1; Level 31 is similar to Level 35, except that eyes with SE are placed in Level 41; Level 41 is similar to Levels 43 and 47 combined; and Level 51 is similar to Level 53

Retinopathy and blood glucose control

Clinical trials

Although the findings of Klein and co-workers, like those of many other studies, leave little doubt that retinopathy is more prevalent, more severe, and more likely to progress in groups of patients who have higher blood glucose levels, *i.e.*, more severe and/or less well controlled diabetes, it has been difficult to determine whether poorer control causes more severe retinopathy, or whether both more severe retinopathy and greater difficulty in achieving good control are parallel effects of diabetes that is "more severe", perhaps because of genetic factors. The best means for differentiating between these two possibilities is a clinical trial in which participants are randomly assigned to two different levels of blood sugar control. Random assignment may be expected to establish two groups that are essentially the same in regard to diabetes severity and in all other respects except the treatment to which they are assigned. If the trial is large enough and participants are followed long enough, and if the assigned treatments are adhered to and produce substantial differences in glycemic control, a firm answer to the question may be anticipated.

Unfortunately, such an answer is not yet available, in spite of many attempts, four which are summarized in Table 4. Each of these trials enrolled patients with type I diabetes and compared intensive treatment, *i.e.*, home blood glucose monitoring combined with either continuous subcutaneous insulin infusion (CSII) or multiple daily insulin injections, with conventional treatment, generally two insulin injections per day without home blood glucose monitoring[32-40]. In each study patients were allocated randomly and analyzed according to that assignment, assessment of retinopathy status was masked, compliance was good, follow-up was nearly complete, and the difference in mean glycosylated hemoglobin between intensively and conventionally treated groups was about 1.5 to 2.0 percentage points. All these studies suffer from small numbers of patients and brief periods of observation.

Table 4. Summary of four randomized trials comparing intensive and conventional insulin treatment in individuals with type I diabetes

Trial	*Århus*[36]	*Oslo*[35,37,40]			*Kroc*[33,38]		*Steno*[32,34]	
A. *Patient characteristics*								
Mean duration of diabetes (years)	10	13			17		19	
Retinopathy severity	50% none 50% < 5 Ma	24% none 27% 1-3 Ma 33% ≥ 4 Ma 16% exudates			Level* 2/<2 to 4/4		Worse eye: 13% Level 3 60% Level 4 27% Level 5 or 6	
HbA_1 difference between groups (percentage points)	2.1	1.5			2.0		1.6	
B. *Number of patients with retinopathy progression/number at risk*								
Follow-up (months)	12	3-6	12	41	8	24**	12	24
Intensive treatment	3/12	15/18	4/28	15/28	13/32	4/29	10/15	6/15
Conventional treatment	4/12	0/12	0/12	12/15	9/33	7/31	5/15	10/15

*Level designations (from ref. 27) correspond closely to those in Table 3 (2=21, 3=31, 4≈41, 5≈51) and Table 1 (6=61 through 72). **At this visit progression was defined as ≥ 2 levels worse, rather than ≥ 1 as at the eight-month visit. The analysis was by original randomization, ignoring several crossovers that occurred after the eight-month visit

In the Århus Study, two ophthalmologists masked to treatment group compared baseline and one-year follow-up photographs and fluorescein angiograms and found progression of retinopathy (mainly an increase in numbers of microaneurysms in the angiograms) in three of 12 patients in the CSII group and in four of 12 in the conventional treatment group. Neither in the photographs nor in an ophthalmoscopic examination at the six-month follow-up visit were cotton-wool spots seen to develop in any patient.

In the intensive treatment group of the Oslo Study, cotton-wool spots had developed at the three- or six-month visit in 15 of 28 patients free of them at the beginning of the study, compared with none of 12 such patients in the conventional treatment group. All but one patient developing spots belonged to the subgroup with some degree of retinopathy on enrollment. Retinopathy had improved again at the one-year visit, with disappearance of the cotton-wool spots in all but four cases. After 41 months of follow-up there was a trend towards more frequent progression in the conventionally treated group.

In the Kroc Study, after eight months of follow-up, 13 of the 32 patients in the CSII group showed retinopathy progression of at least one level, compared with nine of 33 patients in the conventional treatment group. Development of cotton-wool spots and/or IRMA accounted for the worsening in most cases. This trend for an adverse effect of CSII was of borderline statistical significance at eight months and had reversed direction at the 24-month visit. Similarly, in the Steno study at 12 months there was a trend towards more frequent progression in the CSII group, but at 24 months the trend had reversed. Progression was mainly development of cotton-wool spots, but occasional eyes developed proliferative retinopathy.

The Oslo Study found the degree to which control improved to be important: within the intensively treated group the average fall in glycosylated hemoglobin between baseline and three-month follow-up visits was 3.3 percentage points in the 15 patients who developed cotton-wool spots, 1.3 percentage points in the 13 who did not[35]. In 11 of the 15 patients, cotton-wool spots had disappeared at the 12-month visit and did not seem to be of clinical importance, leading to the term transient worsening for this phenomenon. Possible mechanisms that have been suggested are decrease in nutrient substrate, decreased ability of the retinal circulation to autoregulate, and increase in growth factors[35,41-43].

Alloxan diabetes in dogs

In a randomized trial in alloxan diabetic dogs, Engerman and co-workers have presented impressive evidence that good control, when initiated within a few weeks of the onset of diabetes, can almost completely inhibit the retinopathy that regularly develops after five years of poorly controlled diabetes in this animal model[44]. Subsequently, Engerman and Kern found that when 30 months of good control were preceded by 30 months of poor control, retinopathy was almost as severe as it was in dogs under poor control for the entire five-year period, even though retinopathy was not yet present when the switch from poor to good control was made (Table 5)[45]. To the extent that these results may apply to human diabetes, they suggest that good control may be effective only if instituted early in the course of diabetes, as suggested earlier by Constam and Caird, or alternatively that, if improving control after several years of poor control is of benefit, there may be a considerable delay before beneficial effects become apparent[46,47]. The study of Klein and co-workers discussed above is more consistent with the second alternative, because it suggests that improved control may prove to be beneficial even in patients with established retinopathy. Furthermore, that study did not suggest a threshold level of glycemia which must be reached before a beneficial effect might be observed. The studies summarized in Table 4 support the concept that there may be a delay of many months after switching to good control before a beneficial effect can be expected, and that such an effect may even be preceded by "transient worsening" in some cases.

Table 5. Inhibition of retinopathy in alloxan diabetic dogs by good glycemic control: impaired effectiveness following poor control (mean ± SEM)

	Group				
	Poor control (n=8)	*Good control (n=7)*	*Poor →*	*Good (n=6)*	*Non-diabetic (n=14)*
Duration (years)	5	5	2 1/2[a]	5[b]	5
Plasma glucose (mmol/L)					
8:00 am	21±0.7	5.9±0.5	19±0.7	5.7±0.7	4.4±0.1
8:00 pm	21±0.9	3.9±0.3	21±2.3	3.4±0.3	4.3±0.2
Glycosuria (g/day)	104±8	<2	107±7	<2	0
Sugar-free days (%)	0	65	0	64	100
Hemoglobin A_1 (%)	11.1±0.4	6.6±0.3	11.2±0.9	6.7±0.3	6.5±0.2
Retinopathy					
Microaneurysms per eye	42±10	2±1.3	0±0.3	29±16	1±0.2
Capillary atrophy[c]	264±25	80±20	48±8	224±29	39±6
Pericyte loss	+++	0 to +	0 to +	++	0
Hemorrhage	++	0	0	+	0
Basement membrane thickness (nm)	319±34	186±14	164±12	227±14	168±8

SEM: standard error of the mean. [a]Left eye obtained surgically (after 2 1/2 years of poor control). [b]Right eye obtained at autopsy (after 5 years, 2 1/2 years of poor control followed by 2 1/2 years of good control). [c]Acellular capillaries/11 mm^2 of trypsin digested vasculature (From: Engerman RL, Kern TS: Progression of incipient diabetic retinopathy during good glycemic control. Diabetes 36:808-812, 1987.)

Diabetes Control and Complications Trial

The Diabetes Control and Complications Trial (DCCT), in which persons with type I diabetes are being randomly assigned to either intensive or conventional insulin treatment, has now been underway for several years[48]. It includes both primary prevention and secondary intervention components. The former enrolls patients with diabetes duration of one to five years and no retinopathy, the latter patients with one to 15 years of diabetes and very mild to moderate NPDR. This study has reached its enrollment goal of 1400 patients, some of whom have now been followed for more than five years, and should provide reliable information on the possible value of improved control from intensive insulin treatment.

Worsening of retinopathy with rapid improvement of control

Of the trials summarized in Table 4, only the Steno Study included patients with severe NPDR or PDR, in whom worsening of retinopathy following rapid improvement in control might be of immediate clinical importance, but several uncontrolled case series including such patients have been published. Following two isolated case reports of remarkable improvement of retinopathy shortly after CSII was begun in such patients, three small case series appeared reporting continued, perhaps accelerated, progression of retinopathy in similar cases[49-53]. In the latter three studies combined there were 12 patients who had severe NPDR in one or both eyes and had substantial improvement in glycosylated hemoglobin maintained for six to 22 months. Progression to PDR occurred within four months of beginning CSII in six patients, and during the next five months in three more. No patient improved. Six of these cases apparently underwent rapid and dramatic worsening, with development of macular edema, extensive new vessels, and/or vitreous hemorrhage, and are reminiscent of reports (mostly concerning pubertal children) of rapid development of PDR or severe NPDR soon after improvement of long-standing poor control in patients with mild or no retinopathy[54-56]. The best comparison groups are provided by the DRS and the ETDRS, in which about 50% of untreated eyes with severe NPDR developed PDR within the first 15 months of follow-up[25,57], and the study by Klein and co-workers summarized in Table 3, in which about 40-50% of patients with severe NPDR developed PDR during a four-year period.

Two of the three reports mentioned above include 12 patients who had PDR in at least one eye and had substantial improvement of glycosylated hemoglobin maintained for four to 23 months[51,52]. In five patients, new vessels continued to grow and in another four vitreous hemorrhages continued to occur while on CSII. Eight of the 12 patients had had photocoagulation prior to beginning CSII and this was repeated in six because of retinopathy progression while receiving CSII. Three patients had photocoagulation for the first time while on CSII, for increasing new vessels. Although none of these cases apparently had the dramatic progression described in the patients with severe NPDR, the authors' conclusions that CSII was, at best, of no benefit seem justified. Reports of retinopathy progression following successful pancreatic transplantation and in diabetic women brought rapidly under good control as a part of prenatal care provide additional support for the probable clinical importance of the "transient worsening" concept[58,59].

On the basis of the reports cited above, it would appear desirable to proceed cautiously when improvement of long-standing poor control is undertaken in patients with severe NPDR or active PDR, maintaining careful ophthalmologic monitoring during this period and perhaps aiming at gradual rather than rapid improvement. Photocoagulation of at least one eye of such patients prior to initiating better control would seem prudent.

References

1. Larsen HW: Diabetic retinopathy: an ophthalmoscopic study with a discussion of the morphologic changes and the pathogenetic factors in this disease. Acta Ophthalmol (Copenh) 60:1-89, 1960
2. Beetham WP: Visual prognosis of proliferating diabetic retinopathy. Br J Ophthalmol 47:611-619, 1963
3. Dobree JH: Proliferative diabetic retinopathy: evolution of the retinal lesions. Br J Ophthalmol 48:637-649, 1964
4. Davis MD: Vitreous contraction in proliferative diabetic retinopathy. Arch Ophthalmol 74:741-751, 1965
5. Tolentino FI, Lee PF, Schepens CL: Biomicroscopic study of vitreous cavity in diabetic retinopathy. Arch Ophthalmol 75:238-246, 1966
6. Davis MD: The natural course of diabetic retinopathy. In: Kimura SJ, Caygil WM (eds) Vascular Complications of Diabetes Mellitus, pp 139-169. St Louis: Mosby 1967
7. Davis MD, Myers FL, Engerman RL et al: Clinical observations concerning the pathogenesis of diabetic retinopathy In: Goldberg MF, Fine SL (eds) Symposium on the Treatment of Diabetic Retinopathy, pp 569-592. Washington, DC: US Government Printing Office (Public Health Service Pub No 1890) 1969
8. Jonas JB, Gusek GC, Guggenmoos-Holzmann I, Naumann GOH: Variability of the real dimensions of normal human optic discs. Graefe's Arch Clin Exp Ophthalmol 226:332-336, 1988
9. Mansour AM, Walsh JB, Henkind P: Optic disc size in central vein occlusion. Ophthalmology 97:165-166, 1990
10. de Venecia G, Davis M, Engerman R: Clinicopathologic correlations in diabetic retinopathy. I. Histology and fluorescein angiography of microaneurysms. Arch Ophthalmol 94:1766-1773, 1976
11. Davis MD, Norton EWD, Myers FL: The Airlie classification of diabetic retinopathy In: Goldberg MF, Fine SL (eds) Symposium on the Treatment of Diabetic Retinopathy, pp 7-22. Washington, DC: US Government Printing Office (Public Health Service Pub No 1890) 1969
12. Deckert T, Simonsen SE, Poulsen JE: Prognosis of proliferative retinopathy in juvenile diabetes. Diabetes 16:728-733, 1967
13. The Diabetic Retinopathy Study Research Group: Preliminary report on the effects of photocoagulation therapy. Am J Ophthalmol 81:383-396, 1976

14. British Multicentre Study Group: Photocoagulation for proliferative diabetic retinopathy: a randomized controlled clinical trial using the xenon arc. Diabetologia 26:109-115, 1984
15. Rand LI, Prud'homme GJ, Ederer F, Canner PL, the Diabetic Retinopathy Study Research Group: Factors influencing the development of visual loss in advanced diabetic retinopathy. Invest Ophthalmol Vis Sci 26:893-991, 1985
16. The Diabetic Retinopathy Study Research Group: A modification of the Airlie House classification of diabetic retinopathy. DRS Report No 7. Invest Ophthalmol Vis Sci 21:210-226, 1981
17. Early Treatment Diabetic Retinopathy Study Research Group: Grading diabetic retinopathy from stereoscopic color fundus photographs: an extension of the modified Airlie House classification. ETDRS Study Report No 10. Ophthalmology 98:786-806, 1991
18. Bresnick GH, Haight B, De Venecia G: Retinal wrinkling and macular heterotopia in diabetic retinopathy. Arch Ophthalmol 97:1890-1895, 1979
19. Tasman W: Diabetic vitreous hemorrhage and its relationship to hypoglycemia. Mod Probl Ophthalmol 20:413-414, 1979
20. Anderson B: Activity and diabetic vitreous hemorrhages. Ophthalmology 87:173-175, 1980
21. Klein R, Davis MD, Moss SE, Klein BEK, DeMets DL: The Wisconsin Epidemiologic Study of Diabetic Retinopathy: a comparison of retinopathy in younger and older onset diabetic persons. In: Vranic M, Hollenberg C, Steiner G (eds) Comparison of Type I and Type II Diabetes, pp 321-325. New York: Plenum Publishing Corp 1985
22. The Diabetic Retinopathy Study Research Group: Design, methods, and baseline results. DRS Report No 6. Invest Ophthalmol Vis Sci 21:149-209, 1981
23. Aiello LM, Rand LI, Briones JC et al: Diabetic retinopathy in Joslin Clinic patients with adult-onset diabetes. Ophthalmology 88:619-623, 1981
24. Early Treatment Diabetic Retinopathy Study Research Group: Early photocoagulation for diabetic retinopathy. ETDRS Study Report No 9. Ophthalmology 98:766-785, 1991
25. Early Treatment Diabetic Retinopathy Study Research Group: Fundus photographic risk factors for progression of diabetic retinopathy. ETDRS Study Report No 12. Ophthalmology 98:823-833, 1991
26. Early Treatment Diabetic Retinopathy Study Research Group: Effects of aspirin treatment on diabetic retinopathy. ETDRS Study Report No 8. Ophthalmology 98:757-765, 1991
27. Klein BEK, Davis MD, Segal P et al: Diabetic retinopathy: assessment of severity and progression. Ophthalmology 91:10-17, 1984
28. Klein R, Klein BEK, Moss SE et al: The Wisconsin Epidemiologic Study of Diabetic Retinopathy: IX. Four-year incidence and progression of diabetic retinopathy when age at diagnosis is less than 30 years. Arch Ophthalmol 107:237-243, 1989
29. Klein R, Klein BEK, Moss SE et al: The Wisconsin Epidemiologic Study of Diabetic Retinopathy: X. Four-year incidence and progression of diabetic retinopathy when age at diagnosis is 30 years of age or more. Arch Ophthalmol 107:244-249, 1989
30. Klein R, Klein BEK, Moss SE, Davis MD, DeMets DL: Glycosylated hemoglobin predicts the incidence and progression of diabetic retinopathy. JAMA 260:2864-2871, 1988
31. Klein R, Klein BEK, Moss SE, Davis MD, DeMets DL: Is blood pressure a predictor of the incidence or progression of diabetic retinopathy? Arch Intern Med 149:2427-2432, 1989
32. Lauritzen T, Frost-Larsen K, Larsen HW, Deckert T, Steno Study Group: Effect of one year of near-normal blood glucose levels on retinopathy in insulin-dependent diabetics. Lancet 1:200-204, 1983
33. The Kroc Collaborative Study Group: Blood glucose control and the evolution of diabetic retinopathy and albuminuria. N Engl J Med 311:365-372, 1984
34. Lauritzen T, Frost-Larsen K, Larsen HW et al: Two-year experience with continuous subcutaneous insulin infusion in relation to retinopathy and neuropathy. Diabetes 34:74-79, 1985
35. Dahl-Jorgensen K, Brinchmann-Hansen O, Hanssen KF, Sandvik KF, Aagenaes O, Aker Diabetes Group: Rapid tightening of blood glucose control leads to transient deterioration of retinopathy in insulin-dependent diabetes mellitus: the Oslo Study. Br Med J 290:811-815, 1985
36. Beck-Nielsen H, Rickelsen B, Mogensen CE et al: Effect of insulin pump treatment for one year on renal function and retinal morphology in patients with IDDM. Diabetes Care 8:585-589, 1985
37. Brinchmann-Hansen O, Dahl-Jorgensen K, Hanssen KF, Sandvik L, and the Oslo Study Group: Effects of intensified treatment on various lesions of diabetic retinopathy. Am J Ophthalmol 100:644-653, 1985
38. The Kroc Collaborative Study Group: The Kroc Study patients at two years: a report on further retinal changes. Diabetes 34:39, 1985

39. Dahl-Jorgensen K, Brinchmann-Hansen O, Hanssen KF, Ganes T, Kierulf P, Smeland E, Sandvik L, Aagenaes O: Effects of near normoglycaemic for two years on progression of early diabetic retinopathy, nephropathy, and neuropathy: The Oslo Study. Br Med J 293:1195-1199, 1986
40. Brinchmann-Hansen O, Dahl-Jorgensen K, Hanssen KF, Sandvik L: The response of diabetic retinopathy to 41 months of multiple insulin injections, insulin pumps, and conventional insulin therapy. Arch Ophthalmol 106:1242-1246, 1988
41. Ernest JT, Goldstick TK, Engerman RL: Hyperglycemia impairs retinal oxygen autoregulation in normal and diabetic dogs. Invest Ophthalmol Vis Sci 24:985-989, 1983
42. Kohner EM, Sleightholm M, Fallon T; Why does retinopathy deteriorate when diabetic control is improved? Invest Ophthalmol Vis Sci (Suppl) 29:244, 1987
43. Grunwald JE, Brucker AJ, Schwartz SS et al: Diabetic glycemic control and retinal blood flow. Diabetes 39:602-607, 1990
44. Engerman RL, Bloodworth JMB, Nelson S: Relationship of microvascular disease in diabetes to metabolic control. Diabetes 26:760-769, 1977
45. Engerman RL, Kern TS: Progression of incipient diabetic retinopathy during good glycemic control. Diabetes 36:808-812, 1987
46. Constam GR: Zur Spätprognose des Diabetes mellitus. Helv Med Acta 32:287, 1965
47. Caird FI: Diabetes and the Eye, p 84. Oxford: Blackwell 1968
48. The DCCT Research Group: Diabetes Control and Complications Trial (DCCT): Update. Diabetes Care 13:427-433, 1990
49. Irsigler K, Kritz H, Najemnik C: Reversal of florid diabetic retinopathy. Lancet 2:1068, 1979
50. White MC, Kohner EM, Pickup JC, Keen H: Reversal of diabetic retinopathy by continuous subcutaneous insulin infusion: a case report. Br J Ophthalmol 65:307-311, 1981
51. Pucklin JE, Tamborlane WV, Felig P et al: Influence of long-term insulin infusion pump treatment of type I diabetes on diabetic retinopathy. Ophthalmology 89:735-747, 1982
52. Lawson PM, Champion MC, Canny C et al: Continuous subcutaneous insulin infusion does not prevent progression of proliferative and preproliferative retinopathy. Br J Ophthalmol 66:762-766, 1982
53. Van Ballegooie E, Hooymans JM, Timmerman Z et al: Rapid deterioration of diabetic retinopathy during treatment with continuous subcutaneous insulin infusion. Diabetes Care 7:236-242, 1984
54. Daneman D, Drash AL, Lobes LH et al: Progressive retinopathy with improved control in diabetic dwarfism (Mauriac's syndrome). Diabetes Care 4:360-365, 1981
55. Lawrence JR, Bedford GJ, Thomson R.: Rapid development during puberty of proliferative retinopathy after strict control. Lancet 2:322, 1985
56. Dandona P, Bolger JP, Boag F, Fonesca V, Abrams JD: Rapid development and progression of proliferative retinopathy after strict diabetic control. Br Med J 290:895-896, 1985
57. The Diabetic Retinopathy Study Research Group: Photocoagulation treatment of proliferative diabetic retinopathy: the second report of Diabetic Retinopathy Study findings. Ophthalmology 85:82-106, 1978
58. Ramsay RC, Goetz FC, Sutherland DER, Mauer SM et al: Progression of diabetic retinopathy after pancreas transplantation for insulin-dependent diabetes mellitus. New Engl J Med 318:208-214, 1988
59. Phelps RL, Sakol P, Metzker BE et al: Changes in diabetic retinopathy during pregnancy: correlations with regulation of hyperglycemia. Arch Ophthalmol 104:1806-1810, 1986

HISTOPATHOLOGY OF DIABETIC RETINOPATHY

W. Richard Green and David J. Wilson

Eye Pathology Laboratory, The Johns Hopkins Hospital, Baltimore, MD, USA

Professor Norman Ashton contributed much to our knowledge of the pathology of diabetic retinopathy. In 1963 he stated that our knowledge of the morbid anatomy of this condition is nearing completion, and future discoveries are likely to come from dynamic studies on the retinal vessels[1]. Indeed, current research on diabetic retinopathy primarily involves cell molecular biological and biochemical studies on the retinal vasculature. We would like to review some of the pathologic aspects of diabetic retinopathy and how these features relate to the clinical findings and the theories of neovascularization and regression of new blood vessels.

Diabetic retinopathy is primarily a disease of the retinal blood vessels with basement membrane thickening, loss of pericytes, capillary closure, microaneurysm formation and neovascularization. Other changes, including edema, exudates, and cotton wool spots are secondary to the retinovascular changes. One of the earliest and most dramatic changes in the vessels is the thickening of the vascular basement membrane. Ashton suggested that the thickened basement membrane of the precapillary arterioles leads to capillary occlusion and thereby to proliferative diabetic retinopathy. Fig. 1 is one of Ashton's preparations in which India ink was injected into the retinal vasculature. The precapillary arteriole lumen has been narrowed by the thickened vessel wall. Fig. 2 illustrates the ultrastructural appearance of a capillary from a diabetic patient. There is marked basement membrane thickening and lipid vacuoles are present in the wall of the capillary. Similar

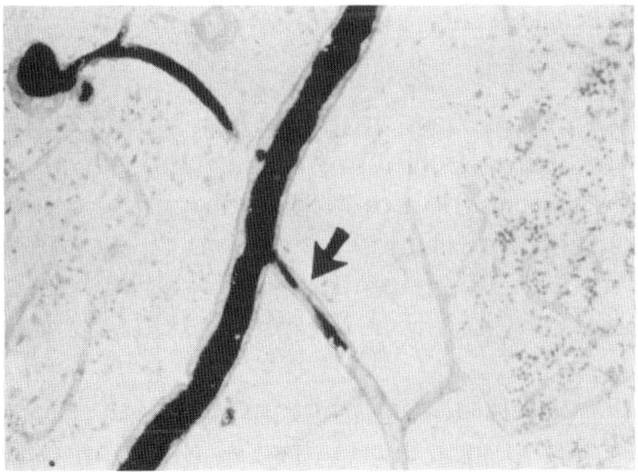

Fig. 1. India ink flat preparation of the retina showing narrowing of the lumen of a prepapillary arteriole (arrow). (From: Ashton N: Studies of the retinal capillaries in relation to diabetic and other retinopathies. Br J Ophthalmol 47:521-538, 1963. Published courtesy *British Medical Association.*)

Address for correspondence: W. Richard Green, MD, Eye Pathology Laboratory, The Johns Hopkins Hospital, 600 N. Wolfe Street, Baltimore, MD 21287-9248, USA

Retina and Vitreous, pp. 63-81
Proceedings of the Symposium on Retina and Vitreous,
organized by the New Orleans Academy of Ophthalmology
New Orleans, LA, USA, March 12-15, 1992
edited by Rudolph M. Franklin

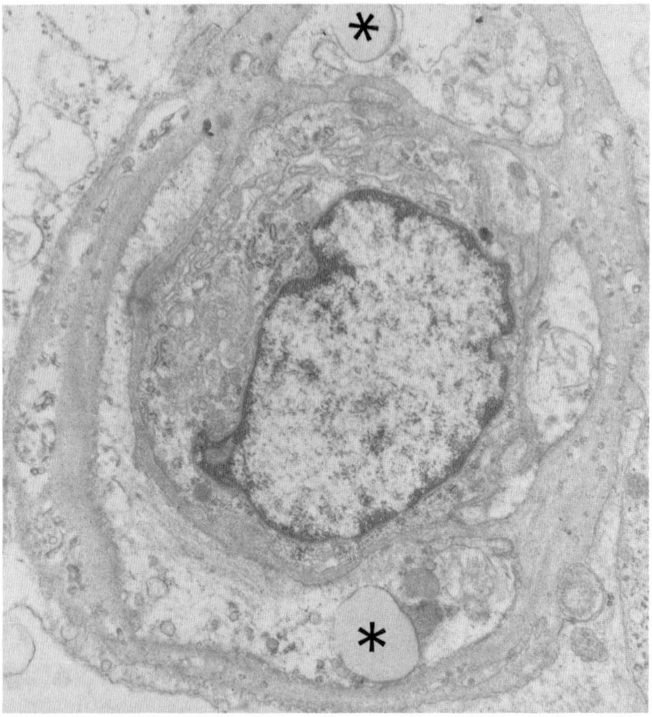

Fig. 2. The ultrastructural appearance of a retinal capillary from a patient with background diabetic retinopathy has marked basement membrane thickening and deposition of lipid vacuoles (asterisks) and other lipid deposits between layers of basement membrane (×18,200).

basement membrane thickening occurs in the retinal vessels and retinal internal limiting membrane of galactosemic animals[2]. In these animals, basement membrane thickening can be prevented by the administration of aldose reductase inhibitors. This evidence suggests that aldose reductase inhibitors may be able to prevent some of the retinovascular changes in diabetes. The multicenter trial of the aldose reductase inhibitor, sorbinil, however, showed no effect of this inhibitor on the progression of diabetic retinopathy[3]. Other studies are being considered.

The common clinical usage of fundus photography and fluorescein angiography has made possible good clinicopathologic correlation of the retinovascular changes present in patients with diabetes. The pathologic technique most comparable to fluorescein angiography is trypsin digestion, which provides a microscopic preparation very similar to the fluorescein angiogram. Using this technique, two types of cells can be identified in retinal capillaries: endothelial cells which have oval pale staining nuclei, and pericytes which have round darker staining nuclei (Fig. 3). Normally, there is an approximately equal number of pericytes and endothelial cells. Cogan *et al.*[4] and Kuwabara and Cogan[5] observed a relative loss of pericytes when compared to the endothelial cells in diabetes. The function of pericytes is still not known, but these cells contain contractile elements and have been shown *in vitro* to inhibit endothelial cell proliferation[6]. It is possible that the selective loss of pericytes results in the formation of hypercellular microaneurysms (Figs. 4 and 5) and dilated retinal vessels which are clearly present in trypsin digest preparations. However, microaneurysms are a common vascular abnormality in diabetics and are important because leakage from microaneurysms contributes to diabetic macular edema.

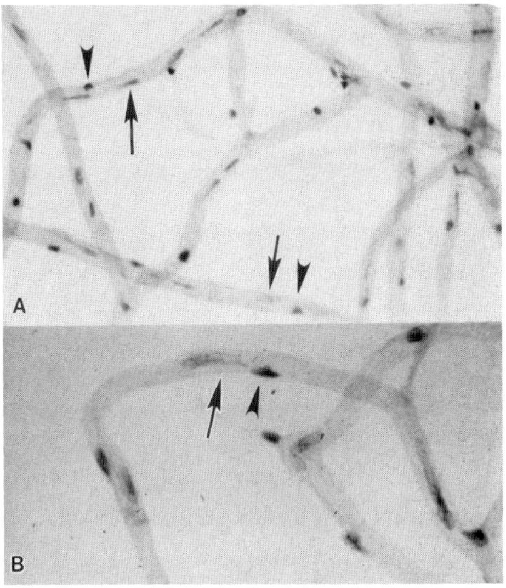

Fig. 3. Trypsin digest preparation of a normal retina with one-to-one ratio of endothelium (arrows) to pericytes (arrowheads) (hematoxylin and eosin and periodic acid-Schiff: A, ×137; B, ×325).

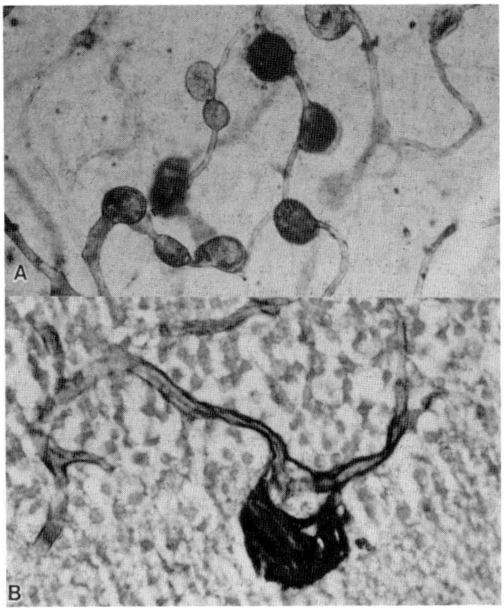

Fig. 4. Undigested flat preparation of a retina illustrates capillary microaneurysms (periodic acid-Schiff: A, ×137; B, ×328).

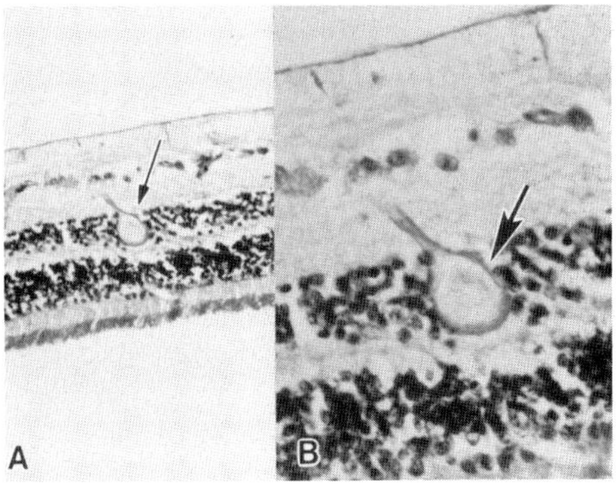

Fig. 5. Section of capillary that has a bullous dilation (arrows) (periodic acid-Schiff: A, ×137; B, ×328).

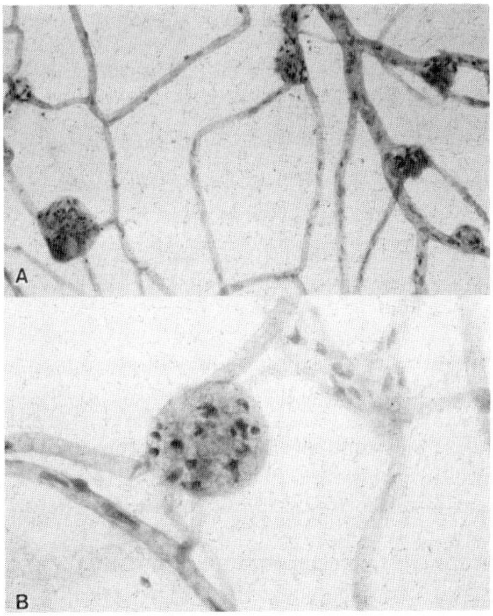

Fig. 6. Trypsin digest preparation of retina from a patient with diabetic retinopathy demonstrates hypercellular capillary microaneurysms. Adjacent capillaries are relatively acellular (hematoxylin and eosin and periodic acid-Schiff: A, ×328; B, ×525).

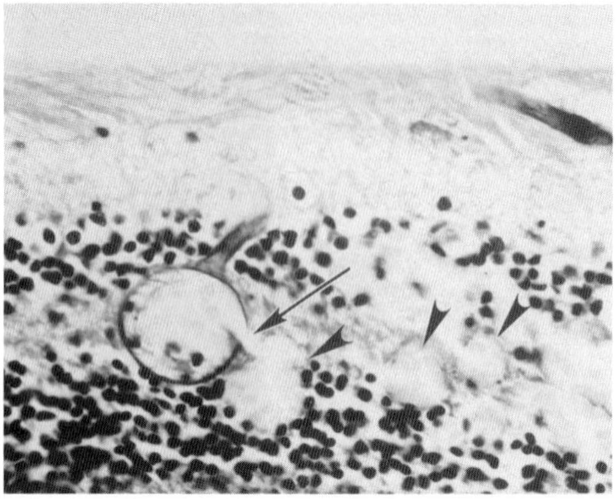

Fig. 7. (left) Capillary microaneurysm with break in its wall (arrow) and associated hemorrhage (arrowheads) (periodic acid-Schiff ×575).

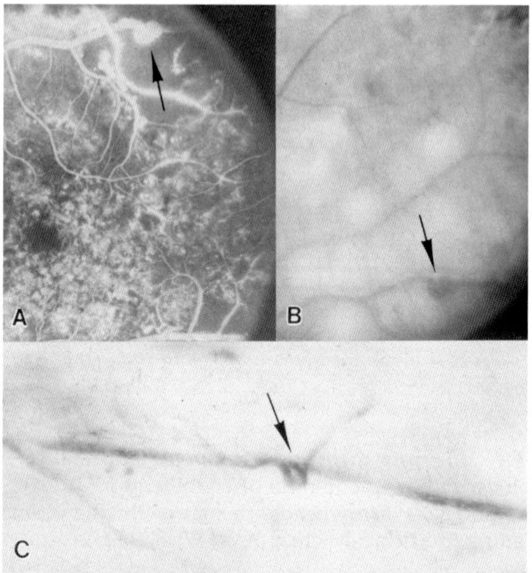

Fig. 8. (right) Fluorescein (A) ophthalmoscopic (B) and gross (C) appearance of tractional venous loops in diabetic retinopathy. (From: Hersh PS, Green WR, Thomas JA: Tractional venous loops in diabetic retinopathy. Am J Ophthalmol 92:661-671, 1981. Published with permission from *The American Journal of Ophthalmology*. Copyright by The Ophthalmic Publishing Company.)

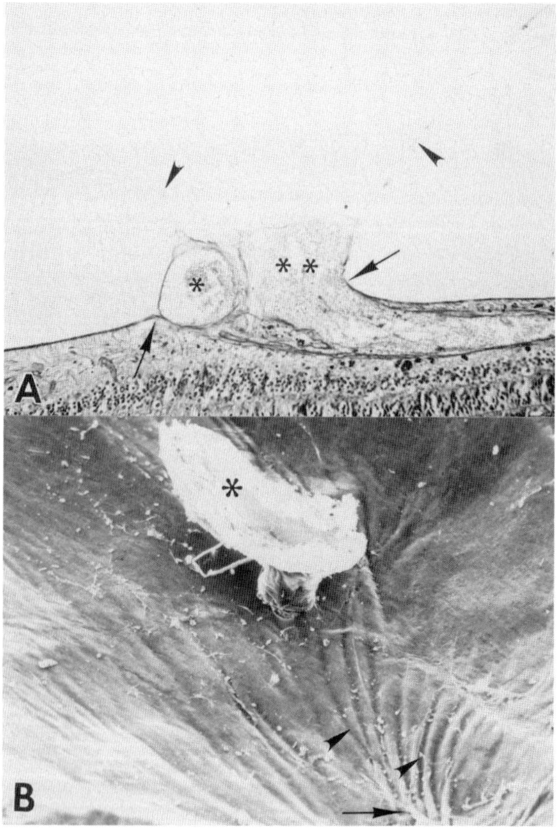

Fig. 9. A. Section through a venous loop and parallel to the axis of the vein shows the anterior (asterisk) and posterior (double asterisk) components of the loop as it extends through a discontinuity in the internal limiting membrane (between arrows). The wall of the loop is thin and tented at the points of attachments of thin delicate vitreous strands (arrowheads) (periodic acid-Schiff ×100). B. Scanning electron microscopic appearance of mushroom-shaped venous loop (asterisk) passing through the internal limiting membrane. Ridges in the membrane (arrowheads) are related to a localized preretinal membrane (arrow) (×60). (From: Hersh PS, Green WR, Thomas JA: Tractional venous loops in diabetic retinopathy. Am J Ophthalmol 92:661-671, 1981. Published with permission from *The American Journal of Ophthalmology*. Copyright by The Ophthalmic Publishing Company.)

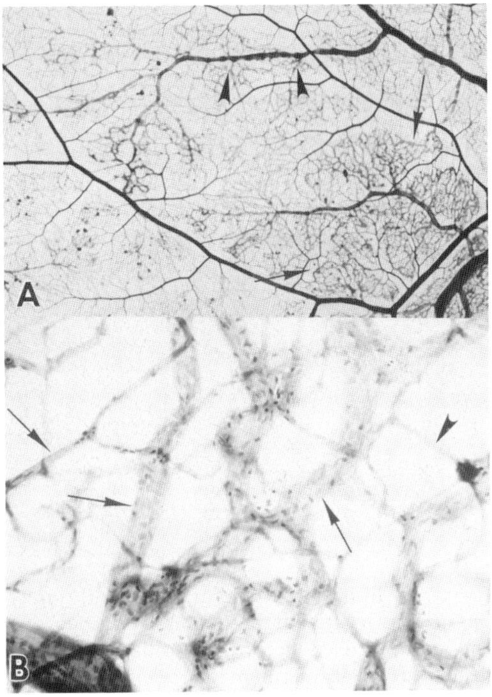

Fig. 10. A. Retinal trypsin digestion preparation showing venous beading (arrowhead) and areas of intraretinal microvascular abnormalities (IRMA) (arrows) in a diabetic patient (hematoxylin, PAS, ×13). B. Higher power view of IRMA shows some capillaries which have become larger and dilated (arrows). These vessels have prominent endothelium but few or no pericytes. Other capillaries in the area are small and hypocellular (arrowheads) (hematoxylin, PAS, ×215). (From: Green WR: Retina. In: Spencer WH (ed) Ophthalmic Pathology, Ch 8, pp 589-1291. Philadelphia: WB Saunders 1985. Permission courtesy of WB Saunders Co.)

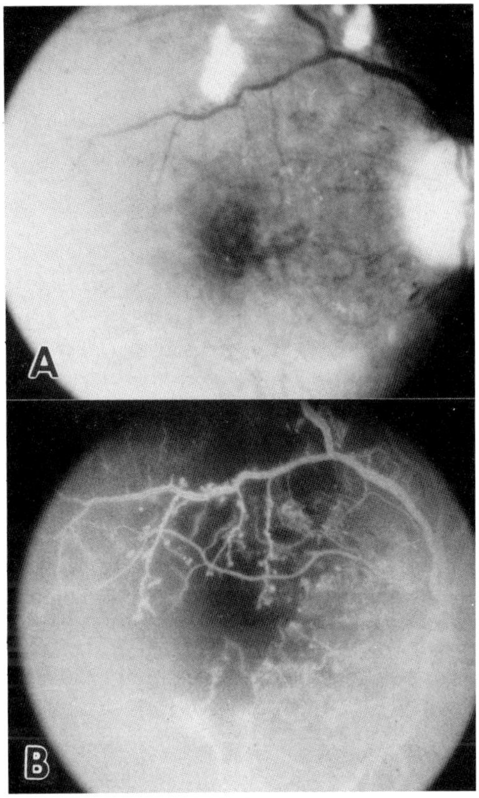

Fig. 11. Ophthalmoscopic (A) and fluorescein angiographic (B) appearance of non-perfusion of macular area of right eye of a 46-year-old woman with insulin-dependent diabetes mellitus.

By trypsin digestion (Fig. 6), it appears there is a progression of microaneurysms from thin walled hypercellular outpouchings occurring at the sites of pericyte loss to thick walled hyalinized structures. Fig. 7 illustrates a thin walled microaneurysm which has ruptured producing a hemorrhage. Ultrastructurally, microaneurysms are endothelially lined but the presence of blood elements, including degenerated platelets, fibrin, and lipid in the wall of the microaneurysm is evidence of extravasation of serum constituents through the microaneurysms wall. While microaneurysms are mostly located in the posterior pole they can occur more peripherally as shown by Niki *et al.*[7].

Venous traction loops may occur in diabetics and may be a source of vitreous hemorrhage. Hersh and co-workers[8] provided a clinicopathologic study and noted that, with partial posterior vitreous detachment, venous loops were pulled into the vitreous cavity by vitreous traction (Fig. 8). By light and electron microscopy, we can see this venous loop extending through internal limiting membrane into the vitreous cavity (Fig. 9).

Capillary non-perfusion is a well recognized feature of diabetic retinopathy. A compensatory change may take place. Some capillaries become dilated and are called intraretinal vascular abnormalities (IRMA) (Fig. 10) while other capillaries become acellular. In some

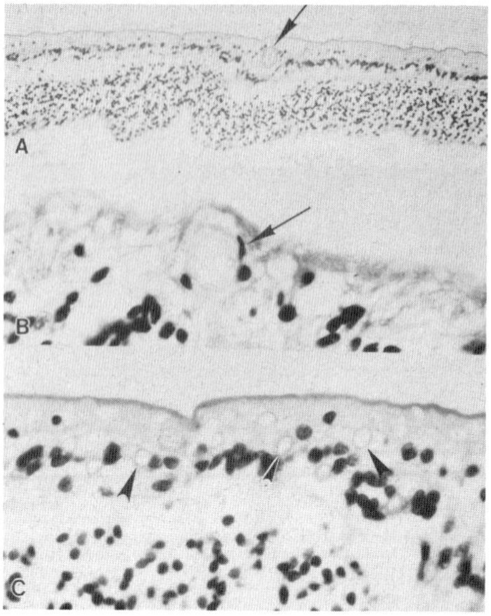

*Fig. 12.*A. Post-mortem examination of the right macular area of patient illustrated in Fig. 11 discloses inner retinal ischemic atrophy with loss of all layers down to and including the inner portion of the inner nuclear layer. An acellular precapillary arteriole is present (arrow) (hematoxylin and eosin ×137). B and C: Higher power illustrates an acellular arteriole (arrow) and acellular capillaries (arrowheads) (hematoxylin and eosin ×538).

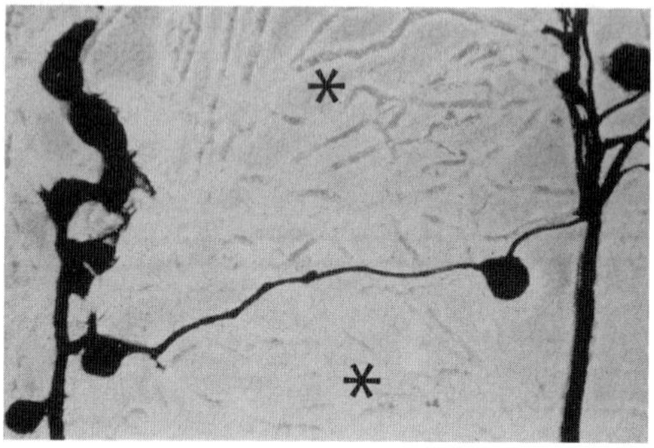

Fig. 13. India ink preparation with microaneurysms located along patent capillaries, while the non-perfused acellular capillaries (asterisk) are mostly free of microaneurysms (phase contrast ×170). (From: Ashton N: Studies of the retinal capillaries in relation to diabetic and other retinopathies. Br J Ophthalmol 47:521-538, 1963. Published courtesy of British Medical Association.)

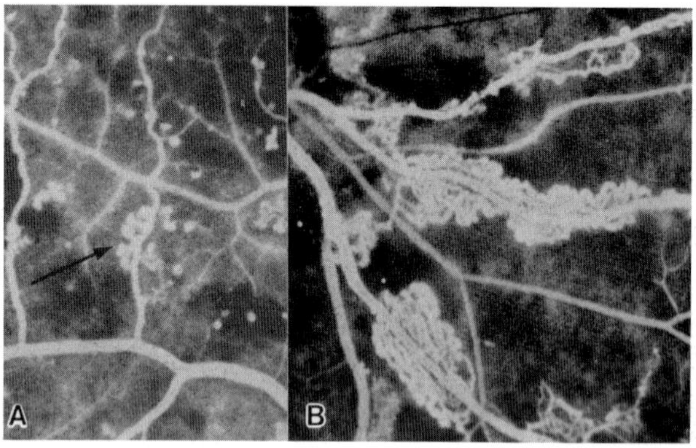

Fig. 14. Fluorescein angiographic appearance of intraretinal neovascularization. A. Six neovascular buds (arrow) from a venule extend into the non-perfused area. B. There are clusters of capillaries along veins in a background of capillary non-perfusion. (From: Muraoka K, Shimizu K: Intraretinal neovascularization in diabetic retinopathy. Ophthalmology 91:1440-1446, 1984. Published courtesy of *Ophthalmology*.)

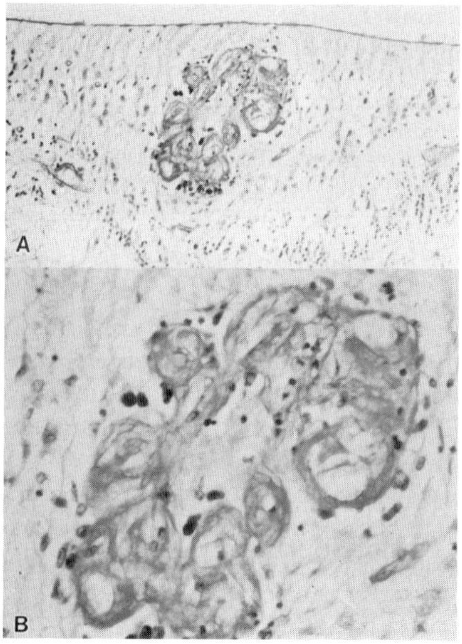

Fig. 15. Area of intraretinal neovascularization in eye with diabetic retinopathy (periodic acid-Schiff: A, ×137; B, ×328).

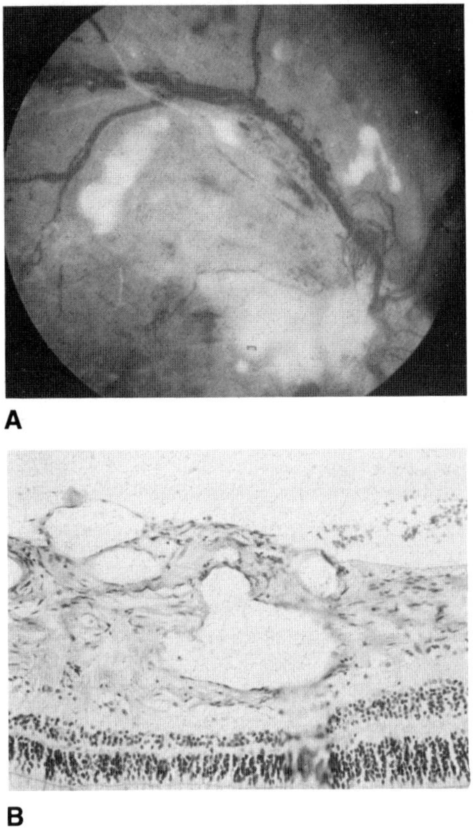

Fig. 16. (left) A. Clinicopathologic correlation of venous beading. B. Section discloses the dilated vein (asterisk) with several surrounding vessels (arrows). (From: Henkind P: Retinal neovascularization in diabetic retinopathy. Presented at the Verhoeff Society, Washington DC, April 27, 1978.)

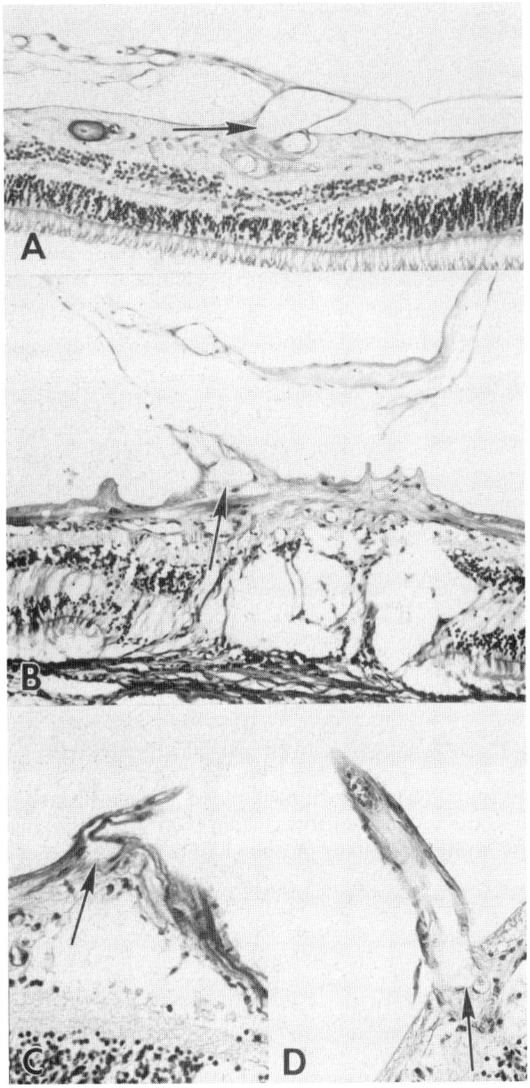

Fig. 17. (right) Examples of new vessels (arrows) extending from the retina, through a defect in the internal limiting membrane where the vessels become intimately associated with the vitreous (periodic acid-Schiff: A, ×165; C, ×260; B, Van de Griff, ×110; D, hematoxylin and eosin, ×230).

areas the entire capillary bed is non-perfused. By careful correlation of fluorescein angiograms with trypsin digest specimens, it has been shown that the areas of non-perfusion correspond to acellular capillary beds and inner retinal ischemic atrophy (Figs. 11 and 12). With the India ink preparation technique, Ashton[1] noted that the ink fails to fill acellular capillaries (Fig. 13). Electron microscopy of such acellular capillaries reveals they are bare basement membrane tubes which may be filled with Müller cell processes.

In proliferative diabetic retinopathy, neovascularization develops in the retina and optic nerve head and extends into the vitreous. The intraretinal phase is not often recognized clinically and histopathologically. Muraoka and Shimizu[9] have presented striking examples of intraretinal neovascularization (Fig. 14). Fig. 15 may be the histopathologic correlate of such intraretinal neovascularization. Intraretinal neovascularization may ac-

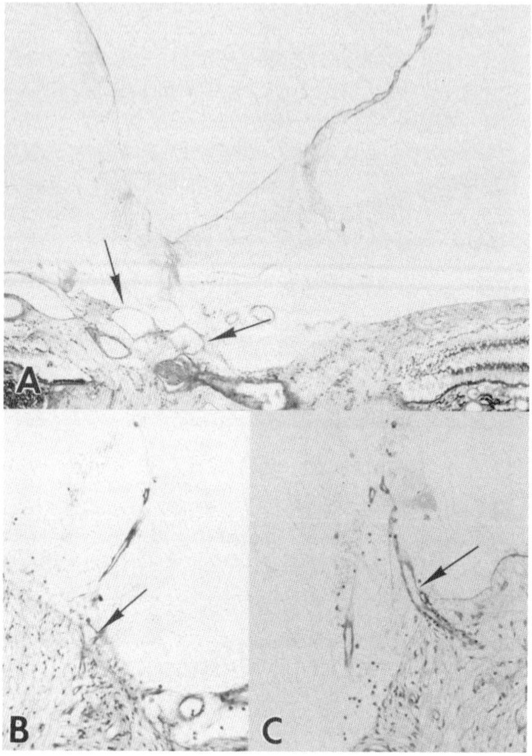

Fig. 18. Examples of new blood vessels extending into the vitreous (arrows) from the optic nerve head (periodic acid-Schiff: A, ×60; B and C, ×100).

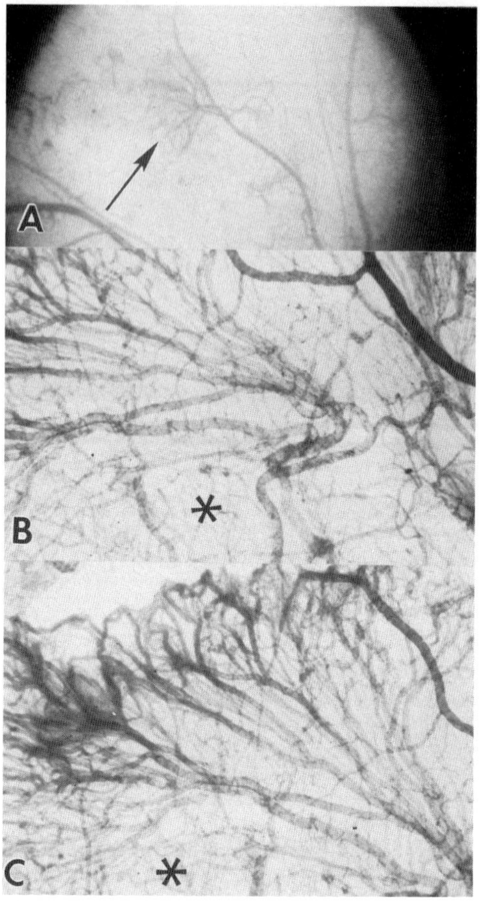

Fig. 19. A. Proliferative diabetic retinopathy with a rete mirabeli-like area of neovascularization of the retina (arrow). B and C. Trypsin digest of similar lesion from a different case, the new vessels form a fan-like configuration from a vein and developed in an area of acellular capillary bed (asterisk). B and C: (hematoxylin and eosin and periodic acid-Schiff ×137).

count for some venous beading as in the case studied by the late Dr. Paul Henkind (Fig. 16).

The neovascular tissue extends into the vitreous from the retina (Fig. 17) and the optic nerve head (Fig. 18) and becomes intimately associated with the cortical vitreous. Some retinal neovascularization may have a rete mirabile-like tuft of retinal neovascularization (Fig. 19). An excellent study of the association of vitreous collagen with preretinal vessels was provided by Faulborn and associates[10] who used a special embedding technique to prevent vitreous shrinkage (Figs. 20 and 21). It is easy to understand how vitreous detachment can cause hemorrhage from these blood vessels which are intimately associated with the cortical vitreous.

Fibrous astrocytes and other cells accompany the new vessels into the vitreous. Cellular contraction contributes to traction on the retina (Fig. 22) and leads to cystic degeneration (Fig. 23), traction retinoschisis and traction retinal detachment (Fig. 24).

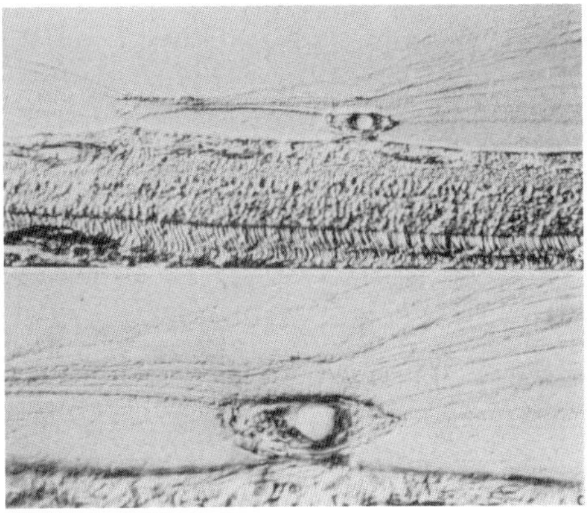

Fig. 20. Area shows new blood vessel with vitreous attached. (From: Faulborn J, Bowald S: Microproliferations in proliferative diabetic retinopathy and their relationship to the vitreous: corresponding light and electron microscopic studies. Graefe's Arch Clin Exp Ophthalmol 223:130-138, 1985. Published courtesy of Springer Verlag.)

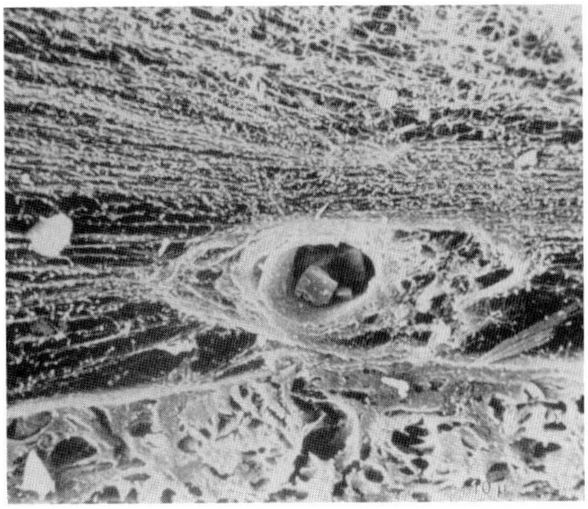

Fig. 21. Scanning electron microscopic view shows intimate association of vitreous to the neovascular tissue. (From: Faulborn J, Bowald S: Microproliferations in proliferative diabetic retinopathy and their relationship to the vitreous: corresponding light and electron microscopic studies. Graefe's Arch Clin Exp Ophthalmol 223:130-138, 1985. Published courtesy of Springer Verlag.)

A characteristic of the new vessels present in diabetic retinopathy is that they leak fluorescein. Fluorescein leakage does not occur from normal retinal vessels because of the continuous tight junctions joining the capillary endothelium. However, in neovascularization membranes, the endothelium has reduced tight junctions and may have fenestrations (Fig. 25). These features account for the fluorescein leakage noted clinically.

The vascular changes we have reviewed result in other clinically apparent lesions including edema, exudates, hemorrhages, and cotton wool spots. Leakage of plasma through microaneurysms and other vascular abnormalities produces retinal edema (Fig. 26). Some components of the leakage such as water and electrolytes are removed by the transport mechanisms of the retinal pigment epithelium and retinal vascular endothelium, but lipid may remain in the retina in the form of exudate residues (Fig. 27). Hard exudates, which are densely PAS positive and rich in lipid, are typically located in

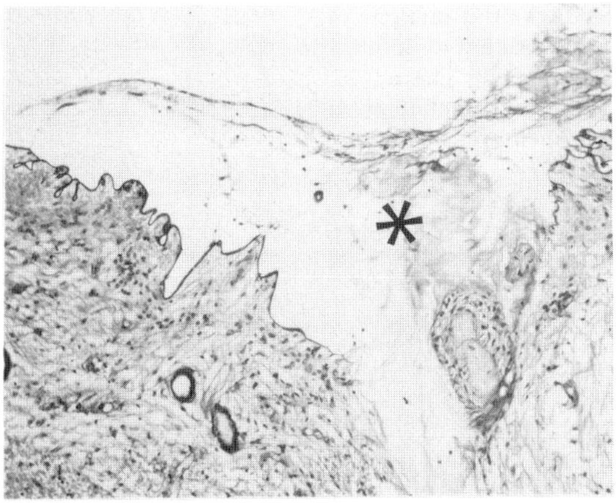

Fig. 22. Fibrovascular tissue (asterisk) at optic nerve head has apparently contracted and drawn the peripapillary retina towards the nerve head (periodic acid-Schiff ×115).

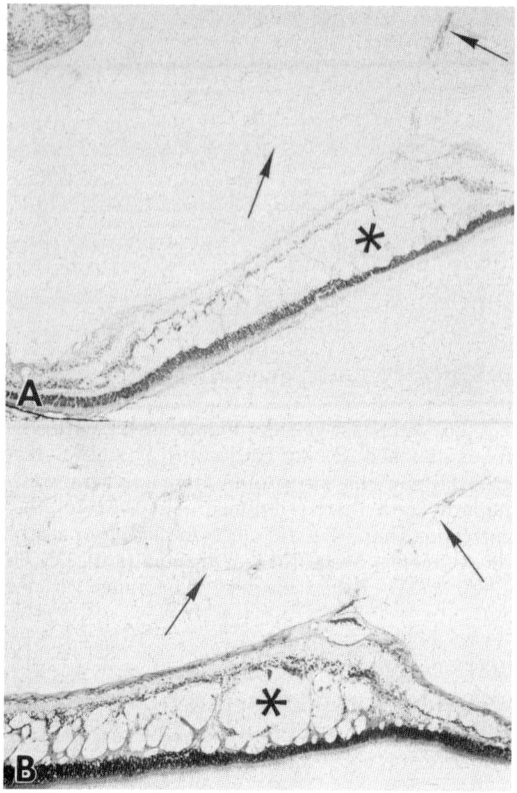

Fig. 23. Examples of proliferative diabetic retinopathy with partial posterior vitreous detachment, remaining vitreous attachment (arrows) at points of retinal neovascularization with traction on retina and cystic degeneration of retina (asterisk) (hematoxylin and eosin: A, ×35; B ×55).

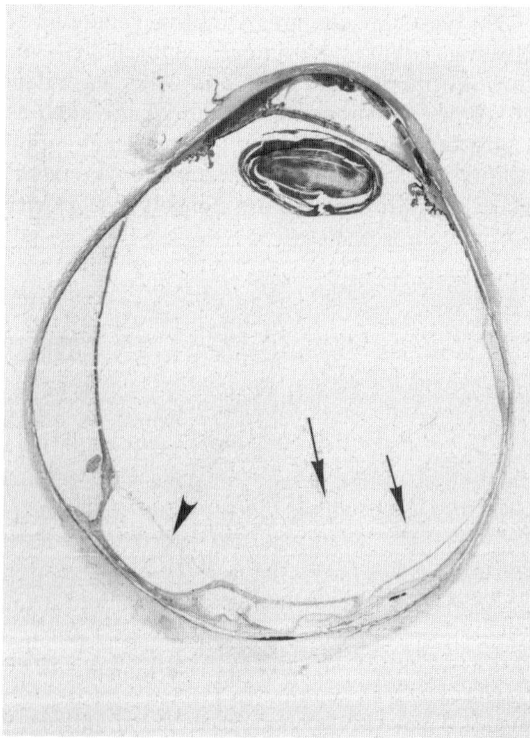

Fig. 24. Proliferative diabetic retinopathy with anterior posterior (arrows) and tangential (arrowhead) traction on a retina with four areas of traction retinal detachment. The retina is tented up at each point of attachment of these tractional vitreous membranes. (hematoxylin and eosin ×45).

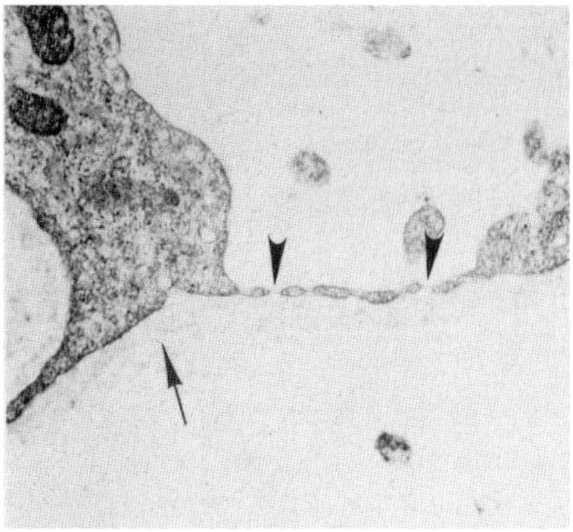

Fig. 25. Endothelium of a new blood vessel in vitreous has endothelium with fenestrae (arrowheads), basement membrane (arrow) and no pericytes.

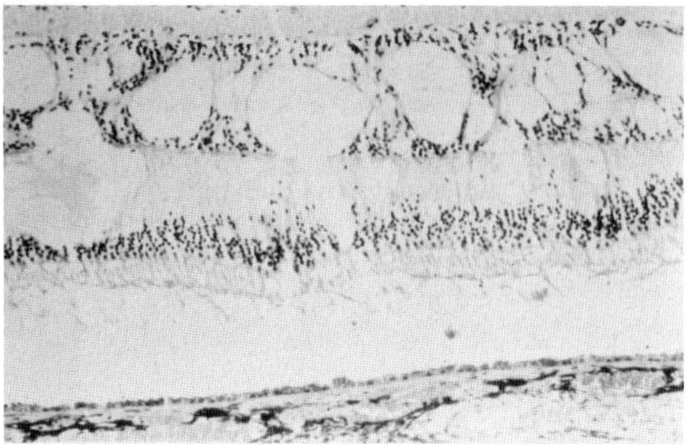

Fig. 26. Parafoveal area of an eye with background diabetic retinopathy with cystic spaces containing a light proteinaceous material in the inner nuclear and outer plexiform layers (hematoxylin and eosin ×137).

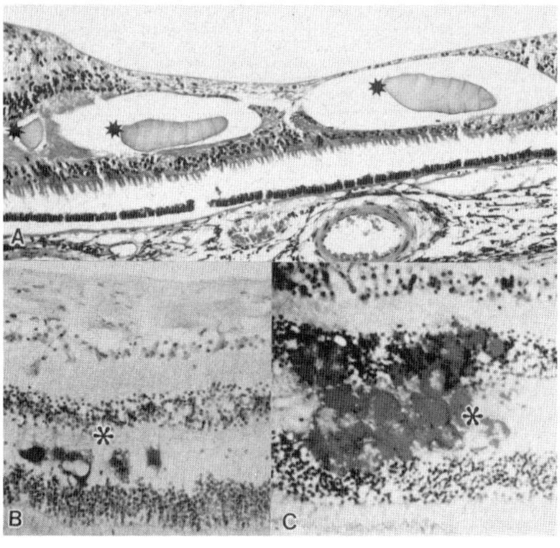

Fig. 27. Lipid-rich exudate residues (hard exudates) (asterisks) in the outer plexiform layer in macular area (A, hematoxylin and eosin ×140; B and C, oil red 0 ×328).

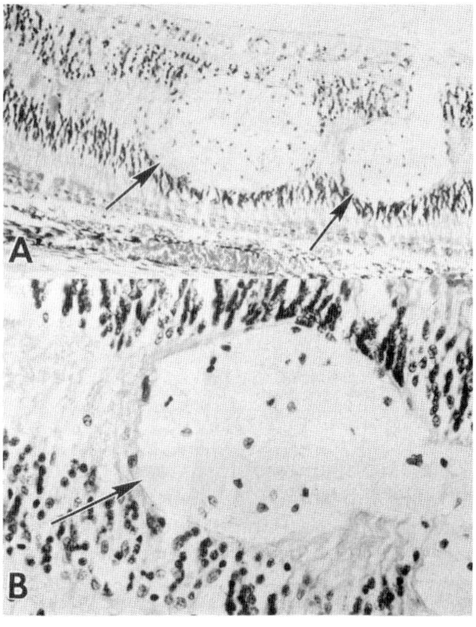

Fig. 28. Aggregates of lipid-laden macrophages (arrows) in outer plexiform layer in macular area (hematoxylin and eosin: A, ×137; B, ×328).

the outer plexiform layer (Fig. 27). The lipid may be phagocytized by macrophages as shown here where numerous lipid-laden macrophages are present in the outer plexiform layer (Fig. 28). Both edema and exudates are most abundant in the outer plexiform layer but they also may be present in the inner nuclear layer.

Hemorrhages present in the nerve fiber layer of the retina are linear since the blood is aligned parallel to the axons (Fig 29). Rounded deep hemorrhages are usually in the outer plexiform layer (Fig. 30) where, like exudates, they may displace neurons and glial cells.

With neovascularization, large preretinal and vitreous hemorrhages occur as shown in Fig. 31 where a large hemorrhage is present, sandwiched between the internal limiting membrane of the retina and the posterior vitreous.

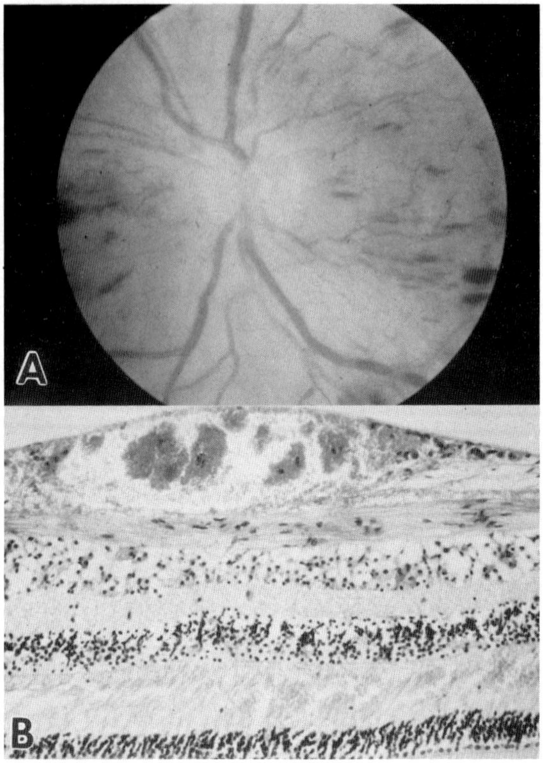

Fig. 29. Ophthalmoscopic (A) and microscopic (B) appearance of splinter-shaped retinal hemorrhage (B, hematoxylin and eosin, ×137).

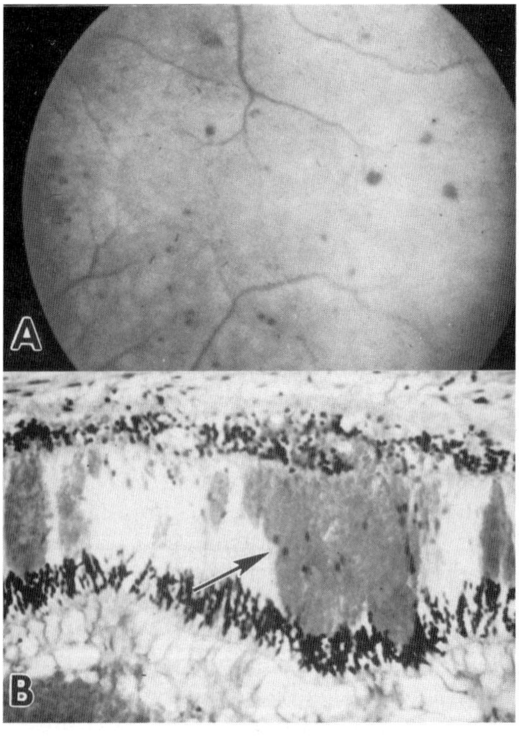

Fig. 30. Ophthalmoscopic (A) and histologic (B) appearance of deep punctate hemorrhages located in the outer plexiform layer (arrow) of different cases (hematoxylin and eosin ×137).

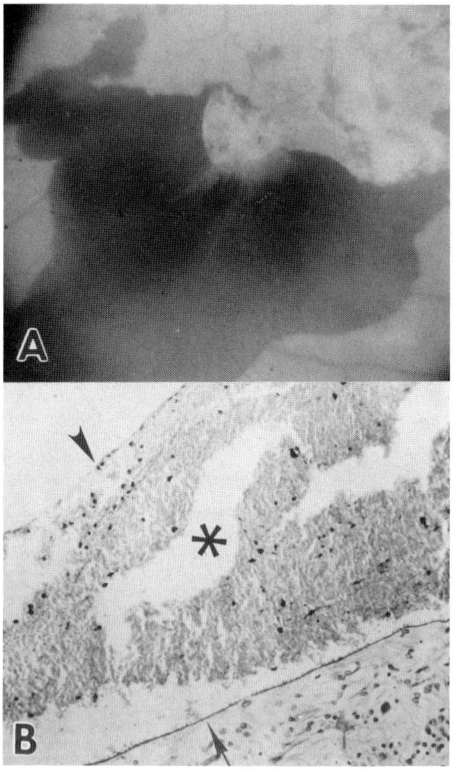

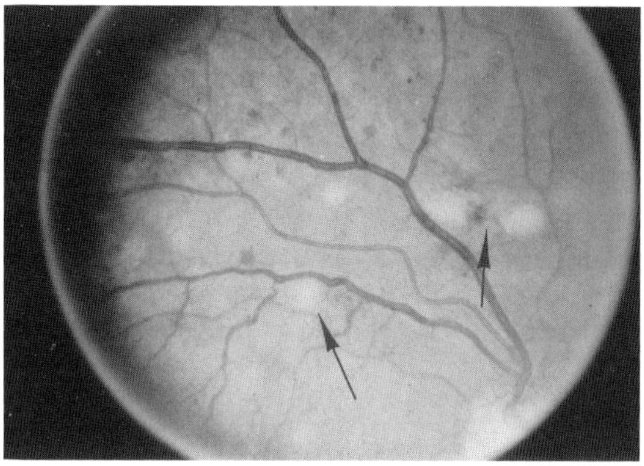

Fig. 31. (left) Ophthalmoscopic (A) and histopathologic (B) correlation of large preretinal hemorrhage in a patient with diabetic retinopathy. The hemorrhage (asterisk) is located between the internal limiting membrane of the retina (arrow) and the posterior vitreous hyaloid (arrowhead) (B, periodic acid-Schiff ×137).

Fig. 32. (right) Background diabetic retinopathy with several cotton wool spots (arrows).

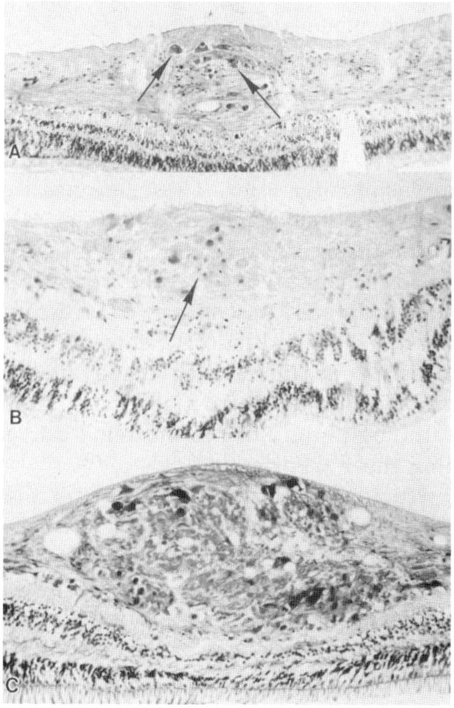

Fig. 33. Examples of cotton wool spots in diabetic retinopathy. There is fusiform thickening of the nerve fiber layer. Axonal enlargements are composed of axoplasmic material and stains like a cell nucleus (arrows) and have been called "cystoid bodies" (hematoxylin and eosin: A, ×137 and B and C ×538).

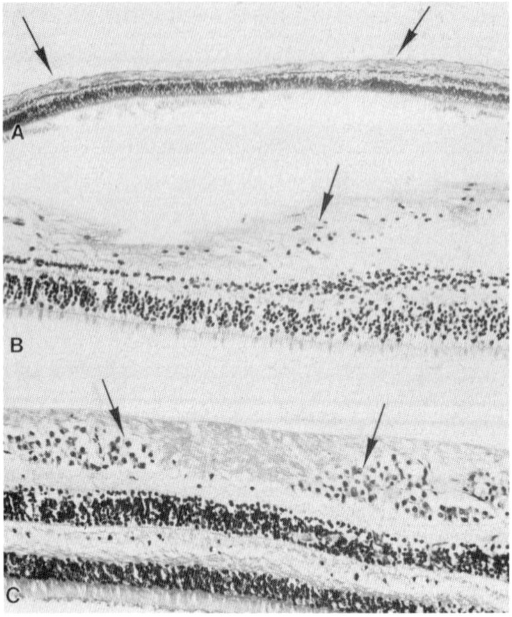

Fig. 34. Areas of inner retinal ischemic atrophy presumed sequelae of cotton wool spots. A. Area where all inner retinal layers, down to and including the inner portion of the inner nuclear layer, are absent (between arrows) (periodic acid-Schiff ×65). B. Margin of area of inner retinal ischemic atrophy (left of arrow) (hematoxylin and eosin ×100). C. Small area of inner retinal ischemic atrophy (between arrows) (hematoxylin and eosin ×225).

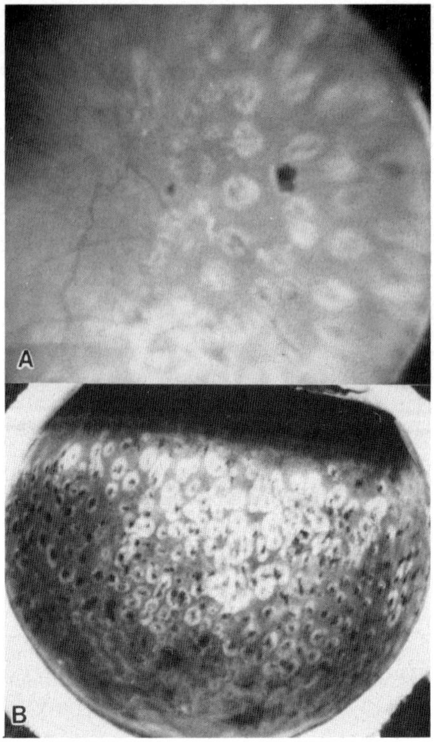

Fig. 35. Ophthalmoscopic (A) and gross (B) appearance of scatter photocoagulation (pan retinal photocoagulation) for proliferative diabetic retinopathy.

Focal infarctions of the nerve fiber layer of the retina (cotton wool spots) are circumscribed areas of thickening in the nerve fiber layer (Fig. 32). The lesion contains globular structures 10-20 μm in diameter (cystoid bodies) (Fig. 33). With electron microscopy, the cystoid body has been shown to be accumulated axoplasmic organelles. These lesions disappear in four to six weeks and leave an area of inner retinal ischemic atrophy (Fig. 34).

It is rare for us to receive postmortem eyes with proliferative diabetic retinopathy which have not had scatter photocoagulations (Fig. 35). There are several theories as to how PRP induces regression of neovascularization including: *1.* destruction of ischemic retina with a resultant decrease in vasoproliferative factors; *2.* production of chorioretinal scars which produce inhibitors of neovascularization; *3.* an increase in the available choroidal oxygen supply due to laser induced retinal thinning or destruction of the outer retina; or combinations of the above mechanisms. Pathologic study of postmortem human eyes provides some useful insight into understanding these theories.

Peripheral laser treatment results in variable destruction of the outer retina and the production of a scar composed of hyperplastic retinal pigment epithelial cells and astrocytes (Fig. 36). Substances produced by these cells may play a role in producing regression of neovascularization[11].

In the area of these laser scars the choriocapillaris is obliterated, as demonstrated by casts made of the choroidal vasculature. Wilson and Green[12] correlated the clinicopathologic features of a 76-year-old man who had his last session of PRP 14 months before death. A plastic cast of the retinal and choroidal vasculatures was made by perfusing the

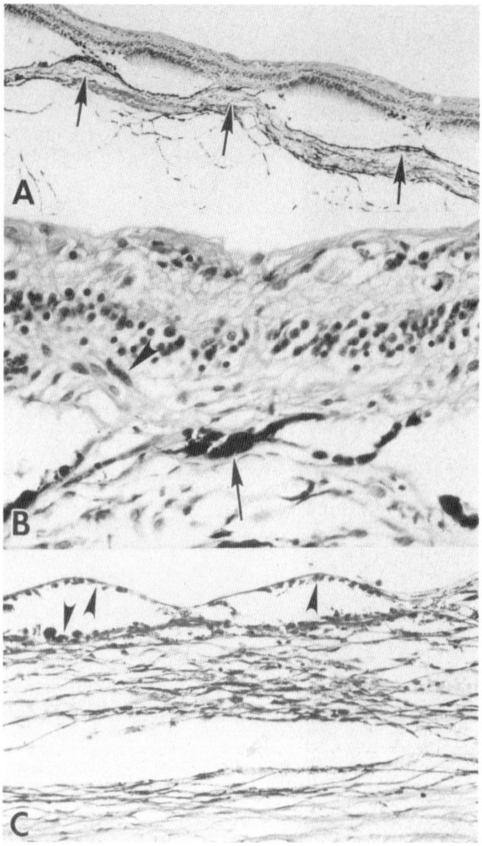

Fig. 36. Examples of peripheral laser scars. In most scars (A and B), there is a chorioretinal adhesion, loss of the photoreceptor cell layer, variable retinal pigment epithelial hyperplasia (arrows), mild gliosis (arrowhead), mild scarring in the choroid and an intact Bruch's membrane. In overlapping areas of treatment and in xenon arc areas, the entire retina may be destroyed and choroidal scarring is more marked (C). Hyperplastic retinal pigment epithelium (arrowheads) is usually present (hematoxylin and eosin: A, ×55; B, ×350; C, ×225).

ophthalmic artery with a plastic material. The surrounding tissue was then removed by digestion. This provided a cast which can be correlated with the antemortem fluorescein angiogram (Fig. 37). The portion of the fluorescein angiogram bordered by these retinal vessels is shown in the cast. It can be seen that there are circular defects in the cast which correspond to the laser lesions (Fig. 37). At higher magnification (Fig. 38), it can be seen that the choriocapillaris is absent, but that medium-sized choroidal vessels remain. In areas of confluent laser, large defects in the choriocapillaris are present (Fig. 39). It is apparent that healing of the choriocapillaris after peripheral laser photocoagulation which has been reported in the cat, does not occur in the human. Only rare laser lesions were crossed by patent vessels and these vessels appeared atrophic. If the underlying choriocapillaris is destroyed, it seems unlikely that an increase in oxygen supply from the choroid is the sole explanation of how scatter photocoagulation induces regression of neovascularization in diabetics.

Accumulation of fluid in the macular area is now known to be a major factor in reduction of vision in diabetic retinopathy (Fig. 26). Macular photocoagulation is now employed for the treatment of diabetic macular edema. This can be applied as a grid or focally to leaking microaneurysms. Wilson and co-workers[13] studied the effect of argon grid photocoagulation in the monkey (Fig 40). There were two findings from that study which were clinically relevant to the use of macular photocoagulation in diabetics. The first was that the retinal vessels did not appear to be directly occluded by the laser (Fig. 41). However, between three days and one month after laser treatment, occluded capillaries became apparent in the retinal capillary bed (Figs. 42 and 43). The loss of capillary bed following photocoagulation may play a role in the reduction of macular edema.

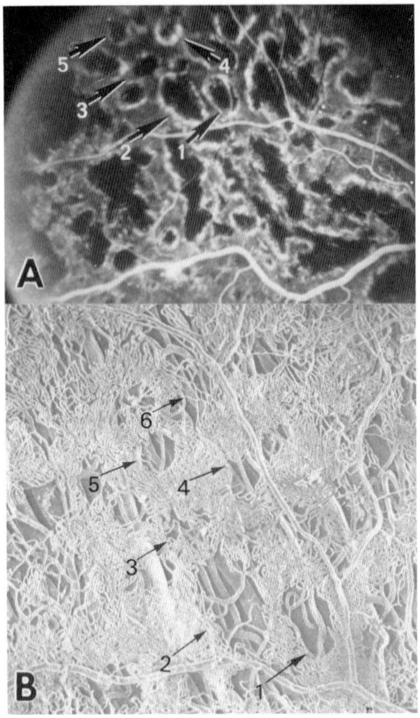

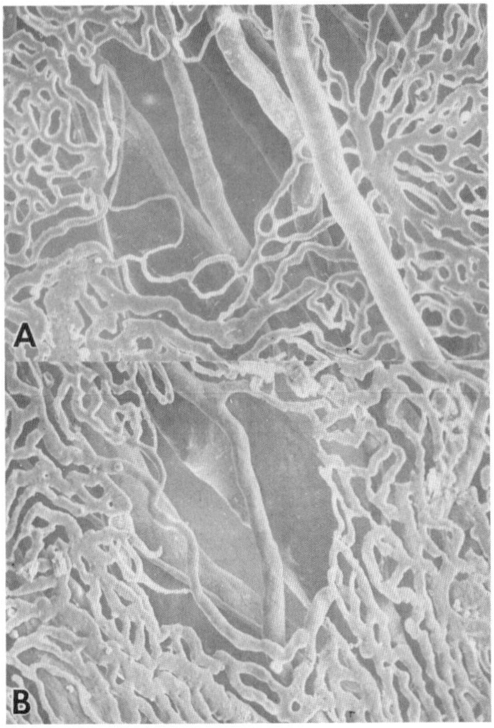

Fig. 37. (upper left) Fluorescein angiographic (A) and scanning microscopic (B) appearance of laser lesions. Retinal vessels shifted slightly in digestion process so that the relation between retinal vessels and laser lesions is slightly different in cast compared with fluorescein angiogram. Five corresponding lesions are indicated (arrows) (B, vascular cast, ×20).

Fig. 38. (upper right) Higher power view of laser lesions 4 (A) and 5 (B). No choriocapillaris is present in the treated area (vascular cast; A, ×140; B, ×170).

Fig. 39. (right) Area of confluent laser photocoagulation just below inferotemporal vein. Arrows mark temporal margin of laser treatment on fluorescein angiogram and margin of choriocapillaris on vascular cast (A, fluorescein angiogram at 50.5 s; B, vascular cast, ×50). (Figs. 37-39 are from: Wilson DJ, Green WR: Argon laser panretinal photocoagulation for diabetic retinopathy: scanning electron microscopy of human choroidal vascular casts. Arch Ophthalmol 125:239-242, 1987. Copyright 1987, American Medical Association.)

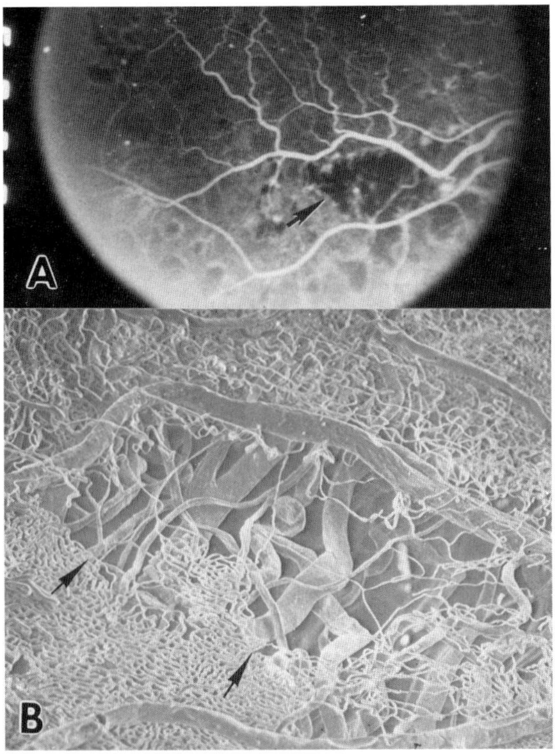

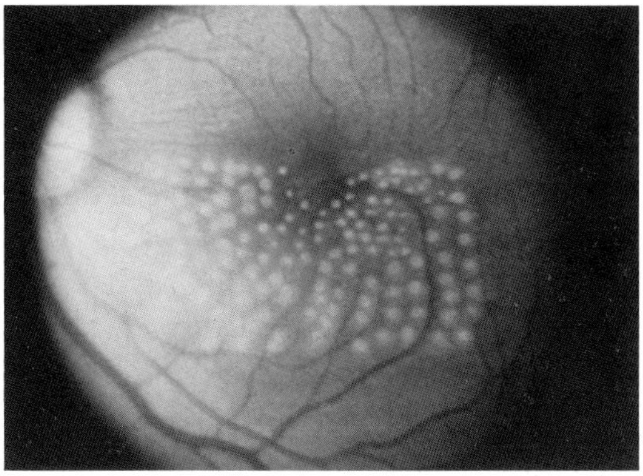

Fig. 40. Appearance of argon laser lesions immediately after treatment.

The second finding was that, in areas between photocoagulation, there was some disorientation of the photoreceptors (Fig. 44). These areas did not return to normal until sometime between one and five months after laser treatment. This may explain why vision initially decreases in some patients and why visual improvement lags behind the resolution of macular edema in some patients.

Summary

In summary, the principal pathologic changes in diabetic retinopathy occur in the retinal blood vessels and consist of thickening of the basement membrane, loss of pericytes, microaneurysms, capillary closure, and new vessel formation. Secondary changes include edema, exudates, hemorrhages and traction cystic degeneration, schisis and retinal detachment.

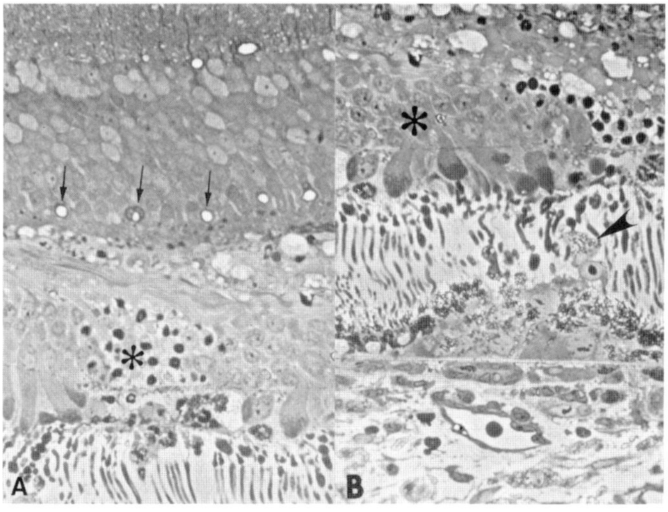

Fig. 41. Appearance of retina three days after grid laser photocoagulation. A. Photoreceptor cell nuclei are pyknotic (asterisk) and there is partial destruction of inner and outer segments. Overlying capillaries in inner nuclear layer are intact (arrows) (paraphenylenediamine, ×480). B. Between laser lesions photoreceptor cell bodies are intact (asterisk). Outer segments are distorted and are no longer in close apposition to retinal pigment epithelium, cells of which are large and multilayered. Occasional pigment-containing cells (arrowhead) are present in subretinal space (paraphenylenediamine, ×480).

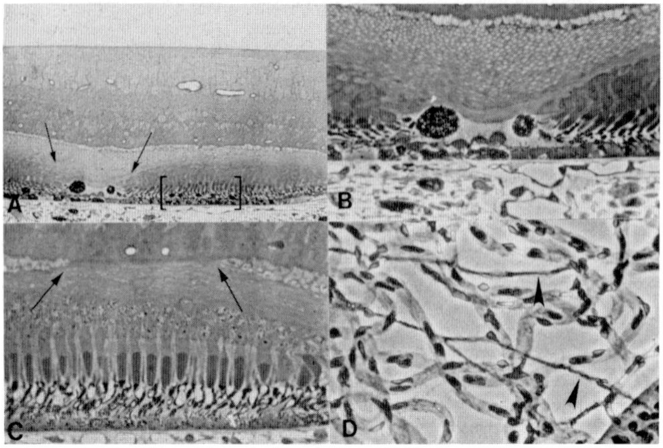

Fig. 42. Light microscopic appearance of a retina one month after argon grid photocoagulation. A. Healed laser lesion (arrows), with total loss of photoreceptor cell layer, minor hyperplastic retinal pigment epithelium (RPE) and pigmented cells in sub-RPE area. In the adjacent, untreated area (brackets), photoreceptor outer segments are in close approximation to RPE but are shorter than normal and pigment containing cells are present in subretinal space (paraphenylenediamine, ×70). B. RPE in area of laser lesion is multilayered, with outer layer consisting of spindle-shaped cells, and inner layer of dome-shaped cells. Photoreceptors are absent, substituted by material resembling interphotoreceptor matrix and pigment containing cells (paraphenylenediamine, ×290). C. Area at junction of outer plexiform and outer nuclear layers lacks photoreceptor synapses (between arrows) (paraphenylenediamine, ×290). D. Trypsin digest preparation showing collapsed acellular capillaries (arrowheads) (hematoxylin eosin, ×290).

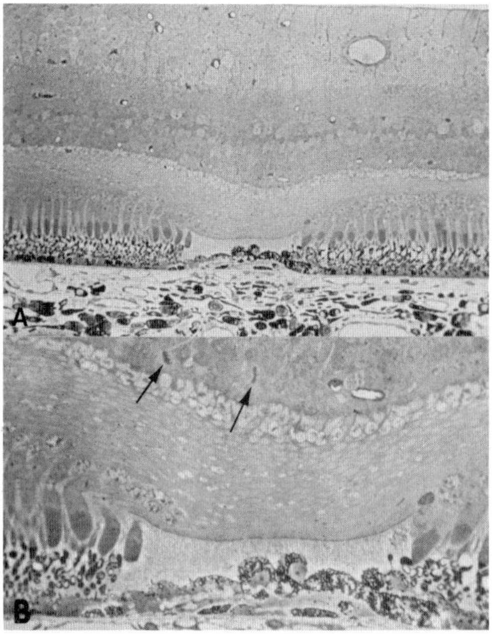

Fig. 43. Appearance of retina five months after argon laser photocoagulation. A. Between laser lesions photoreceptor outer segments are of normal length (paraphenylenediamine, ×120). B. Retinal pigment epithelium is multilayered, with outermost layers consisting of spindle-shaped cells. Inner layers are dome-shaped and at the periphery of the laser lesions some dome-shaped cells touch photoreceptor outer segments. Two occluded capillaries are present in inner nuclear layer (arrows) (paraphenylenediamine ×480).

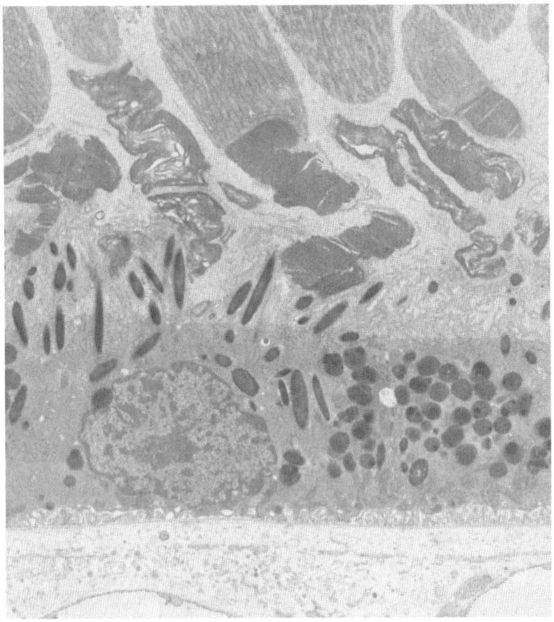

Fig. 44. Electron photomicrograph of a retina and retinal pigment epithelium between laser lesions one month after argon grid photocoagulation. Photoreceptor outer segments are enveloped in retinal pigment epithelium microvilli, but outer segments are shorter than normal. Outer segment discs lack their normal parallel arrangement (×5400). (Figs. 40-44 are from: Wilson DJ, Finkelstein D, Quigley HA, Green WR: Macular grid photocoagulation: an experimental study on the primate retina. Arch Ophthalmol 106:100-105, 1988. Copyright 1988, American Medical Association.)

References

1. Ashton N: Studies of the retinal capillaries in relation to diabetic and other retinopathies. Br J Ophthalmol 47:521-538, 1963
2. Robison WG, Nagata M, Laver N, Hohman TC, Kinoshita JH: Diabetic-like retinopathy in rats prevented with an aldose reductase inhibitor. Invest Ophthalmol Vis Sci 38:2285-2292, 1989
3. Sorbinil Retinopathy Trial Research Group: A randomized trial of sorbinil an aldose reductase inhibitor, in diabetic retinopathy. Arch Ophthalmol 108:1234-1244, 1990
4. Cogan DG, Toussaint D, Kuwabara T: Studies of retinal vascular patterns. IV. Diabetic retinopathy. Arch Ophthalmol 66:100-112, 1961
6. Kuwabara T, Cogan DG: Studies of retinal vascular patterns. VI. Mural cells of the retinal capillaries. Arch Ophthalmol 69:492-502, 1963
6. Orlidge A, D'Amore P: Inhibitor of capillary endothelial cell growth by pericytes and smooth muscle cells. J Cell Biol 37:277-299, 1987
7. Niki T, Muraoka K, Shimizu K: Distribution of capillary nonperfusion in early stage diabetic retinopathy. Ophthalmology 91:1431-1439, 1984
8. Hersh PS, Green WR, Thomas JA: Tractional venous loops in diabetic retinopathy. Am J Ophthalmol 92:661-671, 1981
9. Muraoka K, Shimizu K: Intraretinal neovascularization in diabetic retinopathy. Ophthalmology 91:1440-1446, 1984
10. Faulborn J, Bowald S: Microproliferations in proliferative diabetic retinopathy and their relationship to the vitreous: corresponding light and electron microscopic studies. Graefe's Arch Clin Exp Ophthalmol 223:130-138, 1985
11. Glaser BM, Campochiaro PA, Davis JL Jr, Sabo M: Retinal pigment epithelial cells release an inhibitor of neovascularization. Arch Ophthalmol 103:1870-1875, 1985
12. Wilson DJ, Green WR: Argon laser panretinal photocoagulation for diabetic retinopathy: scanning electron microscopy of human choroidal vascular casts. Arch Ophthalmol 125:239-242, 1987
13. Wilson DJ, Finkelstein D, Quigley HA, Green WR: Macular grid photocoagulation: an experimental study on the primate retina. Arch Ophthalmol 106:100-105, 1988

EVALUATION AND MANAGEMENT OF PROLIFERATIVE AND SEVERE NON-PROLIFERATIVE DIABETIC RETINOPATHY

Matthew D. Davis

Department of Ophthalmology, University of Wisconsin-Madison, Madison, Wisconsin, USA

Evaluation

Much of the discussion in the following article (pp. 93-100) regarding the use of ophthalmoscopy and stereoscopic fundus photography in the evaluation of macular edema also applies to assessment of overall retinopathy severity. Binocular indirect ophthalmoscopy is very useful for scanning the fundus in search of new vessels and for making a brief fundus diagram to document the location and extent of new vessels and other important lesions. *This diagram should be made during, not at the conclusion of, the examination.* A meticulous, unhurried examination is necessary if small patches of new vessels are not to be overlooked, and should be followed by an examination that provides greater magnification, either direct ophthalmoscopy or slit-lamp biomicroscopy, concentrating on the disc and posterior retina and giving special attention to any areas of possible new vessels noted on indirect ophthalmoscopy. I prefer direct ophthalmoscopy for this purpose, but slit-lamp examination with high plus precorneal lens is also quite satisfactory. Slit-lamp and contact lens examination can be used instead, with the added advantage that it affords an assessment of vitreoretinal relationships that is, in my experience, better than that achievable with a high plus precorneal lens. Use of the contact lens should be deferred until after photography, but this has the disadvantage of interfering with smooth patient flow. Whenever retinopathy has reached or passed the moderate non-proliferative stage, it is desirable to obtain stereoscopic color fundus photographs of the seven standard fields at the baseline examination, and to repeat selected fields during follow-up when any substantial change has occurred. When retinopathy is mild, baseline photographs of the disc and macula are usually sufficient, and none are needed when only occasional microaneurysms are present.

Management

As discussed in the article on pp. 43-61, there is little evidence to suggest that improving blood sugar control or undertaking any other systemic treatment, such as blood pressure reduction, will favorably influence retinopathy once the severe non-proliferative or proliferative stage has been reached. Photocoagulation and vitrectomy, therefore, are the only measures available. This chapter will be limited to photocoagulation.

Address for correspondence: Matthew D. Davis, MD, Department of Ophthalmology, University of Wisconsin-Madison, 610 N. Walnut Street, P.O. Box 5240, Madison, WI 53705, USA

Retina and Vitreous, pp. 83-91
Proceedings of the Symposium on Retina and Vitreous,
organized by the New Orleans Academy of Ophthalmology
New Orleans, LA, USA, March 12-15, 1992
edited by Rudolph M. Franklin

Mechanisms of photocoagulation

Initially photocoagulation was used to destroy directly patches of new vessels on the surface of the retina[1,2]. It soon became apparent that extensive photocoagulation seemed to have a beneficial indirect effect, since it was sometimes followed by regression of new vessels and diminution of retinal edema and vascular congestion in areas of the retina not directly treated[3]. Such indirect treatment, in which hundreds of burns are scattered throughout the fundus in a pattern that usually leaves about one-half to one burn width between burns (scatter or panretinal photocoagulation), is now the principal way in which photocoagulation is used when the aim is to induce regression or prevent growth of new vessels (see Fig. 5 on page 46 and Fig. 7 on page 49)[4].

Clinical trials have documented the efficacy of scatter photocoagulation in proliferative diabetic retinopathy (PDR), but its mechanism is not clear. One theory proposes that areas of the inner retina that have become partially ischemic from capillary loss produce a new vessel stimulating factor capable of diffusing through the vitreous to other areas of the retina and into the anterior chamber. It is suggested that scatter photocoagulation may reduce production of the factor by destroying some of the ischemic retina[5,6]. A second theory suggests that photocoagulation improves oxygenation of the ischemic inner retinal layers by destroying some of the metabolically highly active photoreceptor cells and allowing the oxygen normally diffusing from the choriocapillaris to supply these cells to continue on into the inner layers of the retina[7-9]. The latter theory is appealing because it is principally the photoreceptor cells that are destroyed by mild argon laser burns, but fails to explain why stronger burns sometimes seem more effective clinically. This theory is consistent with reports that retinal blood flow decreases, and autoregulatory response to breathing 100% oxygen improves, following scatter photocoagulation, as might be expected if more oxygen were reaching the inner retina from the choroid[10]. However, the choriocapillaris, which presumably is the source of the oxygen postulated to be relieving inner retinal ischemia, has been found to be destroyed beneath at least some scatter burns[11]. A third theory proposes that the cells of the retinal pigment epithelium produce a new vessel inhibiting factor, and that the response of these cells to photocoagulation injury may favor production of this factor[12].

Initial photocoagulation for proliferative or severe non-proliferative retinopathy

Diabetic Retinopathy Study

The efficacy of photocoagulation for PDR has been demonstrated in three randomized clinical trials, each of which found that treatment reduced the rate of severe decrease of vision to less than 50% of the rate observed in untreated eyes[13-17]. The largest of these trials was the Diabetic Retinopathy Study (DRS), conducted from 1971 to 1979 by the National Eye Institute. The DRS enrolled patients with unequivocal new vessels in at least one eye (PDR) or severe non-proliferative retinopathy (NPDR) in both eyes, and a visual acuity of 20/100 or better in each eye. Patients were randomly assigned to either the argon laser or xenon arc treatment group; one eye of each patient was randomly assigned to photocoagulation treatment and the other to a control group in which no photocoagulation was to be carried out (unless the protocol were to be modified during the trial because of evidence that treatment was beneficial). Patients were followed at four-monthly intervals according to a protocol that provided for measurement of best corrected visual acuity with different charts for each eye by specially trained and certified examiners who did not know the identity of the treated eye or type of treatment, and who attempted to reduce patient bias by urging the patient to read as far down the chart as possible with each eye, guessing at letters until more than one in a line was missed. All patients gave written informed consent and understood that the information being col-

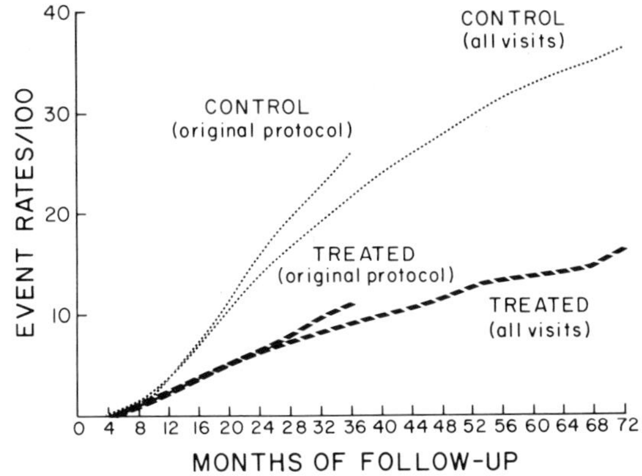

Fig. 1. Cumulative rates of severe visual loss, including and excluding observations made after the 1976 protocol change, argon and xenon groups combined.

lected would be analyzed at frequent intervals and used, if possible, for their benefit.

Both the argon and xenon photocoagulation protocols included scatter treatment extending from the posterior pole to the equator, often completed in a single sitting. The argon technique specified 800 to 1600 500-µm scatter burns of 0.1 seconds' duration and direct treatment of new vessels on or within one disc diameter of the disc (NVD) and elsewhere (NVE), whether flat or elevated. Direct treatment was also applied to microaneurysms or other lesions thought to be causing macular edema. Follow-up treatment was applied as needed at four-month intervals. The xenon technique was similar, but burns were fewer, of longer duration, and stronger, and direct treatment was not applied to elevated new vessels or those on the surface of the disc.

The DRS chose as its principal outcome measure "severe visual loss", defined as a visual acuity of less than 5/200 at each of two consecutively completed follow-up visits. Figs. 1 to 3 depict cumulative rates of severe visual loss for eyes assigned to treatment and control groups[17]. In Fig. 1, the argon and xenon groups are combined and separate analyses are shown including and excluding visits made after the protocol was changed in 1976 (on the basis of analyses similar to those to be discussed shortly) to encourage treatment of control group eyes that were then at high risk of severe visual loss. All eyes were classified in the group to which they were originally randomly assigned, ignoring treatment of control group eyes. In the analysis including all visits, 44% of the two-year visits and all the four-year visits were carried out after the protocol change; by the two-year visit 12% of control group eyes had been treated and by the five-year visit 40% had

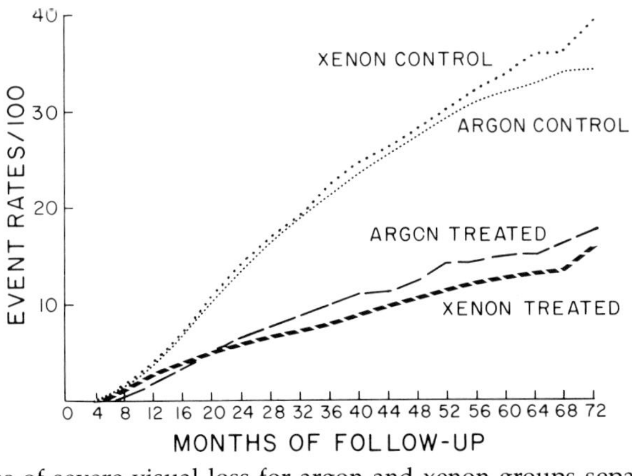

Fig. 2. Cumulative rates of severe visual loss for argon and xenon groups separately.

been treated. The two curves for control group eyes are very similar over the first 20 months of follow-up and those for treated eyes are similar over at least the first 28 months. The difference between the two control group curves is probably due, at least in part, to the beneficial effect of treatment experienced by some of these eyes after the protocol change, and the treatment effect after three years is probably underestimated somewhat. In each of these analyses, treatment reduced the risk of severe visual loss by 50% or more at and after the 16-month visit.

In Fig. 2, the Fig. 1 analysis including all visits is presented separately for the argon and xenon groups. The treatment effect, *i.e.*, the difference between treatment and control groups, appears somewhat greater in the xenon group, but this difference is small, its statistical significance borderline, and its clinical importance outweighed by the greater harmful effects of the xenon treatment used in the DRS (Table 1).

Table 1. Estimated percentages of eyes with harmful effects attributable to Diabetic Retinopathy Study treatment

	Argon	*Xenon*
Constriction of visual field (Goldmann IVe4 test object) to an average of		
≤45°, >30° per meridian	5	25
≤30° per meridian	0	25
Decrease in visual acuity		
1 line	11	19
≥2 lines	3	11

In Fig. 3, the Fig. 1 analysis including all visits is presented for three subgroups defined by retinopathy severity in baseline stereoscopic fundus photographs. These three groups correspond approximately to Levels 53, 65, and 70 in Table 1 on page 51 (see also Fig. 14 on page 53). In each group, treatment reduced the risk of severe visual loss to about one-half that observed in control group eyes, but this effect became apparent later and the

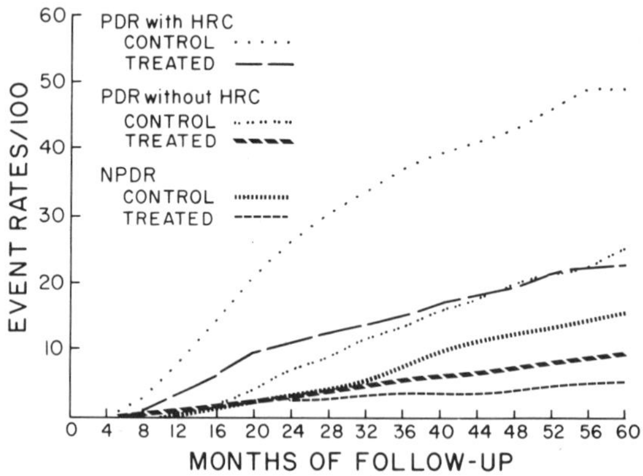

Fig. 3. Cumulative rates of severe visual loss for eyes classified by presence of proliferative retinopathy (PDR) and high-risk characteristics (HRC) in baseline fundus photographs, argon and xenon groups combined. HRC were defined as either of the following: 1. new vessels on or within one disc diameter of the disc (NVD) equalling or exceeding those in Standard Photograph 10A (see Fig. 14 on page 53); 2. NVD less than those in Standard Photograph 10A and/or new vessels elsewhere at least one-half disc area in extent in at least one of the seven standard photographic fields, if vitreous or preretinal hemorrhage was present. NPDR: non-proliferative diabetic retinopathy.
(*Figs. 1-3* from: The Diabetic Retinopathy Study Research Group: Photocoagulation treatment of proliferative diabetic retinopathy: clinical application of DRS findings. DRS Report No 8. Ophthalmology 88:583-600, 1981. Courtesy of the Diabetic Retinopathy Study Research Group.)

percentage of eyes treated that benefitted (the arithmetic treatment difference) became smaller as retinopathy severity decreased. On the basis of this analysis and the harmful effects of treatment summarized in Table 1, the DRS confirmed its earlier conclusion that for eyes with high-risk characteristics ("high risk PDR") the chance of benefit from treatment (for example, reduction of the two-year risk of severe visual loss from about 26% to 11%) clearly outweighed its risks of harm and recommended prompt photocoagulation for most such eyes.

For eyes with severe NPDR or early (non high-risk) PDR, the DRS concluded that either of two alternatives was satisfactory, and that DRS results were not helpful in choosing between them:

1. immediate photocoagulation; or
2. frequent follow-up and prompt initiation of photocoagulation if high-risk PDR developed.

Early Treatment Diabetic Retinopathy Study

One of the goals of the Early Treatment Diabetic Retinopathy Study (ETDRS), a randomized clinical trial sponsored by the National Eye Institute, was to compare these alternatives (designated "early photocoagulation" and "deferral of photocoagulation", respectively) in patients with mild to severe NPDR or early PDR, with or without macular edema. Between 1980 and 1985, 3711 such patients were enrolled. One eye of each patient was randomly assigned to early photocoagulation and the other to deferral. Follow-up ranged from three to eight years.

Eyes assigned to early photocoagulation were randomly assigned to either of two scatter treatment protocols, full or mild. The full scatter protocol called for 500 μm, 0.1 second argon blue-green or green laser burns of moderate intensity, placed one-half burn apart, extending from the posterior pole to the equator. Between 1200 and 1600 burns were applied, divided between two or more episodes. The mild scatter protocol was the same, except that a total of 400-650 more widely spaced burns were applied to the same area in a single episode. Direct (local) treatment was specified for patches of surface NVE that were two disc areas or less in extent (the area of a circle about 1.4 times the diameter of the disc), using confluent, moderately intense burns that extended 500 μm beyond the edges of the patch. For larger patches or several small ones close together, full scatter alone to this area was an acceptable alternative. No direct treatment was carried out for NVD[4].

One important outcome measure used in the ETDRS was the first occurrence of either severe visual loss, as defined in the DRS, or vitrectomy[18]. These events were combined because progression to a stage requiring vitrectomy may rightly be considered a bad out-

Table 2. Cumulative five-year rates of severe visual loss or vitrectomy, and relative risks for entire period of follow-up, by baseline retinopathy status and treatment group (From: Early Treatment Diabetic Retinopathy Study Research Group: Early photocoagulation for diabetic retinopathy. ETDRS Report No 9. Ophthalmology 98:766-785, 1991. Courtesy of the ETDRS Research Group.)

Baseline retinopathy	*Treatment group*				*Relative risk for entire follow-up period (99% confidence interval)*
	Early photocoagulation		*Deferral*		
	No. at baseline	*Five-year rate*	*No. at baseline*	*Five-year rate*	
Mild to moderate NPDR with macular edema	1448	2%	1429	4%	0.55 (0.33-0.94)
Severe NPDR or early PDR with macular edema	1090	6%	1103	10%	0.68 (0.47-0.99)
Moderate to severe NPDR or early PDR without macular edema	1173	4%	1179	5%	0.78 (0.47-1.29)

come for ETDRS-eligible eyes, and because presumably most eyes selected for vitrectomy before the occurrence of severe visual loss (68% of the 243 ETDRS eyes undergoing vitrectomy) would have developed severe visual loss within several months if vitrectomy had not been carried out. Five-year life-table rates of severe visual loss or vitrectomy, and relative risks for early photocoagulation compared to deferral over the entire follow-up period, are shown in Table 2. The first two rows include eyes with macular edema, subdivided by retinopathy severity. As would be anticipated, the outcome was more frequent in eyes with more severe retinopathy (in the deferral group, 10% in eyes with severe NPDR or early PDR *versus* 4% in eyes with mild to moderate NPDR). In both these retinopathy subgroups, early treatment reduced the event rate to about one-half that in the deferral group, but the percentage of eyes treated that benefitted was only 2-4%. The third row of the table includes all eyes without macular edema regardless of retinopathy severity (eyes with mild NPDR were not eligible unless macular edema was present) and, as might be expected, outcome here was intermediate between that in rows 1 and 2. There was little difference between full and mild scatter for this outcome measure.

Some harmful effects of scatter photocoagulation were observed in the ETDRS, an early decrease in visual acuity (a doubling or more of the visual angle at the four-month visit in about 10% of eyes assigned to early full scatter, compared to about 5% of eyes assigned to deferral) and some decrease in visual field. It was recommended that scatter treatment not be used in eyes with mild to moderate NPDR, but that it be considered for eyes approaching the high-risk stage, *i.e.*, eyes with very severe NPDR or moderate PDR (Levels 53E and 65 in Fig. 15 on page 53), in which 50% of deferral group eyes developed high-risk PDR within about 18 months, and that it usually should not be delayed when the high-risk stage is present[18].

Application of ETDRS results to clinical practice and personal preferences

Figs. 3 and 4 on page 45 provide examples of eyes with very severe NPDR. When seeing a patient for the first time in whom retinopathy of this severity is present in both eyes, I am inclined to recommend either very close follow-up, with re-examination after a month or so, or initiation of photocoagulation in one eye. If one waits for unequivocal new vessels to develop before recommending photocoagulation, both eyes may enter a rapidly progressive proliferative phase simultaneously and optimal timing of all of the necessary treatment episodes may not be possible. When new vessels are already present in an eye with the lesions of very severe NPDR (see Fig. 5. on page 46), I have no hesitation in recommending prompt initiation of photocoagulation. For eyes with new vessels but without the lesions of severe NPDR, however, I am inclined to recommend an initial period of observation, even if NVE are extensive. Many such eyes remain asymptomatic for many years, with little growth and often substantial regression of the new vessels. If new vessels are demonstrated to be actively growing, photocoagulation is usually recommended.

I prefer to use the green only wave length and to follow the ETDRS guidelines for full scatter and local treatment, dividing treatment between two or three episodes usually two weeks apart. Many experienced clinicians use scatter treatment alone, without any local treatment, and I have little doubt that it is probably equally effective. For most patients I prefer topical anesthesia, because excessively strong burns are avoided. However, for the occasional patient who experiences more than mild discomfort and photophobia, failure to use retrobulbar or peribulbar anesthesia may result in under-treatment. I do not use the cumulative number of burns applied at all previous treatment episodes as an index of the extent of treatment, because the size of burns varies not only with the spot size setting but also with the power and duration of exposure, the plane of focus of the slit-lamp, and the degree to which lens opacities defocus the laser beam. It is better to estimate the extent of past treatment by the amount of retina remaining free of scars.

Additional photocoagulation when initial response is inadequate

There is general agreement that when regression of new vessels is induced by scatter photocoagulation it usually occurs rapidly, sometimes being apparent in a day or two, and reaches a maximal level within a month or so, but few data have been published to support these generalizations. It is also generally recognized that additional scatter photocoagulation is often effective in inducing regression of new vessels when they do not regress after initial treatment or when they recur after initial partial or complete regression[19].

Blankenship[20] observed 31 eyes with NVD 1/4 disc area or more in extent one and six months following extensive scatter photocoagulation applied in a single episode[20]. NVD had regressed to less than 1/4 disc area in 30/31 eyes (97%) at one month, but regression to this level persisted at six months in only 23 of 30 eyes (77%). Rogell used an incremental approach to scatter photocoagulation, initially applying, with retrobulbar anesthesia, 1100 to 1500, 500-μm, moderately intense argon laser burns, divided between two episodes about one week apart[21]. Patients were seen at monthly intervals and 300 to 400 additional burns were applied at each visit until "substantial regression" of new vessels had occurred. In about 40% of 55 eyes with PDR, the initial treatment was sufficient; in 50%, one or two and in 10%, three to five follow-up treatments were required. Additional treatment is required more frequently in younger patients, who tend to have more severe retinopathy[22].

My usual custom is to evaluate the degree of regression one or two months after completion of the initial treatment, hoping for complete regression but accepting a 50% reduction in new vessels as sufficient to continue observation without additional treatment. If there has been no regression, additional scatter treatment is usually recommended, while if some regression is present but not as much as 50%, the decision may be difficult.

The ETDRS protocol suggested guidelines for follow-up treatment, specifying six factors to be considered[4]:

1. change in new vessels since the last visit and/or since the last photocoagulation treatment;
2. appearance of the new vessels (caliber, degree of network formation, extent of accompanying fibrous tissue);
3. frequency and extent of vitreous hemorrhage since the last visit and/or since the last photocoagulation treatment;
4. status of vitreous detachment;
5. extent of photocoagulation scars; and
6. extent of traction retinal detachment and fibrous proliferations[4].

Additional treatment is more likely to be recommended when new vessels appear active, as suggested by formation of tight networks and a paucity of accompanying fibrous tissue, and are increasing in extent, or when vitreous hemorrhages are occurring repeatedly. If the caliber of new vessels has decreased and fibrous proliferations are developing, this suggests that retinopathy is entering a quiescent stage in which additional treatment may be unnecessary. Additional photocoagulation may be less urgent after occurrence of extensive posterior vitreous detachment because additional growth of new vessels (whether along the detached posterior hyaloid surface or, much less commonly, along the surface of the retina) does not increase the extent of vitreoretinal adhesions. If the previous scatter burns appear widely spaced, or if there are areas where scatter was omitted, additional photocoagulation is considered more seriously, but if little untreated retina remains outside of the posterior pole it may be better to defer additional photocoagulation in order to preserve the visual field. If severe vitreous hemorrhage occurs in such eyes, vitrectomy can be done, with a good chance of restoration of both central and peripheral vision.

When additional scatter treatment is carried out, burns are placed between treatment scars, anterior to them, and/or in the posterior pole, sparing the area within 500 to 1500 μm of the center of the macula. The areas chosen for treatment are generally those in which new vessels are present or toward which they appear to be growing, or in which scars are less tightly spaced. It is the clinical impression of some experienced observers that priority should be given to the posterior pole, particularly the area temporal to the center of the macula, where extensive capillary loss is common and small new vessel patches sometimes occur, and where the posterior extent of the original scatter treatment is sometimes three to four disc diameters or more from the center of the macula.

Special situations

Severe retinal ischemia

The presence of extensive retinal hemorrhages, venous beading, and opaque small arteriolar branches, often accompanied by prominent soft exudates, suggests rapidly progressive closure of the retinal capillary bed and severe retinal ischemia[23]. New vessels are usually present in such eyes, but may be relatively unimpressive. Severe retinal ischemia increases the urgency to initiate scatter photocoagulation, whether or not high-risk PDR is present, because these eyes appear to be at greater risk of anterior segment neovascularization. Patients should be aware of this risk and the risk of a sudden decrease in central vision that may occur with occlusion of the remaining arterioles supplying the macula. The clinical impression that scatter photocoagulation may precipitate such an occlusion has led to the suggestion that initial scatter treatment be divided between three or four episodes in the hope of reducing this risk.

High-risk PDR with extensive fibrous proliferations and/or localized extramacular traction retinal detachment

Progressive contraction of fibrous proliferations and extension of localized traction retinal detachment into the center of the macula sometimes follow scatter photocoagulation for high-risk PDR in eyes with extensive fibrous proliferations. Early experience with such cases led to some reluctance to advise photocoagulation in this situation. Few such eyes were included in the DRS, but analyses of them indicated that outcome was better with photocoagulation than without it and suggested that it is only excessively heavy treatment that should be avoided. Only in the xenon group was a severe adverse treatment effect found in these eyes, and even here the benefit of treatment outweighed its risks[24]. When high-risk characteristics are definitely present, scatter photocoagulation should usually be carried out, in spite of the presence of fibrous proliferations and/or localized traction retinal detachment. Areas of fibrous proliferations and retinal detachment should be avoided, and treatment strength should be mild to moderate. It may be desirable to divide treatment between several episodes.

Which eye to treat first

When both eyes of a patient are in need of scatter photocoagulation and the prognosis in one eye is obviously poorer, because of severe ischemia, extensive fibrous proliferations and/or traction retinal detachment, or severe macular edema, it may often be wiser to treat the better eye first. This provides a better opportunity to preserve the best possible visual acuity for the patient and avoids the possibility that the patient may refuse treatment for the eye with the better prognosis following a disappointing outcome in the poorer eye.

References

1. Meyer-Schwickerath G: Drance SM (trans) Light Coagulation. St Louis: Mosby 1960
2. Wetzig PC, Worlton JT: Treatment of diabetic retinopathy by light coagulation. Br J Ophthalmol 47:539-541, 1963
3. Beetham WP, Aiello JM, Balodimos NC, Konca L: Ruby laser photocoagulation of early diabetic neovascular retinopathy. Trans Am Ophthalmol Soc 67:39-67, 1969
4. The Early Treatment Diabetic Retinopathy Study Research Group: Techniques for scatter and local photocoagulation treatment of diabetic retinopathy: ETDRS Report No 3. Int Ophthalmol Clin 27:254-264, 1987
5. Patz A: Clinical and experimental studies on retinal neovascularization. Am J Ophthalmol 94:715-743, 1982
6. Little HL, Zweng C, Jack RL, Vassiliadis A: Techniques of argon laser photocoagulation of diabetic disc new vessels. Am J Ophthalmol 82:675-683, 1976
7. Wolbarsht ML, Landers MB: The rationale of photocoagulation therapy for proliferative diabetic retinopathy: a review and a model. Ophthalmic Surg 11:235-245, 1980
8. Weiter JJ, Zuckerman R: The influence of the photoreceptor-RPE complex on the inner retina; an explanation for the beneficial effects of photocoagulation. Ophthalmology 87:1133-1139, 1980
9. Molnar J, Poitry S, Tsacopoulos M et al: Effect of laser photocoagulation on oxygenation of the retina in miniature pigs. Invest Ophthalmol Vis Sci 26:1410-1414, 1985
10. Grunwald JE, Brucker AJ, Petrig BL, Riva CE: Retinal blood flow regulation and the clinical response to panretinal photocoagulation in proliferative diabetic retinopathy. Ophthalmology 96:1518-1522, 1989
11. Wilson DJ, Green WR: Argon laser panretinal photocoagulation for diabetic retinopathy: scanning electron microscopy of human choroidal vascular casts. Arch Ophthalmol 105:239-242, 1987
12. Glaser BM, Campochiaro PA, Davis DL Jr, Sato M: Retinal pigment epithelial cells release an inhibitor of neovascularization. Arch Ophthalmol 103:1870-1875, 1985
13. The Diabetic Retinopathy Study Research Group: Preliminary report on the effects of photocoagulation therapy. Am J Ophthalmol 81:383-396, 1976
14. British Multicentre Study Group: Photocoagulation for proliferative diabetic retinopathy: a randomized controlled clinical trial using the xenon arc. Diabetologia 26:109-115, 1984
15. Hercules BL, Gayed II, Lucas SB, Jeacock J: Peripheral retinal ablation in the treatment of proliferative diabetic retinopathy: a three-year interim report of a randomized, controlled study using the argon laser. Br J Ophthalmol 61:555-563, 1977
16. The Diabetic Retinopathy Study Research Group: Photocoagulation treatment of proliferative diabetic retinopathy: the second report of Diabetic Retinopathy Study findings. Ophthalmology 85:82-106, 1978
17. The Diabetic Retinopathy Study Research Group: Photocoagulation treatment of proliferative diabetic retinopathy: clinical application of DRS findings. DRS Report No 8. Ophthalmology 88:583-600, 1981
18. Early Treatment Diabetic Retinopathy Study Research Group: Early photocoagulation for diabetic retinopathy. ETDRS Report No 9. Ophthalmology 98:766-785, 1991
19. Early Treatment Diabetic Retinopathy Study Research Group: Case reports to accompany Early Treatment Diabetic Retinopathy Study Reports 3 and 4. Int Ophthalmol Clin 27:273-333, 1987
20. Blankenship GW: A clinical comparison of central and peripheral argon laser panretinal photocoagulation for proliferative diabetic retinopathy. Ophthalmology 95:170-177, 1988
21. Rogell GD: Incremental panretinal photocoagulation: results in treating proliferative diabetic retinopathy. Retina 3:308-311, 1983
22. Meyer-Schwickerath G, Gerke E: Treatment of diabetic retinopathy with photocoagulation: results of photocoagulation therapy of proliferative retinopathy in childhood-onset and maturity-onset diabetes and an approach to the dosage in photocoagulation. Acta Ophthalmol 61:756-768, 1983
23. Bresnick CH, de Venecia G, Myers FL, Harris JA, Davis MD: Retinal ischemia in diabetic retinopathy. Arch Ophthalmol 93:1300-1310, 1975
24. Diabetic Retinopathy Study Research Group: Photocoagulation treatment of proliferative diabetic retinopathy: relationship of adverse treatment effects to retinopathy severity. DRS Report No 5. Dev Ophthalmol 2:248-261, 1981

EVALUATION AND MANAGEMENT OF DIABETIC MACULAR EDEMA

Matthew D. Davis

Department of Ophthalmology, University of Wisconsin-Madison, Madison, Wisconsin, USA

Evaluation

Definitions and natural course

As discussed on pp. 43-61, excessive permeability of the retinal vasculature is one of the pathophysiologic processes characteristic of diabetic retinopathy. Three clinical signs of this excessive permeability are:
1. leakage of fluorescein;
2. deposition of hard exudates; and
3. thickening of the retina.

These signs tend to occur together and, when the posterior pole is involved, have been called, loosely, "macular edema". The extent of capillary loss is also often taken into consideration when evaluating and classifying the macular abnormalities of diabetic retinopathy and three principal categories of "diabetic maculopathy" have been proposed: focal, cystoid (diffuse edema), and ischemic[1]. However, it has been difficult to develop precise definitions for these categories and for the intermediate categories required for cases that have features of two or more of them. Because of this problem and a paucity of data on the natural course of macular edema, no generally accepted classification has emerged. There is, however, general agreement on two principles. The first of these is that the term retinal edema should be reserved for actual thickening of the retina, and should not include fluorescein leakage without visible thickening. In this chapter, macular edema will be defined as retinal thickening within one disc diameter of the center of the macula. The second principle is that the most important clinical feature of macular edema is the degree to which the center of the macula is involved or threatened by retinal thickening or associated hard exudates.

Little detailed information has been published regarding the natural course of diabetic macular edema. Clinical impression suggests considerable variability. When hard exudates are part of the picture, they tend to increase gradually over periods of months to years and then to decrease, sometimes disappearing entirely. However, if a large plaque of hard exudate develops at the center of the macula, it may be converted to a permanent subretinal fibrous scar. Retinal thickening may also increase gradually over many months, and then decrease again. Long-standing macular edema is sometimes accompanied by fine pigment mottling in the macular area. Unfortunately, when the center of the macula has been thickened for many months the resultant impairment of visual acuity usually remains, even if thickening subsequently decreases or resolves.

Address for correspondence: Matthew D. Davis, MD, Department of Ophthalmology, University of Wisconsin-Madison, 610 N. Walnut Street, P.O. Box 5240, Madison, WI 53705, USA

Retina and Vitreous, pp. 93-100
Proceedings of the Symposium on Retina and Vitreous,
organized by the New Orleans Academy of Ophthalmology
New Orleans, LA, USA, March 12-15, 1992
edited by Rudolph M. Franklin

Ophthalmoscopy

Thickened retina usually retains normal or near-normal transparency and, thus, it is the increased thickness itself that must be recognized. Thickening should be suspected within a ring of hard exudates, but is not always present here, and may be present in the absence of hard exudates. Similarly, fluorescein leakage within the retina is suggestive of edema, but is often present in areas that do not appear thickened. Retinal thickening is not easy to perceive with either conventional direct or binocular indirect ophthalmoscopy, because of lack of stereopsis with the former method and insufficient magnification with the latter. Use of the slit-lamp and high plus precorneal lens is not much better, because stereoscopic effect and magnification are limited. When direct ophthalmoscopy is carried out through a widely dilated pupil thickening can be detected using monocular clues, *i.e.*, the shifting of relationships between superficial retinal structures and the retinal pigment epithelium (RPE) observed as these structures are viewed alternately through opposite sides of the pupil. This shifting increases proportionally with increasing retinal thickness and is quite apparent when thickness approaches or exceeds twice normal.

Photography

The most sensitive techniques for detecting subtle retinal thickening are slit-lamp examination with contact lens and examination of good quality 30° stereoscopic color fundus photographs with a viewer that provides at least 5× magnification. Thirty-degree photographs, particularly those taken with the standard Zeiss fundus camera using the technique of Allen, provide a substantially better stereoscopic effect than wider angle photographs, probably chiefly because of the greater magnification[2]. The Zeiss camera is superior because an acceptable stereoscopic effect can often be obtained through pupils as small as 4 or 5 mm, the maximum attainable in some patients with diabetic retinopathy. Retinal thickness often seems somewhat greater in stereoscopic fluorescein angiograms than in the corresponding color photographs, perhaps because the distance estimated in the angiogram is that between the superficial retinal vascular bed and the choriocapillaries, while in the color photographs it is the distance between vessels or abnormalities in the inner retina and the RPE. However, thickness at the center of the macula usually cannot be directly assessed in an angiogram, because retinal capillaries are usually absent here and the position of the inner retinal surface must be inferred from the position of the capillary network bordering the foveal avascular zone. In addition to the excellent stereoscopic assessment provided by photographs at any single visit, good quality stereophotographs also provide a record with unequalled accuracy for comparisons at future visits. However, changes in elevation between visits must be interpreted cautiously, because they may be due to differences in the amount the camera was moved between the left and right members of the stereopair at the two visits. The stereoseparator, which produces the same optical effect as lateral displacement of the camera by tilting a thick plate of glass suspended in front of the camera alternately to the left and right by a standard amount, reduces but does not eliminate this problem.

Slit-lamp and contact lens examination

The contact lens examination is best initiated by using the slit-lamp as a binocular ophthalmoscope, with a short broad illuminating beam set on the lowest intensity and positioned centrally, between the right and left optical systems. This illumination, combined with 10× or 16× magnification, provides large, sharp images with adequate magnification and excellent stereoscopic effect. Retinal thickness is perceived directly, assuming the examiner has normal stereopsis, and findings in a fairly large area are easily integrated in the examiner's mind. It is important to be able to guide the patient's fixation slowly and smoothly while observing the fundus, so that the whole posterior pole can be examined, and for this it is helpful to have the focusable Haag-Streit bull's eye fixation target that automatically retains its orientation towards the pupil of the patient's fellow eye as it is moved. As a second step, it is sometimes useful to study selected areas with a narrow, bright slit beam positioned to one side of the optical system, *i.e.*, to use the slit-lamp as a slit-lamp. Subtle degrees of thickening are sometimes more easily seen with this technique, but it is difficult to integrate many narrow images into a coherent overall impression. When fundus photography or angiography are to be carried out, this should be done before the contact lens examination, so that corneal clarity is unimpaired, and this may lead to problems with smooth patient flow through a busy clinic.

Management

Although clinical experience indicates that macular edema in patients with fluid retention and/or uncontrolled hypertension sometimes resolves dramatically with diuretics or other antihypertensive treatment, or sometimes spontaneously, such cases are infrequent and the principal treatment currently available for macular edema is photocoagulation. Two techniques have been used, direct ("focal") treatment to occlude leaking microaneurysms or other sources of focal leakage and indirect ("grid") treatment, which aims to reduce diffuse leakage by mechanisms that are not well understood. Theoretical rationales proposed for indirect treatment are modification of fluid transit across the RPE and improvement of retinal capillary function. Suggested mechanisms by which capillary function might be improved include (1) relief of inner retinal hypoxia by increased diffusion of oxygen from the choriocapillaries following destruction of some of the metabolically highly active photoreceptors; and (2) facilitation of endothelial cell renewal, mediated perhaps by growth factors reaching the capillaries via the altered RPE[3-11].

Early Treatment Diabetic Retinopathy Study

The most complete information on photocoagulation treatment of macular edema comes from the Early Treatment Diabetic Retinopathy Study (ETDRS), a randomized clinical trial sponsored by the National Eye Institute. In this study patients with mild to severe non-proliferative or early (non-high-risk) proliferative retinopathy with or without macular edema were randomly assigned to aspirin (650 mg per day) or placebo. One eye of each patient was randomly assigned to early photocoagulation with one of four combinations of focal/grid and/or scatter (panretinal) photocoagulation, using a blue-green or green only argon laser, and the other eye was assigned to deferral of photocoagulation. Patients were followed at frequent intervals, with photocoagulation to be carried out in the eye assigned to deferral only if high-risk proliferative retinopathy developed[12].

In eyes with macular edema, focal and diffuse leakage and capillary loss were identified by stereoscopic fluorescein angiography. Lesions thought to be contributing to retinal thickening and/or hard exudates were treated if between 500 and 3000 µm from the center of the macula. Treatment 300-500 µm from center was optional initially, but was required during follow-up for focal leaks, if thickening persisted after other lesions had been treated, visual acuity was 20/40 or worse, and the treating ophthalmologist did not believe that such treatment would destroy the remaining perifoveal capillary network. The principal lesions treated focally were microaneurysms, usually using 50 µm, 0.1 second burns. The endpoint aimed for was a color change in the microaneurysm, if it was 40 µm or more in diameter, or whitening of adjacent retina, if it was smaller (Fig. 1). Grid treatment was applied to thickened areas with diffuse leakage or capillary loss, usually

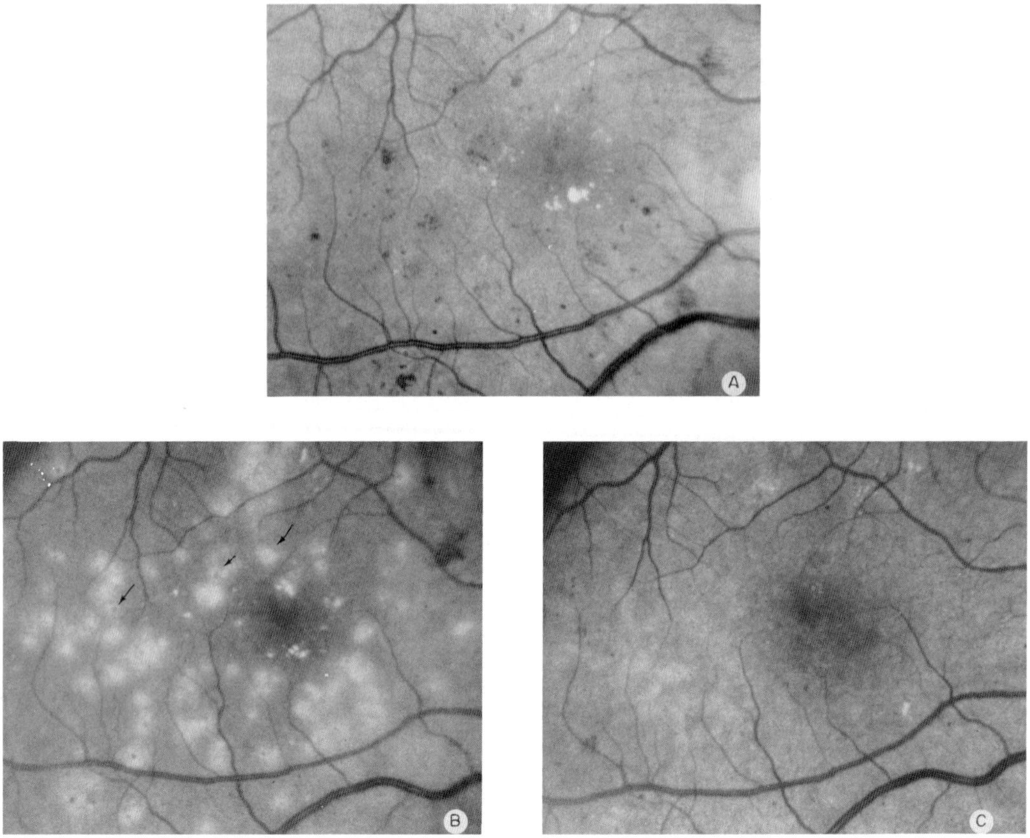

Fig. 1A. Microaneurysms are scattered throughout the posterior pole of this right eye. There is a faint hard exudate ring surrounding the center of the macula and perhaps another fainter one above the first. Although not visible in this non-stereoscopic photograph, the retina was mildly thickened throughout the area within 1.5 disc diameters of the center of the macula, including the center itself. Visual acuity was 20/25. *B.* The same eye shortly after focal photocoagulation. Arrows indicate some of the treated microaneurysms that have had their color changed by treatment (turned brown or white). *C.* One year later the retina was no longer thickened and most of the microaneurysms and hard exudates had disappeared. Photocoagulation scars were faint. Visual acuity remained at 20/25. (Courtesy of the ETDRS Research Group.)

using mild 50 to 100 μm burns placed one burn diameter apart (Fig. 2). The need for follow-up treatment was assessed at four-month intervals; re-treatment was to be carried out if retinal thickening involved or threatened the center of the macula and treatable lesions were present. Focal and grid treatment were not compared with each other, but were used singly or in combination as was considered appropriate for each eye assigned to early treatment. Many eyes received focal treatment only, some eyes a combination of focal and grid treatment, and very few eyes grid treatment alone.

In one group of ETDRS eyes, which had mild to moderate non-proliferative retinopathy and macular edema, early photocoagulation was limited initially to focal/grid treatment for macular edema (scatter treatment was withheld unless severe non-proliferative or early proliferative retinopathy developed). Comparisons between all eyes assigned to this treatment group and a control group consisting of all similar eyes assigned to deferral of photocoagulation provided the only assessment in the ETDRS of focal/grid treatment without concurrent or antecedent scatter treatment[13,14]. The principal outcome measure

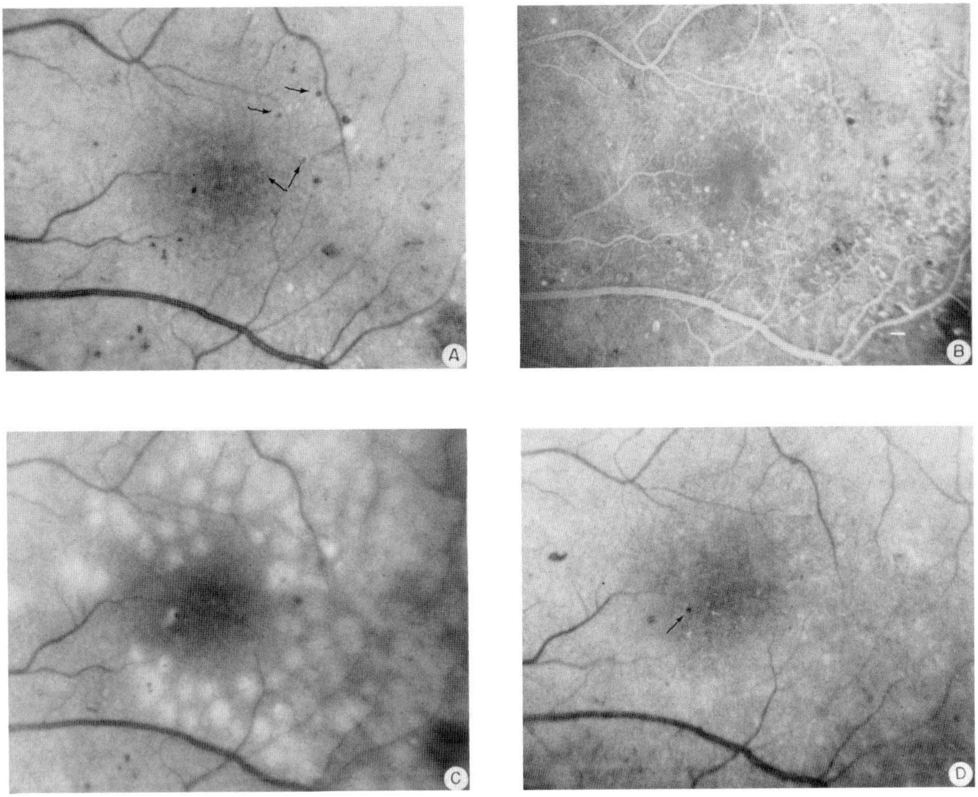

Fig. 2A. Microaneurysms and hard exudates in the posterior pole. Although not visible in this non-stereoscopic photograph, the retina was thickened at the center of the macula and temporally for about two disc diameters. Arrows indicate fairly large microaneurysms with visible walls. Visual acuity was 20/40. *B.* Early-phase fluorescein angiogram showing many dilated capillaries and early diffuse leakage. *C.* Because most of the leakage came from dilated capillaries, photocoagulation was applied mainly in a grid pattern (but three of the four microaneurysms indicated by arrows in part A of the figure were treated focally, all but the one closest to the center of the macula). *D.* Four months later most of the microaneurysms and hard exudates had disappeared. The retina was no longer thickened. Photocoagulation scars were inconspicuous. Arrow indicates moderately large microaneurysm that was incompletely treated focally and remains patent. Visual acuity had improved to 20/25. (Courtesy of the ETDRS Research Group.)

Table 1. Macular edema as defined in the Early Treatment Diabetic Retinopathy Study (in order of increasing severity) (From: Early Treatment Diabetic Retinopathy Study Research Group: Photocoagulation for diabetic macular edema: ETDRS Report No 4. Int Ophthalmol Clin 27:265-272, 1987. Courtesy of the ETDRS Research Group.)

Not clinically significant	
1.	Hard exudate ≥ Standard Photograph No. 3 within Field 2, some of which is within one disc diameter of the center of the macula (without retinal thickening)
2.	Retinal thickening within Field 2, but not fulfilling criteria for "clinically significant"
Clinically significant	
1.	An area of retinal thickening at least one disc area in size, some of which is within one disc diameter of the center of the macula
2.	Retinal thickening (or hard exudate adjacent to thickened retina) present within 500 μm of the center of the macula, but not involving the center
3.	Center of macula involved by retinal thickening (or hard exudate adjacent to thickened retina)

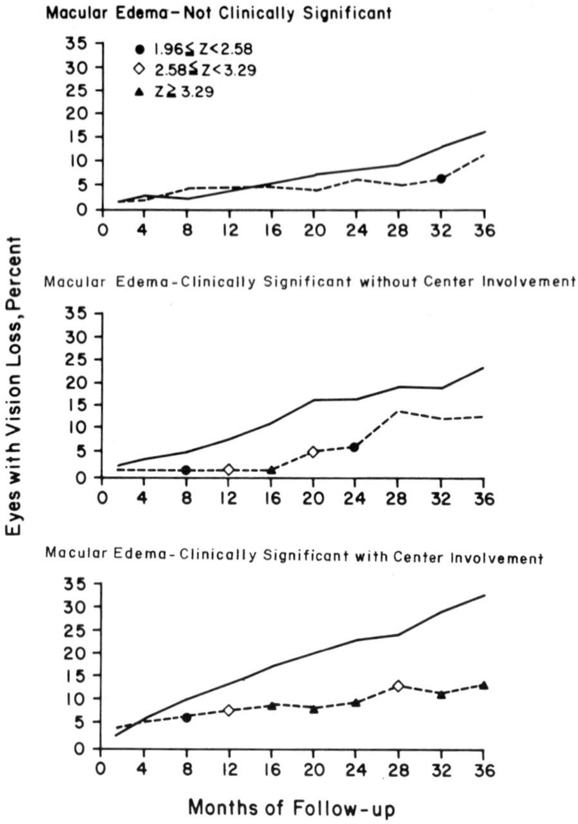

Fig. 3. Comparison of percentages of eyes that experienced visual loss of three or more lines (equivalent to at least doubling of the visual angle) in eyes classified by severity of macular edema in baseline fundus photographs and assigned either to immediate focal/grid photocoagulation for macular edema (broken line) or to deferral of photocoagulation unless high-risk characteristics developed (solid line). (From: Early Treatment Diabetic Retinopathy Study Research Group: Photocoagulation for diabetic macular edema: ETDRS Report No 4. Int Ophthalmol Clin 27:265-272, 1987. Courtesy of the ETDRS Research Group.)

for this comparison was moderate visual loss, defined as a decrease of three or more lines on a specially designed eye chart, on which a three-line decrease in any part of the chart amounts to a doubling of the visual angle, for example, a change from 20/20 to 20/40, or from 20/50 to 20/100. After three years of follow-up, 24% of 526 control group eyes had experienced moderate visual loss, compared with 12% of 268 treated eyes. Among eyes entering the study with visual acuity of worse than 20/40, about 40% of treated eyes showed improvement of one line or more, compared with 20% of control group eyes, but few eyes in either group improved by as much as three lines. No adverse effects of focal/grid photocoagulation on visual acuity, visual field, or color vision were detected.

Fig. 3 shows the percentages of treated and control group eyes with moderate visual loss at each follow-up visit for three subgroups of the group discussed above, defined by severity of macular edema in baseline stereoscopic fundus photographs. In the mildest subgroup (upper panel), eyes with macular edema which was not clinically significant (see Table 1), there was little difference between treated and control groups until after 24 months, when presumably some eyes had developed clinically significant macular edema, but in the other two subgroups treatment reduced the rate of moderate visual loss by more than 50% at most visits. The risk of visual loss in untreated eyes was greater when the center of the macula was involved (lower panel). Prompt photocoagulation is usually indicated for such eyes. When the center is threatened, but not involved, visual acuity is usually good. Either prompt treatment or deferral of treatment with careful follow-up is appropriate for such eyes.

Application of ETDRS results to clinical practice

In applying the ETDRS results summarized above it is important to emphasize that the ETDRS comparison was, essentially, one between focal/grid treatment applied at Study entry *versus* no such treatment ever. In clinical practice, the choice is between prompt treatment *versus* deferral of this decision until the next follow-up visit. Because progression is usually slow, and because the patient can help monitor for unexpected worsening by checking his/her vision regularly between scheduled follow-up visits, initiation of treatment is never urgent.

Because the principal benefit of treatment is to prevent further decrease in visual acuity, treatment should be considered even in eyes with normal visual acuity, if clinically significant macular edema is present. Factors favoring prompt treatment are summarized in Table 2. The most important consideration is the degree to which the center of the macula is involved or threatened. When the center is obviously thickened visual acuity is usually reduced and there is little reason to delay treatment. If hard exudates along the posterior edge of a zone of thickening are close to the center of the macula and threaten to extend into it, prompt treatment may be the safer alternative, even if visual acuity is normal, particularly if the principal leaks are large microaneurysms located far from the center. Such leaks are easily closed with little risk. If the center is not threatened by hard exudate and thickening here is slight or equivocal, there is little to lose from deferral, particularly if there has been little or no decrease in visual acuity.

Table 2. Factors favoring prompt photocoagulation for diabetic macular edema

- Center of macula thickened or threatened by adjacent thickening or hard exudate
- Principal sources of leakage far (> 500-700 μm) from center
- Treatable aggravating factors absent (hypertension, fluid retention)
- Complicating factors anticipated soon (scatter photocoagulation, cataract extraction, renal failure)

The location of the principal sources of leakage and the ease with which they can be identified and treated are important, because treatment near the center carries greater risks of an inadvertent burn at the center, late expansion of a perifoveal scar into the center, and annoying paracentral scotomas.

Diabetic patients who are retaining fluid because of hypertension, pregnancy, or other systemic factors sometimes develop extensive macular edema, often without prominent focal leaks. In such cases edema may resolve after treatment with diuretics or other antihypertensive medications (or sometimes spontaneously), and deferral of photocoagulation for several weeks while such treatment is undertaken is usually desirable. Macular edema sometimes worsens following scatter photocoagulation, cataract extraction (particularly if intracapsular), or the onset of renal failure. The likelihood that any of these aggravating factors will occur in the near future provides additional justification for initiating focal/grid treatment.

In eyes with edema involving or imminently threatening the center of the macula that also need scatter treatment for retinopathy at or approaching the high-risk stage, ETDRS results and the observations of other investigators suggest that it may be preferable to do focal/grid photocoagulation first or to combine focal/grid treatment with the first episode of scatter, placed in the nasal quadrants[15-19]. However, other investigators have observed occasional improvement in extensive macular edema following scatter photocoagulation which was applied in a pattern that spared the retina within four disc diameters of the center of the macula[20,21]. This may be an attractive alternative for eyes with markedly thickened retina involving much of the posterior pole, diffuse fluorescein leakage, and poor visual acuity.

Although ETDRS conclusions regarding the value of focal/grid treatment are based mainly on eyes with mild to moderate non-proliferative retinopathy, it seems reasonable to extend them to eyes with more severe retinopathy, with or without prior scatter photocoagulation.

References

1. Whitelock RAF, Kearns M, Blach RK, Hamilton AM: The diabetic maculopathies. Trans Ophthalmol Soc UK 99:314-320, 1979
2. Allen L: Ocular fundus photography. Am J Ophthalmol 57:13-28, 1964
3. Patz A, Schatz H, Berkow JW et al: Macular edema: an overlooked complication of diabetic retinopathy. Trans Am Acad Ophthalmol Otolaryngol 77:34-42, 1973
4. Schatz H, Patz A: Cystoid maculopathy in diabetes. Arch Ophthalmol 94:761-768, 1976
5. Peyman GA, Bok D: Peroxidase diffusion in the normal and laser-photocoagulated primate retina. Invest Ophthalmol 11:35-45, 1972
6. Wallow IH: Repair of the pigment epithelial barrier following photocoagulation. Arch Ophthalmol 102:126-135, 1984
7. Wolbarsht ML, Landers MB: The rationale of photocoagulation therapy for proliferative diabetic retinopathy: a review and a model. Ophthalmic Surg 11:235-245, 1980
8. Weiter JJ, Zuckerman R: The influence of the photoreceptor-RPE complex on the inner retina; an explanation for the beneficial effects of photocoagulation. Ophthalmology 87:1133-1139, 1980
9. Marshall J, Clover G, Rothery S: Some new findings on retinal irradiation by krypton and argon lasers. Doc Ophthalmol 36:21-27, 1984
10. Bresnick GH: Diabetic retinopathy; a clinical review highlighting diffuse macular edema. Ophthalmology 90:1301-1317, 1983
11. Bresnick GH: Diabetic macular edema. Ophthalmology 93:989-997, 1986
12. Early Treatment Diabetic Retinopathy Study Research Group: Early Treatment Diabetic Retinopathy Study design and baseline patient characteristics. ETDRS Report No 7. Ophthalmology 98:741-756, 1991
13. Early Treatment Diabetic Retinopathy Study Research Group: Photocoagulation for diabetic macular edema. ETDRS Report No 1. Arch Ophthalmol 103:1796-1806, 1985
14. Early Treatment Diabetic Retinopathy Study Research Group: Photocoagulation for diabetic macular edema: ETDRS Report No 4. Int Ophthalmol Clin 27:265-272, 1987
15. Early Treatment Diabetic Retinopathy Study Research Group: Early photocoagulation for diabetic retinopathy. ETDRS Report No 9. Ophthalmology 98:766-785, 1991
16. Meyers SM: Macular edema after scatter laser photocoagulation for proliferative diabetic retinopathy. Am J Ophthalmol 90:210-216, 1980
17. McDonald HR, Schatz H: Visual loss following panretinal photocoagulation for proliferative diabetic retinopathy. Ophthalmology 92:388-393, 1985
18. McDonald HR, Schatz H: Macular edema following panretinal photocoagulation. Retina 5:5-10, 1985
19. Ferris FL III, Podgor MJ, Davis MD, and Diabetic Retinopathy Study Research Group: Macular edema in Diabetic Retinopathy Study patients: DRS Report No 12. Ophthalmology 94:754-760, 1987
20. Gardner TW, Eller AW, Friberg TR: Reduction of severe macular edema in eyes with poor vision after panretinal photocoagulation for proliferative diabetic retinopathy. Graefe's Arch Clin Exp Ophthalmol 229:323-328, 1991
21. Blankenship GW: A clinical comparison of central and peripheral argon laser panretinal photocoagulation for proliferative diabetic retinopathy. Ophthalmology 95:170-177, 1988

DISSECTION METHODS IN VITRECTOMY FOR DIABETIC RETINOPATHY

Gary W. Abrams

Associated Retinal Consultants, Royal Oak, Michigan, Eye Research Institute, Oakland University, Rochester, Michigan, USA

Abstract

The major pathoanatomical variants found during vitrectomy for diabetic retinopathy are focal or broad vitreoretinal adhesions associated with vascular epicenters which may be located in the posterior pole or peripheral retina. The posterior hyaloid may be separated from the retina except at vascular epicenters or remain mostly unseparated from the retina. In addition, the posterior hyaloid can sometimes split, giving the appearance of posterior vitreous separation, but leaving cortical vitreous adherent to the retina. The indications for surgery are reviewed, and an approach to surgery for diabetic retinopathy is presented in which separation of the posterior hyaloid and its associated membranes is emphasized.

Introduction

The pathoanatomy of retinal detachment due to diabetic retinopathy can be quite complicated. Various dissection methods have been developed for use during vitrectomy for diabetic retinopathy[1-5]. The major goal of all of the methods of vitrectomy is to relieve vitreoretinal traction. Because of the complexity of the vitreoretinal pathoanatomy, however, it is sometimes difficult to accomplish that goal. Most descriptions of vitrectomy for diabetic retinopathy have emphasized membrane cutting or separation techniques such as those used in membrane sectioning and membrane delamination, respectively. When accomplished, these valuable techniques will usually accomplish the goal of relieving vitreoretinal traction. The major problems encountered by most vitreoretinal surgeons are in obtaining access to the membranes and adequately sectioning or separating the membranes from the retina without causing severe retinal damage. The vitrectomy procedure can be simplified even in complex cases by focusing on separating the posterior hyaloid from the retina. In this paper I will describe the major variations in the pathoanatomy of diabetic retinopathy and a surgical approach emphasizing separation of the posterior hyaloid and its associated vitreoretinal membranes.

This material was presented at the Third International Congress on Vitreoretinal Surgery, Rome, 1991, and published as part of *Advances in Vitreoretinal Surgery*, Mario Stirpe, Editor, The Ophthalmic Communications Society, Publisher, pp 98-104

Address for correspondence: Gary W. Abrams, MD, 632 Wm Beaumont Medical Building, 3535 West Thirteen Mile Road, Royal Oak, MI 48072, USA

Retina and Vitreous, pp. 101-113
Proceedings of the Symposium on Retina and Vitreous,
organized by the New Orleans Academy of Ophthalmology
New Orleans, LA, USA, March 12-15, 1992
edited by Rudolph M. Franklin

Pathophysiology

The pathophysiologic processes leading to vitreoretinal traction, hemorrhage, and retinal detachment have been described elsewhere[6,7]. Briefly, fibrovascular proliferation originates from the major blood vessels of the optic disc and the retina. This fibrovascular proliferation grows in the potential space between the retina and the posterior hyaloid. Contraction of the vitreous caused by the fibrovascular membranes exerts retinal traction at areas where the vitreous is firmly adherent to the retina. Firm adherence is found at the vitreous base and at the areas of fibrovascular proliferation at so-called "epicenters". Vascular epicenters are areas of vitreoretinal adhesion caused by adherence of vitreous to new blood vessels and associated fibrous tissue. Each epicenter was originally supplied by a single feeder vessel which has grown from a retinal blood vessel. The intensity of vitreous contraction, the degree of vitreous separation, the configuration and number of vitreoretinal adhesions at epicenters, the amount of fibrosis, and the presence of retinal breaks will determine the pathoanatomy of the eye for vitrectomy. In addition, vitreous hemorrhage will influence the preoperative and intraoperative ability to analyze the pathoanatomy.

Surgical indications

Vitreous hemorrhage is a relative indication for vitrectomy. Many vitreous hemorrhages clear with time, and may never recur. The Diabetic Retinopathy Vitrectomy Study (DRVS) randomized patients with acute vitreous hemorrhages which reduced the visual acuity to 5/200 or worse for at least one month to early vitrectomy *versus* deferral of vitrectomy one year[8]. Eyes randomized to delayed vitrectomy in which the hemorrhage subsequently cleared did not undergo surgery, and eyes which developed retinal detachment were operated upon when the macula became detached. With 24 months' follow-up, 25% of early vitrectomy *versus* 15% of control eyes had visual acuities of 10/20 or better (p=0.01). However, among a subgroup of patients with type I diabetes who had onset of diabetes at or before 20 years of age and were taking insulin at randomization, 36% of eyes undergoing early vitrectomy regained 10/20 or better visual acuity compared to 12% of those in the deferral group (p=0.0001). The benefit of surgery was even greater in type I diabetics who had a duration of diabetes <20 years at randomization. There was no difference in the percentage of eyes with a poor visual outcome. This benefit of surgery was not significant in patients with onset of diabetes after the age of 20 years, regardless of insulin therapy. The treatment benefit of early vitrectomy may have been a result of more active, progressive fibrovascular proliferation and traction in the younger patient group with a shorter duration of diabetes.

Within the guidelines of the DRVS, a period of observation (several weeks) is reasonable for most eyes with vitreous hemorrhage because sometimes even a dense hemorrhage will clear rapidly enough to allow laser photocoagulation. Ultrasound examination should be done to rule out retinal detachment when the patient with a vitreous hemorrhage is first examined, and if the hemorrhage does not clear enough to allow visualization of the retina, ultrasound examination should be repeated at intervals of four to six weeks. If progressive retinal detachment is found, then early surgery is indicated in most cases. If the patient has bilateral non-clearing vitreous hemorrhages, or if the patient is monocular, earlier surgery may be indicated to allow earlier visual rehabilitation regardless of the patient's age or duration of diabetes.

The major indication for vitrectomy in eyes with diabetic retinopathy is retinal detachment involving the macula[9]. Eyes with recent loss of vision due to retinal detachment involving the macula should be considered for vitrectomy. Surgery should be performed as soon as possible after the onset of macular detachment[10]. However, in eyes with long-standing macular detachment, it is unlikely that vision will improve following surgery, so surgery may not be indicated.

Fibrovascular proliferation in the posterior pole may exert traction which distorts the macula, reducing visual acuity or causing severe metamorphopsia[11]. A common finding is traction retinal detachment nasal to the optic disc with the macula, although not detached, displaced nasally towards the disc. Eyes with documented progressive visual loss due to this type of traction may benefit from surgery.

Extramacular traction retinal detachments with no macular traction may remain stable for long periods of time and so should be observed for progression in most cases[12]. If the macula is threatened by progression of the retinal detachment, surgery while the macula is still attached may be indicated. Progressive traction-rhegmatogenous retinal detachments may threaten to detach the macula, and are candidates for surgery at an earlier stage than similar pure traction retinal detachments. In most cases with the macula still attached, the decision for surgery should include consideration of the difficulty of surgery. Eyes with multiple, wide-spread vitreoretinal adhesions, broad adhesions, chronic traction retinal detachment, and peripheral vitreoretinal adhesions are usually more difficult cases and surgery may reasonably be deferred until visual acuity is affected by the retinal detachment. Other considerations are the health of the patient and the status of the other eye. Patients at high risk for morbidity due to surgery, and patients who had a poor result following surgery in the opposite eye, might best delay surgery until visual acuity is decreased by the retinal detachment. These patients should be followed closely for progression, and instructed to notify the ophthalmologist immediately if progression is noted.

The DRVS showed a benefit of early vitrectomy in eyes with visual acuity at 10/200 or better and severe, active fibrovascular proliferative diabetic retinopathy without retinal detachment involving the macula[13]. Such eyes were randomized to vitrectomy *versus* conventional management (delay of vitrectomy until vision is decreased due to macular retinal detachment or severe vitreous hemorrhage). After four years, 44% of eyes which had early vitrectomy had visual acuity of 10/20 or better *versus* 28% of eyes managed conventionally ($p<0.05$). There was no difference in the percentage of eyes with a poor visual result and the percentage with no light perception. The greatest treatment effect was obtained in eyes with the most severe proliferation, while there was little difference in eyes with the mildest proliferation. While the DRVS included eyes with active retinopathy which had no previous laser treatment, previous studies have shown a major benefit of laser treatment for such eyes. Therefore, it is prudent to use laser as the initial form of therapy if possible in eyes with active retinopathy. In addition, only eyes with moderately severe retinopathy as defined by the study should be considered for early vitrectomy[13,14]. Active retinopathy is required as a criterium for vitrectomy, and eyes with atrophic, primarily inactive retinopathy are usually not candidates for vitrectomy without previously mentioned complications such as macular retinal detachment or traction producing visual loss.

Premacular hemorrhage has been advocated as an indication for early vitrectomy[15]. These eyes may develop fibrosis and traction detachment. Many of these eyes will show resolution of neovascularization and hemorrhage with laser treatment. However, these eyes should be followed closely and vitrectomy may be beneficial if fibrosis is associated with continued dense premacular hemorrhage.

A small subset of patients with macular edema associated with a retracting, taut posterior cortical vitreous may benefit from vitrectomy[16]. These patients have usually had previous laser treatment, and the retraction of the cortical vitreous is usually associated with neovascularization. There is little or no posterior vitreous separation. There may or may not be cystoid spaces associated with the macular edema. Some of the reported patients demonstrated diffuse deep leakage on fluorescein angiography, while others had primarily perifoveal capillary leakage. The posterior hyaloid was thickened and exerted traction on the macula. During surgery, the posterior hyaloid was separated from the posterior pole.

Vitrectomy

The vitrectomy method involves many of the principles of "en bloc" dissection (Fig. 1)[4]. In general, the method entails separation of the posterior hyaloid from the retina and exposure of areas of vitreoretinal adhesion at vascular epicenters which are severed with scissors. In addition, identification and removal of associated epiretinal membranes and treatment of retinal breaks and retinal detachment is required.

Basic instruments needed for membrane dissection are a vitreous cutting instrument and horizontally cutting vitreoretinal scissors. Illuminated picks are very useful in com-

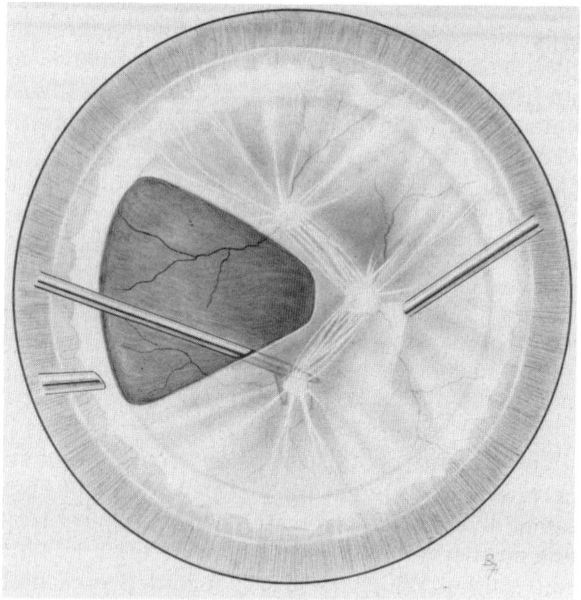

Fig. 1A.

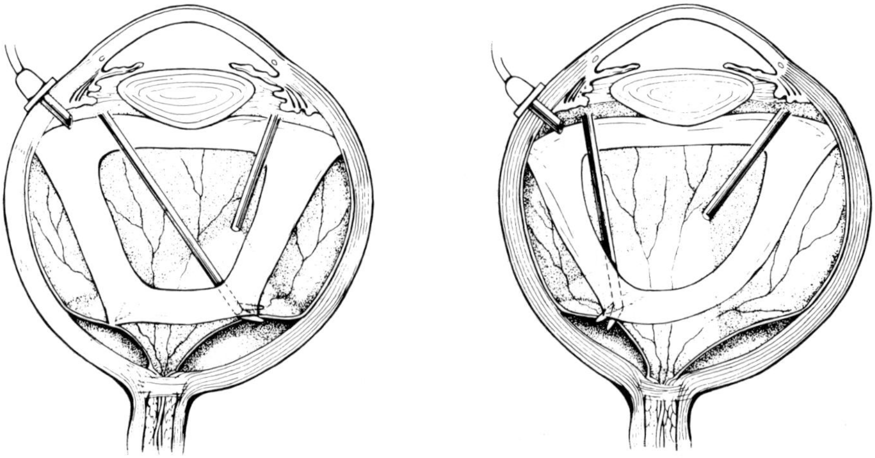

Fig. 1B.

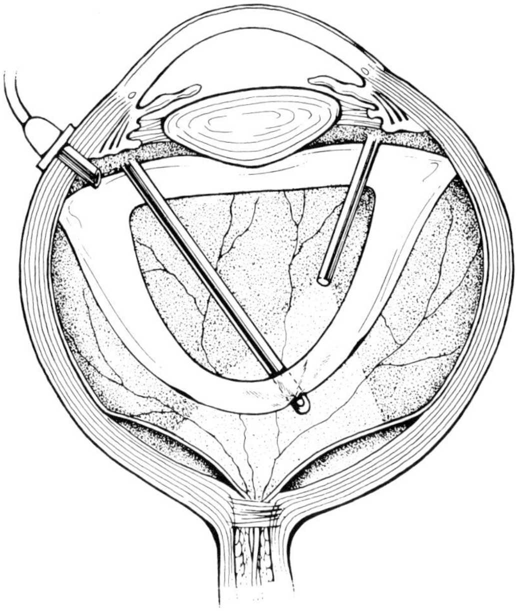

Fig. 1C.

Fig. 1. Basic en bloc dissection technique. *A.* Opening is made in posterior hyaloid adjacent to vascular epicenters. *B.* Focal adhesions are cut parallel to retinal surface. *C.* Posterior hyaloid and membranes removed with vitreous cutting instrument. (From: Abrams GW, Williams GA: "En bloc" excision of diabetic membranes. Am J Ophthalmol 103:302-308, 1987. Published with permission from the American Journal of Ophthalmology. Copyright: Ophthalmic Publishing Company.)

plex cases[17]. In addition, other instruments, such as the fiberoptic tissue manipulator[5], illuminated scissors, and illuminated and non-illuminated vitreoretinal forceps may be useful in some cases.

General vitrectomy principles

Regardless of the pathoanatomy of the vitreous and the retina, following limited vitrectomy, the first surgical maneuver is to make an opening in the posterior hyaloid in order to gain access to the vascular epicenters. If there is complete posterior vitreous separation, then the whole procedure is performed with the vitreous cutter. After opening the posterior hyaloid, blood is often seen covering the posterior pole. Following removal of the blood with a suction or extrusion needle, visualization improves as more light is reflected from the posterior fundus. In the presence of posterior vitreoretinal adhesions, a wide opening is made in the posterior hyaloid, usually temporally, and is then extended posteriorly adjacent to the areas of vitreoretinal adhesion and out to the temporal periphery posterior to the sclerotomy site (Fig. 1A). A wide opening allows better visualization of the epicenters of adhesion, and excising vitreous posterior to the temporal sclerotomy site reduces the likelihood of a peripheral break forming where multiple instruments are passed through the sclerotomy site. In some cases there is no separation of the vitreous from the retina outside the posterior pole (Fig. 2A). An opening should be made in the hyaloid where it is separated from the retina. Sometimes the only area of vitreoretinal separation may be over a preretinal hemorrhage. In other cases, a small area of separation may be found over the posterior pole adjacent to an area of contracted membrane. Some area of vitreoretinal separation is found in virtually every case. The opening is made with a sharp, pointed blade such as the MVR blade. Then a membrane pick or the tip of the closed horizontally cutting vitreoretinal scissors is used to separate the surrounding posterior hyaloid from the retina. The hyaloid can usually be bluntly stripped from the retina, while vascular epicenters usually should be cut. Some immature vascular epicenters can be easily stripped from the retina, but most mature vascular epicenters have fibrous proliferative tissue, causing adherence of the vitreous to the retina and the retina may tear

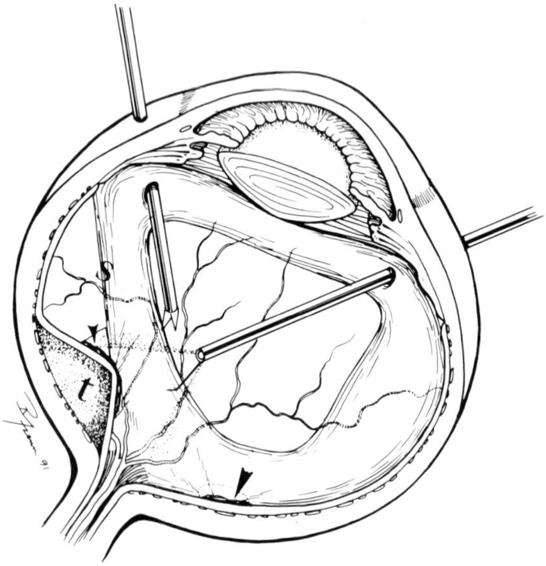

Fig. 2A. Pathoanatomy of complex traction retinal detachment following limited vitrectomy in preparation for *en bloc* dissection. t: traction retinal detachment; S: partially separated posterior hyaloid; small arrow: epiretinal membranes surrounding vascular epicenter; large arrow: flat vascular epicenter with no associated posterior vitreous separation.

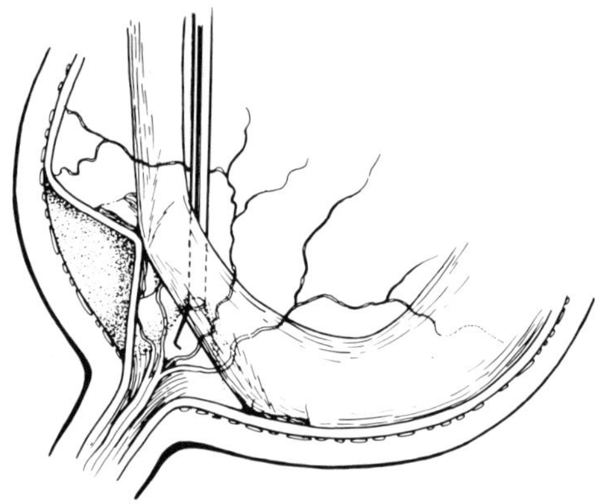

Fig. 2B. Posterior hyaloid bluntly separated from posterior pole and optic disc exposing vascular epicenters of vitreoretinal adhesion. Either pick or closed scissors can be used for stripping hyaloid from retina.

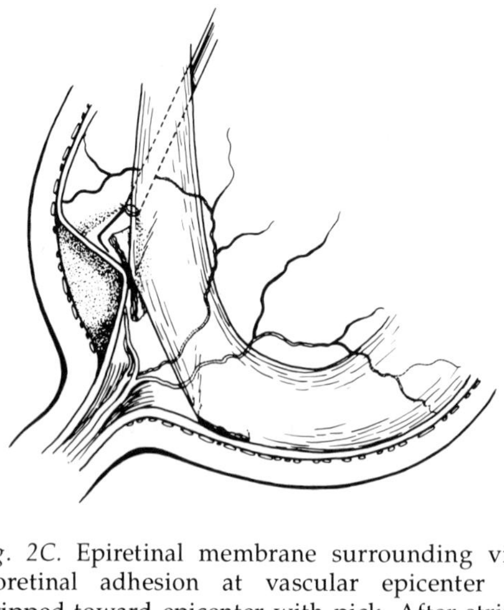

Fig. 2C. Epiretinal membrane surrounding vitreoretinal adhesion at vascular epicenter is stripped toward epicenter with pick. After stripping membrane towards epicenter, only a focal adhesion remains.

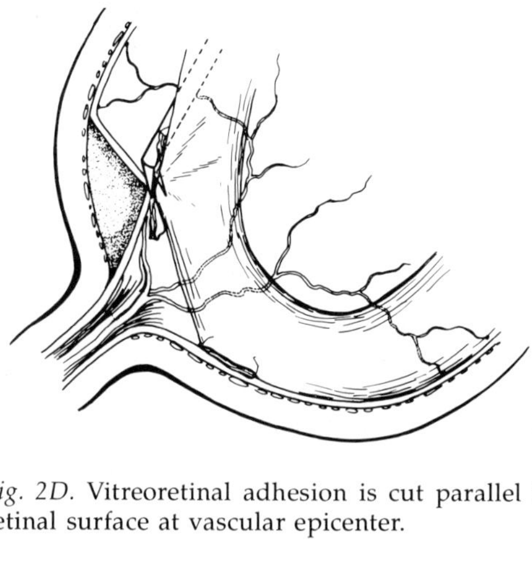

Fig. 2D. Vitreoretinal adhesion is cut parallel to retinal surface at vascular epicenter.

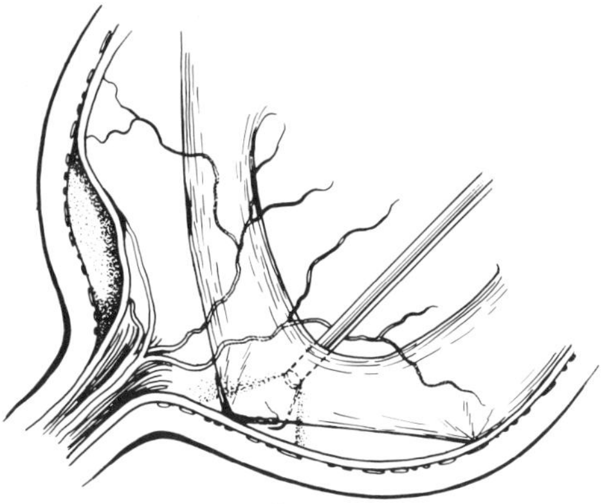

Fig. 2E. Hyaloid and membranes around epicenter on undetached retina are separated with either pick or closed scissors.

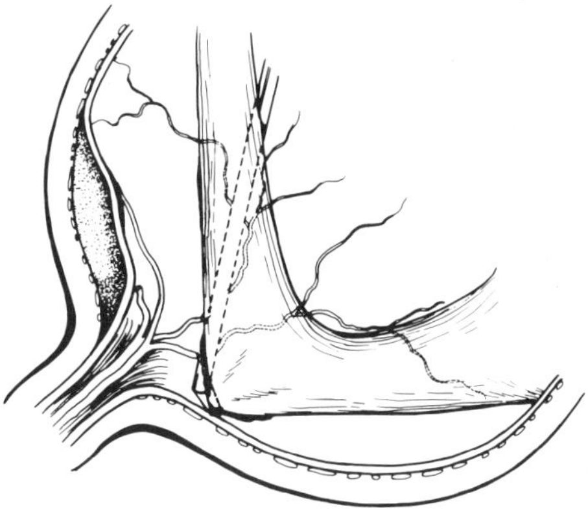

Fig. 2F. Final focal vitreoretinal adhesion is cut. Vitreous and membranes will now be removed with vitreous cutter.

before the fibrous tissue will strip free from the retina; therefore, the adhesion must be cut with scissors. An exception is a fibrovascular membrane adherent to the optic nerve head. Even fibrous membranes which are tightly adherent to the retina will usually strip away from the optic nerve head without complication (Fig. 2B). Minor bleeding is usually easily controlled by raising the intraocular pressure for one to two minutes. A vascularized membrane with both large and small blood vessels without white collagen is indicative of a relatively immature fibrovascular process. The underlying retina is usually relatively healthy and is less likely to tear with traction on the membrane. Because the collagen is not mature, the membrane is often not extremely adherent to the retina and will strip away. On the other hand, a membrane that has less small vessels and has white collagen is indicative of a more chronic, mature process. The retina is often thin beneath and adjacent to the membrane due to chronic traction and is more likely to tear when traction is applied to the membrane. Detached retina in areas of vascular occlusion becomes thin and atrophic and also tears easily.

While it is often advantageous to leave most of the posterior hyaloid intact during dissection, it is best to work adjacent to the opening in the hyaloid rather than reaching far beneath the hyaloid. Therefore, as membranes are separated and vascular epicenters are cut, the opening in the hyaloid is opened wider with scissors or the vitreous cutter to allow access to other areas of adhesion. Following separation of the posterior hyaloid and the membranes from the retina, vitreous is cut back toward the vitreous base 360°. Scleral depression is used during peripheral vitrectomy only if peripheral vitreous adhesions and traction are found.

Surgical method for various common pathoanatomical variants of diabetic retinopathy

Focal vitreoretinal adhesions

With a focal vitreoretinal adhesion, when the vitreous is otherwise separated, it may be adequate to do a vitrectomy and "circumcise" the vitreous around the adhesion. However, some apparently focal adhesions on closer inspection may be broader than expected. There is often an associated epiretinal membrane surrounding the area of vitreoretinal adhesion (Fig. 2A) The origin of the surrounding epiretinal membrane is not clear. The membrane may indicate that the blood vessels at the epicenter invaded lamellar cortical vitreous, and when traction was applied to the epicenter leading to tractional retinal elevation, there was incomplete posterior vitreous separation surrounding the epicenter. The epiretinal membrane may represent residual lamellae of cortical vitreous with associated epiretinal fibrosis. Alternatively, the membrane may simply represent fibrous epiretinal proliferation around the epicenter. Sometimes retinal folds can be hidden by the epiretinal membrane. If no epiretinal membrane is present, then the adhesion between vitreous and retina at the epicenter is easily visualized and cut (Fig. 1B). If an epiretinal membrane is present, sometimes the best access to the vascular epicenter of the membrane is obtained by stripping the epiretinal membrane towards the center of the adhesion (Fig. 2C). After the membrane is stripped, the vascular epicenter, which can now be easily seen, is cut with horizontally cutting vitreoretinal scissors (Fig. 2D).

With multiple focal points of adhesion with separated hyaloid between these epicenters, the method is similar to that described for a single focal adhesion, and each is cut sequentially.

If there is no posterior vitreous separation, focal points of adhesion are identified as the vitreous is separated from the retina (Fig. 2E). If an adhesion is noted, vitreous surrounding the adhesion should be bluntly separated as widely as possible. The adhesion can then be seen and removed in the same manner as in an eye with partial posterior vitreous separation (Fig. 2F).

Broad vitreoretinal adhesions

Broad vitreoretinal adhesions are of two types. The first type is a broad, fibrous plaque-like adhesion in which the thickened fibrous hyaloid is tightly adherent to unfolded underlying retina (Fig. 3). The second type of broad adhesion is formed by multiple, adjacent focal adhesions in which the hyaloid between the epicenters has contracted to bring the epicenters together (Fig. 4). The retina is thrown into folds between the epicenters.

In the former broad, plaque-like adhesion, the posterior hyaloid is adherent to the retina by many fine adhesions. When the membrane is mature (composed of white collagenous tissue), it will not strip away from the retina although it may strip free in the immature state. This type of membrane and associated hyaloid is best lifted with an illuminated pick and each individual small adhesion cut with horizontally cutting scissors (Fig. 3). Alternatively, the membrane can be elevated with a fiberoptic tissue manipulator or illuminated forceps to facilitate cutting it free. The disadvantage of all of the above methods is that the light may be difficult to direct on the adhesions for cutting. Illuminated scissors give excellent illumination at the point to be cut.

A broad vitreoretinal adhesion with multiple focal vitreoretinal adhesions with retinal folds between the adhesions is approached similarly to the approach for a focal adhesion (Fig. 4). First, hyaloid should be separated on all sides if possible. Epiretinal membranes

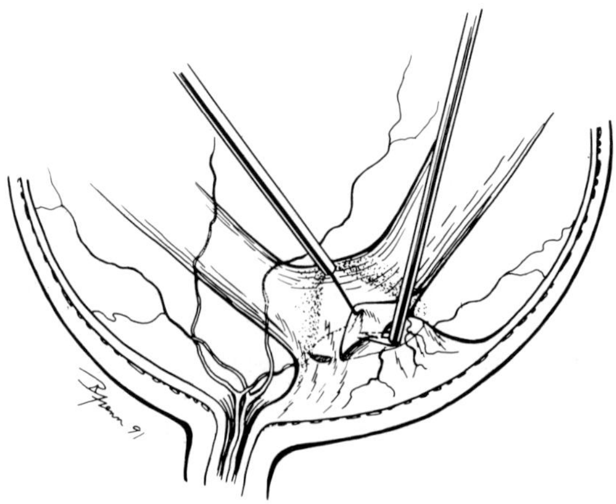

Fig. 3. Broad, plaque-like vitreoretinal adhesion. Multiple fine focal adhesions are often found and must be cut. Bimanual technique with illuminated pick and scissors.

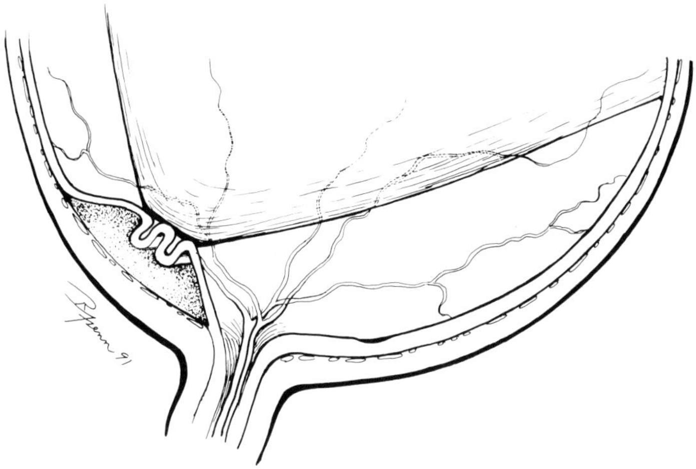

Fig. 4. Broad vitreoretinal adhesion composed of multiple contracted focal adhesions with retinal folds between the adhesions. Surrounding membranes should be stripped toward epicenters, then each adhesion cut individually.

around the adhesions should be stripped towards the adhesions. When the adhesion is exposed, it is cut with horizontally cutting scissors. With chronic traction, the folds may become fixed and differentiation of membrane from retina may be difficult. Each individual epicenter is exposed and cut. Bimanual methods are recommended to give maximal exposure.

Split posterior hyaloid

A split posterior hyaloid occurs when there is lamellar separation of the vitreous from the retina leaving cortical vitreous adherent to the retina (Fig. 5). This may present clinically as a thickened, often hemorrhagic vitreous membrane which looks like posterior hyaloid. The membrane usually remains attached to posterior epicenters and often bridges from the posterior adhesions anteriorly and peripherally to the vitreous base. Closer examination, often at surgery, will reveal an unseparated posterior hyaloid. These eyes have often had severe vitreous hemorrhage, and hemorrhage in the formed vitreous may cause condensation of vitreous collagen which may lead to lamellar separation of the vitreous. A less obvious form of lamellar splitting of the cortical vitreous may be epiretinal membranes surrounding vascular epicenters (Fig. 2A).

Once it is determined that a split hyaloid is present and hyaloid is still adherent to the retina, the hyaloid must be separated. A limited area of residual hyaloid can sometimes be stripped from the retina with a membrane pick towards vascular epicenters where it is usually cut with scissors (Fig. 2C). When widespread unseparated hyaloid is present, an area of separation should be identified (often adjacent to the optic disc or elsewhere in the posterior pole). An opening is made in the residual hyaloid over an area where it is separated from the retina in the same manner as described above. The hyaloid is separated with a membrane pick or the tip of the closed horizontally cutting scissors (Fig. 2E).

Peripheral vitreoretinal adhesions

One of the most difficult problems in vitrectomy for diabetic retinopathy is management of peripheral vitreoretinal adhesions. Peripheral adhesions are due to vascular epicenters outside of the posterior pole. Vascular epicenters are found most commonly at the optic nerve and along the posterior temporal vessels. Nasal epicenters and epicenters located further anteriorly at the equator or anteriorly are sometimes found (Fig. 6). In most

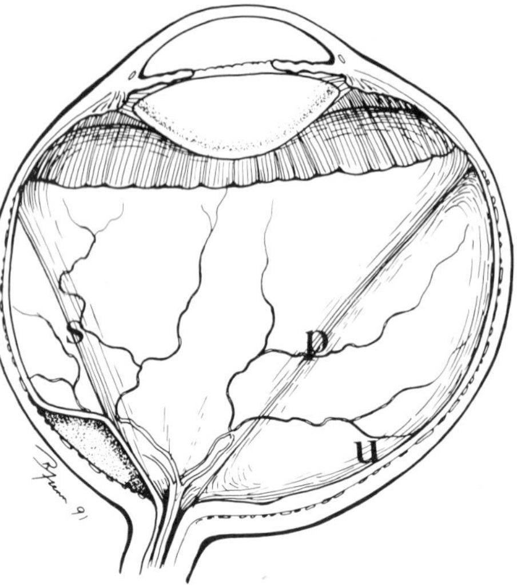

Fig. 5. Split hyaloid with partial posterior vitreous separation. S: separated posterior hyaloid; U: unseparated posterior hyaloid; P: pseudohyaloidal membrane. The pseudohyaloidal membrane is due to condensed vitreous collagen and is often found following hemorrhage in the formed vitreous.

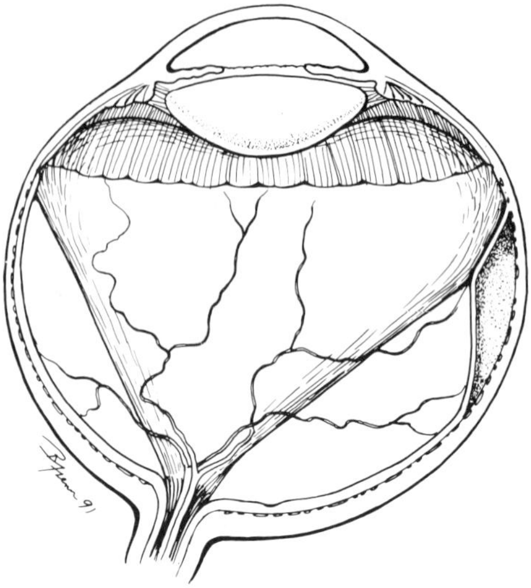

Fig. 6. Peripheral traction retinal detachment. Partially separated posterior hyaloid.

instances the hyaloid should be separated from the retina at these epicenters. A less desirable but acceptable alternative when the retina is not folded or detached at the epicenter is to circumcise the vitreous on all sides of the epicenter to relieve traction.

The major difficulty in separating the hyaloid at peripheral areas of adhesion is in obtaining good visualization and surgical access. These eyes are usually phakic and, if possible, the lens should not be removed. Visualization and surgical access is most difficult and the danger of lens damage is greatest during dissection when the area of vitreoretinal adhesion is located within one clock hour superiorly and two clock hours inferiorly of the instrument sclerotomy sites which are most commonly located at approximately 2 o'clock and approximately 10 o'clock in the horizontal meridians. Bimanual techniques are difficult in these areas because of the likelihood of lens touch when reaching across the eye.

When the peripheral vitreoretinal adhesion is located more than one clock hour superiorly or two clock hours inferiorly from an instrument sclerotomy site, access can be obtained by utilizing external scleral depression. The assistant depresses the sclera to bring the area of vitreoretinal adhesion into view. Vitreous should be separated and excised to the posterior aspect of the adhesion. Then the vitreous around the adhesion can be separated with a membrane pick or the horizontally cutting scissors. An immature vascular epicenter without fibrous tissue may avulse as the vitreous is separated from the retina and hemorrhage can be controlled by raising the pressure of the eye above systolic pressure for one to two minutes. More mature, fibrous adhesions must be separated with scissors or circumcised with the vitreous cutter. When an area is visualized by scleral depression, it is important that the surgeon be cognizant of the area being depressed and that the assistant not move the depressor during dissection in order to avoid inadvertent retinal damage. Also, when working at the equator and anteriorly, there is a significant danger of lens touch when reaching across the eye to an area more than 90° away from the sclerotomy site through which an instrument is placed. In the phakic eye, when working at the equator and anteriorly using standard horizontally placed sclerotomy sites, bimanual techniques can be used only in a limited area. The further anteriorly the adhesion is located, the less access is possible by bimanual techniques, while conversely, the more posteriorly the adhesion is located, the more likely the adhesion can be removed bimanually.

If an adhesion is located in an area not accessible to bimanual techniques, then unimanual techniques will often work. The vitreous around and adherent to the epicenter is cut away using the vitreous cutter placed through the sclerotomy nearest the adhesion. This is usually accomplished while the adhesion is visualized with scleral depression. Alternatively, if the surgeon is skilled in the use of the indirect ophthalmoscope for visualization and manipulation of intraocular instruments, the dissection can be done unimanually under indirect ophthalmoscopic visualization. Because of the problem of a reversed image, for the surgeon inexperienced in the technique this maneuver involves risk for retinal or lens damage. A third alternative is to make one or more new sclerotomy sites which allow bimanual dissection.

When vitreoretinal traction in a phakic eye cannot be adequately relieved by dissection, a decision must be made as to whether a scleral buckle alone will adequately relieve traction or whether lens removal is necessary in order to allow adequate dissection. If there is no retinal detachment except possibly at the focal point of vitreoretinal adhesion, and retinal folding is minimal, an encircling scleral buckle is often adequate to relieve traction. If there is significant retinal detachment or folding due to peripheral vitreoretinal traction that cannot be removed by dissection in the phakic eye, lens removal is necessary in order to relieve traction. Once the lens is removed, good access to the vitreous base for bimanual dissection is easily obtained.

Results

The results of *en bloc* excision of diabetic membranes have been reported previously[18]. Of 69 eyes of 63 patients with traction retinal detachments due to diabetic retinopathy, the retinas of all 69 eyes were re-attached by surgery. With a minimum of six months' follow-up, the maculae remained attached in 61 eyes (88%), while the retinas were completely attached in 57 eyes (83%). Final visual acuity was 5/200 or better in 49 eyes (71%) and 20/100 or better in 30 eyes (43%).

Management of intraoperative complications

Hemorrhage

Hemorrhage is the most commonly encountered intraoperative complication of vitrectomy for diabetic retinopathy. Hemorrhage may originate from cut or torn vascularized membranes, vascular epicenters (which are the "feeder vessels" of neovascular fronds), or from normal retinal vessels. The most profuse bleeding comes from retinal vessels. Retinal vessels may be torn by excessive traction on membranes or cut if tissue is not adequately visualized during cutting. Vascularized membranes tend to bleed and "ooze" when cut and may be obscured by tightly adherent blood clots. Sectioning of vascularized membranes should therefore usually be avoided. In contrast, when vascular epicenters are cut, bleeding usually stops permanently when the pressure in the eye is raised above systolic blood pressure for one to two minutes. This is accomplished by raising the infusion bottles in a gravity system or increasing the pressure in a pressurized system. The time the pressure is elevated should be monitored and pressure should be lowered to normal after a few minutes.

Diathermy is usually not applied to membranes or vascular epicenters prior to cutting. If bleeding persists after the pressure is normalized, unimanual bipolar diathermy is applied directly to the bleeding site. Excessive diathermy can cause retinal necrosis and retinal breaks. In addition, major blood vessels may be permanently occluded by the diathermy. Occasionally there is bleeding from optic disc vessels when proliferative tissue is cut or avulsed from the disc. This is also usually controllable with transient pressure elevation. We do not recommend applying diathermy to the optic disc vessels for fear of optic nerve damage.

Retinal breaks

Retinal breaks occurred in 35% of 69 eyes operated upon with the *en bloc* technique for tractional retinal detachments associated with diabetic retinopathy[18]. Posterior retinal breaks were much more common than peripheral retinal breaks. Retinal breaks could be successfully managed at surgery in all cases in which the breaks were recognized and no cases failed because of re-detachment of the retina from retinal breaks recognized at surgery. Eyes at greatest risk for retinal breaks had chronic traction retinal detachment due to fibrous membranes which were tightly adherent to the retina. Eyes with retinal breaks had a poorer visual prognosis than eyes without breaks, but that may have been because eyes at higher risk for retinal breaks (eyes with chronic traction retinal detachment) had a poorer visual prognosis regardless of the presence of retinal breaks.

If the surgical goal of separating the posterior hyaloid and membranes is accomplished, traction is released and management of retinal breaks is not difficult. Retinal breaks become a serious problem when traction remains. If a retinal break is noted, it is imperative that traction be relieved. For retinal breaks posterior to the equator, no scleral buckle is required. After vitreoretinal traction is relieved by dissection, breaks are marked with diathermy for identification under air, and the retina is re-attached with a fluid-air exchange. Laser endophotocoagulation is applied in one or two confluent rows around the break. A retinal break in attached retina can be treated with laser endophotocoagulation and tamponade of the retina with air or gas is usually not needed. In eyes with retinal detachment, posterior retinal breaks involving the superior 180° can usually be adequately tamponaded with air. We use a non-expansile, longer-acting tamponade (20% SF_6) for breaks in the inferior 180° associated with retinal detachment. The preferred method of gas injection is to flush the air-filled eye with at least 25 ml of the selected gas prior to closing the last sclerotomy site[19].

Peripheral retinal breaks are more problematic. Retinal breaks at the vitreous base should be examined to determine if vitreous traction remains. A retinal break associated with a peripheral epicenter with vitreoretinal traction may be adequate cause to remove the lens and surgically relieve traction if that traction cannot be relieved in the phakic state. A retinal break at the vitreous base or just posterior to the vitreous base is usually best managed with an encircling scleral buckle. This is especially true for most breaks in the inferior 180° which may not be adequately tamponaded with gas. Later vitreous base contraction, frequently seen in eyes of diabetics following vitrectomy, may re-open unsupported breaks. Breaks associated with the sclerotomy sites in the superior 180° can sometimes be safely managed with air or gas without a scleral buckle. If no scleral buckle is placed, it is important that all vitreous around the break be removed. This is difficult in the phakic eye and may require scleral depression or peripheral cutting with indirect ophthalmoscopic visualization to relieve traction. If the vitreous around the break cannot be cut to the surface of the vitreous base, then an encircling scleral buckle should be placed. Peripheral breaks in the phakic eye are usually treated with cryotherapy.

Longer-acting gases such as C_3F_8 are seldom used in phakic eyes because of the fear of severe cataract formation. In aphakic or pseudophakic eyes which have undergone extensive peripheral dissection, long-acting gases are useful. The long-acting gases are used most commonly in re-operations where anterior retinal pathology similar to that found in cases with proliferative vitreoretinopathy is present. However, the experience of minimal, if any, cataract formation following use of C_3F_8in eyes of non-diabetic patients with macular holes has led us to use C_3F_8 in selected phakic eyes of diabetic patients with extensive retinal breaks.

Several of the described variations in the pathoanatomy are often found to co-exist in eyes with severe retinal detachment due to diabetic retinopathy. Widespread vitreoretinal adhesion with posterior pole traction retinal detachment has been called a "tabletop" traction retinal detachment. In addition, peripheral vitreoretinal adhesions and retinal detachments, when found, usually co-exist with posterior traction retinal detachments. An approach aimed at systematically separating the posterior hyaloid and its membranes from the retina will often allow successful management of even these most complex cases.

References

1. Meredith TA, Kaplan HJ, Aaberg TM: Pars plana vitrectomy techniques for relief of epiretinal traction by membrane segmentation. Am J Ophthalmol 89:408-413, 1980
2. Charles S: Delamination. In: Vitreous Microsurgery, p 115. Baltimore: Williams & Wilkins 1981
3. Michels RG: Vitrectomy for diabetic retinopathy: pathophysiology of extraretinal complications and principles of vitreous surgery. Retina 1:1-17, 1981
4. Abrams GW, Williams GA: "En bloc" excision of diabetic membranes. Am J Ophthalmol 103:302-308, 1987
5. McCuen BW II, Hickingbotham D: A fiberoptic diathermy tissue manipulator for use in vitreous surgery. Am J Ophthalmol 98:803-804, 1984
6. Davis MD: Vitreous contraction in proliferative diabetic retinopathy. Arch Ophthalmol 74:741-751, 1965
7. Machemer R: Pathogenesis of proliferative neovascular retinopathies and the role of vitrectomy: a hypothesis. Int Ophthalmol 1:1-3, 1978
8. The Diabetic Retinopathy Vitrectomy Study Research Group: Two-year results of a randomized trial. DRVS report 2: early vitrectomy for severe vitreous hemorrhage in diabetic retinopathy. Arch Ophthalmol 103:1644-1652, 1985
9. Aaberg TM, Abrams GW: Changing indications and techniques for vitrectomy in management of complications of diabetic retinopathy. Ophthalmology 94:775-779, 1987
10. Aaberg TM: Pars plana vitrectomy for diabetic traction retinal detachment. Ophthalmology 88:639-642, 1981
11. Packer AJ: Vitrectomy for progressive macular traction associated with proliferative diabetic retinopathy. Arch Ophthalmol 105:1679-1682, 1987
12. Charles S, Flinn CE: The natural history of diabetic extramacular traction retinal detachment. Arch Ophthalmol 99:66-68, 1981
13. The Diabetic Retinopathy Vitrectomy Study Research Group: Results of a randomized trial. DRVS report 3: early vitrectomy for severe proliferative diabetic retinopathy in eyes with useful vision. Ophthalmology 95:1307-1388, 1988
14. The Diabetic Retinopathy Vitrectomy Study Research Group: Clinical application of results of a randomized trial. DRVS report 4: early vitrectomy for severe proliferative diabetic retinopathy in eyes with useful vision. Ophthalmology 95:1321-1334, 1988
15. Ramsay RC, Knobloch WH, Cantrill HL: Timing of vitrectomy for active proliferative diabetic retinopathy. Ophthalmology 93:283-289, 1986
16. Lewis H, Abrams GW, Blumenkranz MS, Campo R: Vitrectomy for diabetic macular traction and edema associated with posterior hyaloid traction. Ophthalmology 99:753-759, 1992
17. Williams GA, Abrams GW, Mieler WF: Illuminated picks for vitreous surgery. Arch Ophthalmol 107:1086, 1989
18. Williams DF, Williams GA, Hartz A et al: Results of vitrectomy for diabetic traction retinal detachments using the en bloc excision technique. Ophthalmology 96:752-758, 1989
19. Williams DF, Peters MA, Abrams GW et al: A two-stage technique for intraoperative fluid-gas exchange following pars plana vitrectomy. Arch Ophthalmol 108:1484-1486, 1990

ROUND TABLE: EFFECTS OF CATARACT EXTRACTION ON MACULAR AND RETINAL DISEASES

Stuart L. Fine, moderator

Stuart L. Fine: We heard this morning from speakers who reflected on data that they had developed alone or with collaborators. In the case of the diabetic retinopathy studies, several dozen investigators have collaborated over the course of many years. Dr. Davis already has pointed out that clinical experience and clinical judgment are helpful in knowing how to apply data from randomized clinical trials to an individual patient. Most of us recognize that data from large randomized trials are irrefutable and represent the platinum standard in terms of information which can be used in the care of patients. Dr. Franklin asked me to moderate this panel on the relationship between cataract surgery and the subsequent course of retinopathy. On that topic, we have precious little hard data and a multiple of opinions supported by only a few cases. As a matter of interest, I would like to sample some opinions from the audience. Please let us not have the customary American practice where 40 percent of the eligible voters actually vote. Let us have everyone vote on these two questions, even if you are not sure. First, how many have an opinion as to whether there is some causal relationship between cataract surgery and the subsequent course of retinopathy? How many have no opinion about that? About 90% of those who voted have an opinion. Second, how many of you believe that performing planned extracapsular cataract surgery with posterior lens implantation actually will have an adverse effect on the course of pre-existing diabetic retinopathy? For example, if one has a patient who has retinopathy and a cataract, and undergoes surgery with posterior chamber lens implantation, how many believe that the operation will have an adverse effect on the course of that retinopathy? How many do not know? Okay, that is actually about equal. Well, I think those are some questions. We would like answers too. There are some data available. There is one paper from the Medical College of Wisconsin at Milwaukee published by Tom Burton and Glenn Jaffe. Barton and Jaffe described the course of eight patients who had been referred to the retina service in Milwaukee. A couple of weeks ago, Dr. Burton reported preliminary results from 21 patients whom he and his colleagues at Milwaukee had followed prospectively. Perhaps I will begin by asking Dr. Abrams, who is chief of the retina service at the Medical College of Wisconsin, to give his impressions based either on his personal experience or on the data that he no doubt reviewed with Dr. Burton.

Gary W. Abrams: Thanks Stuart. As Stuart has said, this is a group which was prospectively followed. The authors were able to obtain preoperative and postoperative visual acuities in all, and fluorescein angiograms in most, patients. The patients were followed for an average of 15 months after the surgery. Seventeen of 21 operated eyes developed new or recurrent clinically significant macular edema (CSME). All six eyes successfully treated with laser for CSME prior to cataract surgery developed recurrent CSME. Eight eyes developed CSME in the operated eye only, while nine eyes

Retina and Vitreous, pp. 115-123
Proceedings of the Symposium on Retina and Vitreous,
organized by the New Orleans Academy of Ophthalmology
New Orleans, LA, USA, March 12-15, 1992
edited by Rudolph M. Franklin

developed CSME in both eyes, always worse in the operated eye. The four eyes that did not develop CSME all had transient macular edema that resembled the Irvine-Gass syndrome. A substantial number of eyes developed increased retinal hemorrhages, and four eyes developed proliferative diabetic retinopathy in the operated eye. While the operated eye usually had improvement in visual acuity following surgery, in only four eyes was the final visual acuity better than that of the fellow eye. At last follow-up, only four of 21 eyes had a substantial improvement in visual function when the visual acuity of both eyes was considered. If cases have complications such as vitreous loss, or if they have primary posterior capsulotomies, anything that will have the usual effects on vitreous which would normally increase the incidence of cystoid macular edema after cataract surgery, will have an enhanced effect in the diabetic. What I believe is that there is a different standard, there is a different visual standard for cataract surgery in the diabetic *versus* the non-diabetic, that we have to tighten up those standards a bit, and that the patient with 20/30-20/40 visual acuity who is just starting to have problems with a cataract probably should be deferred until he is much more visually involved, in which the visual acuity and his visual function is much more impaired than in the usual non-diabetic patient.

Fine: Gary, let me just push you a little bit on that subject. This morning Dr. Davis emphasized the importance of careful follow-up. There are two components to careful follow-up. One concerns the frequency of the examination, and the other concerns how detailed the examinations are. If one waits until the cataract progresses too far, one could examine the patient frequently, but not be able to assess the retina very well. So how does one take that into consideration? At what point does one's inability to examine the fundus carefully make him want to recommend cataract surgery earlier?

Abrams: Well, actually, I would have to say that that is unusual. Usually, if the patient has enough of a cataract that I cannot do an adequate examination, and I cannot do adequate treatment if I need to do it, the patient has enough visually significant cataract that he has crossed the borderline to where cataract surgery is indicated. There is a threshold where you should go ahead and proceed with the cataract surgery. If the patient has significant reduction in visual acuity, and I cannot give you a definite threshold level, and I am having difficulty examining the fundus, then I think that is an indication for cataract surgery.

Fine: Dr. Aaberg would like to ask a question.

Thomas M. Aaberg, Sr.: Gary, two points. I am not sure you could tell it in those cases, but the first question is whether there is a difference between patients who have cataract and non-proliferative diabetic retinopathy with a posterior vitreous separation already present *versus* those who do not. The first question is which ones progress as far as macular edema goes. And the second is, based on the study that Tom Burton has reported, if a person does not have clinically significant macular edema, but does have extensive microaneurysmal change, should that patient be treated prior to the development of clinically significant edema before the cataract gets so extensive that you cannot treat it?

Abrams: As far as the relationship of posterior vitreous separation is concerned, I do not know the answer to that question, and Dr. Burton did not look at that specific question. So I really cannot answer that question. Certainly, there has been some evidence, or at least some reports, that posterior vitreous separation is somewhat protective. It is certainly protective against proliferative diabetic retinopathy, and it may be at least somewhat protective against diabetic macular edema; but I think that that is much less clear than the effect on proliferative diabetic retinopathy.

Aaberg: I was thinking of those cases you presented where you stripped off the posterior vitreous and the macular edema got better.

Abrams: I think that is a specific group in which there was true posterior hyaloidal traction. I do not think in the usual case with diabetic macular edema that the vitreous contributes a great deal to the diabetic macular edema. There is a very small subset of eyes, usually associated with areas of neovascularization in the posterior pole, which develop taut, contracting hyaloid with foveal traction which causes decompensation of the perifoveal capillaries. That is an unusual situation. What was the second question?

Aaberg: Whether you treat prior to the development of clinically significant edema.

Abrams: That is a difficult question. I think I would certainly have a lower threshold for treating macular edema if the patient is going to have cataract surgery than if he is not. Some of these patients following cataract surgery would have a significant progression of macular edema and develop what looks like an enhanced form of Irvine-Gass syndrome where they have diffuse leakage from the perifoveal capillaries. I do not think that one could manage this sort of edema in any way short of doing an extensive grid treatment, and I would certainly not do that preoperatively unless I had a definite indication. I would not do that prophylactically.

Fine: I interpreted Tom's question slightly differently, but the answer that you gave is a good answer. I thought one of the topics you were addressing was the patient who has macular edema that is not clinically significant, and who also has a few cortical spokes with maybe a little yellowing of the nucleus. Would you then treat this patient, even with non-clinically significant macular edema, because as the retinopathy advances the cataract may also advance, making it more difficult to treat?

Matthew D. Davis: I probably would not treat for the reason that you mention. I think that one of the important things is the patient's expectation, and I think this is sometimes difficult to know. The patient has say 20/50 to 20/70 vision and a nuclear cataract, maybe a little posterior subcapsular, maybe a little thickening in the macula – it is hard to decide how much of this is cataract and how much of this is macular edema. I think it is important for the patient to understand that we are not counting on a substantial improvement following cataract extraction. I agree with Gary that usually one can see well enough to treat if you need to treat with photocoagulation, but if not, then it seems reasonable to me to go ahead and take the cataract out and treat it postoperatively if you need to. I would not treat a patient with photocoagulation who did not have thickening or hard exudate that was at least threatening the center of the macula. If it was threatening the center of the macula, and I could see well enough to treat it, and the cataract looks as though it is progressing and is going to need to be extracted, then I think I would. As Gary said, I would lower my threshold, but I would not lower it a long way.

Fine: I think that my threshold may be just a quarter of a notch lower than yours. I have told patients with crystal clear lenses that I would not consider treating their retinopathy at that stage, but would simply follow it at regular intervals. However, if the patient has the same degree of maculopathy and a cataract, and I obviously do not know how quickly the cataract or retinopathy are going to advance, but I know that it is easy to treat the retinopathy at this stage – and I am not talking about three microaneurysms nasal to the disc – I am talking about mild but perhaps not clinically significant macular edema. I tell them that I can not be sure what the situation will be in four or eight or 12 months. Specifically, I do not know if the retinopathy will be worse, and that the cataract will not be worse, or *vice versa*, thus making it more difficult to treat. Thus, I may treat some patients with non-clinically significant edema and a cataract. About the question of posterior vitreous detachment, I have two pages of notes from Dr. Burton's presentation at a meeting last week. I do not think he mentioned anything about the proportion of those 21 eyes with or without posterior vitreous separation. Any other questions by the panelists on this subject? There is not a lot of information on this issue. I think we can summarize by saying that whereas we might tell a non-diabetic patient that the likelihood of a successful outcome following cataract surgery is 95% or greater, I think we definitely have to modify that for a patient who has even mild retinopathy, because we have two independent reasons, namely, diabetes and intraocular surgery that might cause leakage of capillaries in the posterior pole, thereby adversely affecting the subsequent course of macular edema. I think the diabetic patient with retinopathy deserves all possible considerations. As someone who does not perform cataract surgery, perhaps such a patient should go to the very best cataract surgeon available!

Aaberg: Stuart, could you extend that discussion to proliferative change. Would you manage the patient any differently if proliferative changes and cataract were present, make it both active and involuted?

Fine: Let me ask Dr. Davis if he would like to start out and answer that question.

Davis: Well, certainly, if the proliferative retinopathy has involuted, I would not do any, or any more photocoagulation in anticipation of cataract extraction.

Aaberg: What if there were none so far?

Davis: No proliferative...?

Aaberg: No, no photocoagulation, but an involuted, featureless retina.

Davis: If there were no active new vessels, if the new vessels had pretty much completely regressed, I think I would not recommend treatment. In my mind, the reason to do photocoagulation is either to make new vessels that are there go away, or to prevent them from occurring in someone who has severe intraretinal changes where I expect them to occur. If the new vessels have already been there and regressed, sometimes they come back, but usually not, and I do not have any impression that cataract extraction makes them come back once they have gone away. On the other hand, if this is active proliferative retinopathy, then by all means, I think, it needs to be treated, and if one can not treat it because the cataract is so severe, then I think it needs to be treated very soon postoperatively, not a month postoperatively, but a few days, tomorrow, the day or two or three after cataract extraction. I have seen at least one patient get into very bad trouble when I could not complete scatter photocoagulation because of the cataract and a miscommunication between myself and the ophthalmologist who took the cataract out. I wanted to see the patient a day or two later. I did not see him for a month, and there had already been a lot more proliferation and contraction, and I wished that I had treated the patient two days post-cataract rather than a month.

Fine: Gary, did you want to comment?

Abrams: I have a question for you, Stuart. We have been talking about patients with significant diabetic non-proliferative retinopathy or proliferative retinopathy. What is your opinion on cataract surgery in the diabetic who has no or minimal diabetic retinopathy?

Fine: Again, I personally do not recall any data, but what I would tell a diabetic patient without retinopathy is not a whole lot different from what I would tell a patient who did not have diabetes, except I would say that there is this possibility of leakage after cataract surgery resulting from inflammation. Diabetes also increases the likelihood of leakage from retinal blood vessels. It seems that there are now two reasons why you potentially could have this complication of cataract surgery that is associated with edema, and I think you are just at a slightly increased risk, and I would hope that the cataract surgeon would also tell the patient something similar to that.

Fine: Dinny?

Davis: I agree.

Fine: We have got four or five questions that were sent up and only 15 or 20 minutes for discussion. I would encourage those of you who have questions to address to anyone on the panel to bring them up and give them to Dr. Franklin. First question for Dr. Davis, how soon after initial photocoagulation do you retreat if there is insufficient regression of new vessels; and the second question is, how many burns are given during the first session?

Davis: Well, my custom is to do initial scatter photocoagulation in two sittings about two weeks apart and to put in somewhere between 600 and 1000 burns each time. I hate to stop lower than 600, and I rarely go over 1000; and then, after doing two sittings, which to me is a complete initial treatment, I wait a month. If there has not been any response at all in a month, I do more, I do another sitting, another 500, and wait maybe another month and do another 500. If there has been substantial regression after a month, then I wait and follow the patient maybe a couple of months from then, and then maybe every three or four months. I just sort of keep on going with that initial 600 to 800 to 900 burns, then two weeks later, then again a month later; if things are not going well, then I sort of keep going until the eye is full. Then I stop and then I wait.

Fine: It might be worthwhile to recall, Dinny, you probably have those data on the tip of your tongue, the results that were published I think by George Blankenship and Bernie Doft from Pittsburgh, who actually looked at very short follow-up intervals and found that 75 or 80 percent of the effects of scatter photocoagulation are seen within the first four to six weeks. I know that in the DRS we often waited for, I think, four months, for the effect, and again this was when scatter photocoagulation was in its infancy in the early 1970s, but I think it is the experience of most people that most of what you get, you do get within that first four to six week period.

Aaberg: Dr. Davis, if you found clinically significant macular edema, and the need for panretinal photocoagulation, which would you do first, or would you split it and treat the nasal retina with PRP and focally treat the macula in the first session? Thinking that the macular edema will get worse from the PRP, how would you do the treatment?

Davis: Well, unless the scatter is really urgent, horrible new vessels and vitreous hemorrhage are already present, I would like to get the macular edema treated first. If the intraretinal changes are not severe, or there is not any vitreous hemorrhage, and there is just say, a disc area of new vessels on and adjacent to the disc, then I would like to get the macular edema treated in maybe a couple of sessions and maybe wait two or three months before doing scatter photocoagulation. One has to weigh the macular edema and the severity of the proliferative retinopathy. In the middle of that spectrum I would do as you mentioned, I would start scatter photocoagulation on the nasal side and do focal treatment at the same sitting, and then sort of decide what to do next. If the macular edema was not worse two weeks later, then I might go ahead with more scatter. If the macular edema was substantially worse a couple of weeks later, maybe I would hold off on the scatter and do some more focal treatment or grid treatment of the macular edema, and sort of continue to weigh those two conflicting indications.

Fine: Thank you. Another question, I want to ask Dr. Aaberg to address this. Would you comment on the use of cryotherapy to the peripheral retina to augment PRP or scatter treatment in a patient with persistent proliferative retinopathy and vitreous hemorrhage?

Aaberg: Well, I am very worried about cryotherapy if there is NVE. The papers in the past – one was by Buettner and Robertson from Mayo Clinic – showed significant tractional detachment after using cryotherapy in a panretinal fashion, when there was active NVE, and I have had limited experience with that myself, so that I am very worried about doing cryotherapy. If it is NVD that is present, it is less of a problem. You may have some vitreous hemorrhage from the NVD, but it will not be as big a worry as far as getting tractional detachment and possibly rhegmatogenous detachment. So it would vary, but the other side of the coin is that if you have a very ischemic peripheral retina and cannot give photocoagulation, and that patient may at some time in the future require some form of intraocular procedure, be it cataract surgery or vitrectomy surgery, then I get very worried about the development of anterior hyaloidal fibrovascular proliferation. Prior to doing vitrectomy intervention, in such a case, I would treat that patient with cryotherapy.

Fine: Thank you. Question directed to Dr. Davis. What is the status of studies on aldose reductase inhibitors for diabetic retinopathy?

Davis: Well, as Dr. Green mentioned, the Sorbinil Study was completed and did not show any effect. There is a study of Tolrestat ongoing with no results as yet, but I think they have several hundred, I think perhaps as many as a thousand patients, some of whom have been followed now for two or three years, and some maybe longer, but there are no results reported as yet.

Fine: Question for Dr. Green. What role does the type of lens implant, ACIOL *versus* PCIOL, play in the progression of either non-proliferative or proliferative retinopathy and macular edema? Does the type of lens implant make any difference?

W.R. Green: I am not sure I know the answer to that.

Fine: That is why I asked you. I thought you knew the answer to almost everything.

Green: I really do not know.

Fine: Anyone on the panel have any information about that?

Aaberg: Assuming that the ACIOL has at least the anterior, if not the anterior and posterior capsules removed, there should be forward movement of the vitreous, and I would think that would then worsen the retinopathy?

Green: I can answer that in terms of the vitreous, but am not sure of the answer in relation to diabetes. In our studies of the vitreous, we found up to 70 to 75 percent incidence of posterior vitreous detachment after intracapsular cataract extraction. With extracapsular cataract extraction with posterior chamber IOL, posterior capsule intact, the incidence was much lower. An intermediate level of posterior vitreous detachment was seen after ECCE with posterior chamber IOL and capsulotomy. So there is, with time, after cataract extraction, leeching out of the hyaluronic acid with vitreous collapse and posterior vitreous detachment. If that has an ill effect on diabetic retinopathy, well then I think you could infer that it would be worse with intracapsular and less with procedures in which the posterior capsule was intact.

Fine: Thank you. Question, a type II insulin dependent diabetic has had a complicated cataract extraction with vitreous loss resulting in severe proliferative diabetic retinopathy with vitreous hemorrhage and macular edema. Not a good outcome. The other eye now has a 20/400 cataract without evidence of any background diabetic retinopathy. Prior to cataract extraction, is prophylactic scatter indicated, is there any situation where prophylactic scatter is indicated? So here you had a cataract operation in one eye with vitreous loss and vitreous hemorrhage, presumably from proliferative retinopathy which was pre-existing, the opposite eye now has 20/400 without evidence of even background retinopathy. I think that in itself is an unusual situation, but maybe you would like to...Gary wants to respond to that.

Abrams: I have two reasons I would like to respond. Because I want to say something else too that is related. One, you can have a featureless retina that through a cataract will look almost normal, that in fact is quite ischemic with marked capillary dropout. Even with a significant cataract, sometimes you can get enough evidence from fluorescein angiography to tell if there is a great deal of capillary dropout. Therefore, if you can see well enough through the cataract, it might be worthwhile doing fluorescein angiography. And if they do have marked ischemia with the picture they have had in the other eye, I would consider going ahead and doing prophylactic treatment in that eye. The other point I wanted to make is that you can get an amazing amount of laser treatment through a cataract or a hemorrhage using the longer wave lengths. I have seen quite a number of patients who were referred to me with vitreous hemorrhages in whom referring ophthalmologists have waited too long for referral. These are eyes that I think should receive treatment with either the krypton or the diode laser, either of which can deliver good laser treatment in such situations. If I can see the retina with an indirect ophthalmoscope, I can usually adequately treat it with a krypton or a diode laser. In addition, if one can partially treat the retina, the treatment itself may increase the likelihood of resolution of the hemorrhage, and one is more likely to be able to do a second treatment a few weeks later. If there is a 20/400 cataract, often using either krypton or diode wave lengths, one can still get treatment through. And so I think it is very important that if one has only argon wave length, that one should think in terms of obtaining one of the longer wave length lasers in order to treat in the presence of vitreous hemorrhage or extensive cataract.

Fine: Gary, you said something that may be correct, but I am just not aware of it. What is the evidence that treating actually promotes quicker resolution of vitreous hemorrhage?

Abrams: There have been some studies that show panretinal cryotherapy does enhance resolution of vitreous hemorrhage. How, I am not really sure. It is probably breakdown of the blood-retinal barrier with increased resolution through that mechanism. But I think cryo, no doubt, does increase the resolution, and I am taking the leap in my clinical observation that laser does the same thing.

Fine: You mentioned krypton and diode. Are you talking about a slit lamp delivery system, or have you also had experience with the indirect ophthalmoscope delivery system?

Abrams: My major experience has been with krypton laser using slit lamp delivery, but more recently I have been very impressed with the ability to deliver diode laser using the indirect delivery system. It is a nice way to deliver it in these patients, and you can get through the hemorrhage or the cataract really quite well.

Fine: Tom.

Aaberg: Stuart, anytime you have that degree of asymmetry between the two eyes, you certainly want to look at the carotid status, because that is indeed an unusual situation, and you want to make sure you are not dealing with severe carotid disease, at least on the side of the eye that had the proliferative change.

Fine: Maybe we can take the last two questions quickly and then break for lunch. How does one manage areas of capillary non-perfusion in the posterior pole and areas of adjacent edema?

Davis: Well in the ETDRS, those areas of non-perfusion were included in the grid treatment, whether or not the retina was thickened. I am not sure that it makes sense to treat them, thinking about macular edema, if the retina is not thickened. On the other hand, I think it makes sense to treat them the way you would treat proliferative retinopathy with scatter. I think it is reasonable to include large areas of ischemia, either in the grid treatment or something intermediate between that and scatter, say a 200 micron burn; that is what I would be inclined to do. Not right near the center of the macula, but say a disc diameter away from it.

Fine: Okay, Dinny, thank you. Last question. A patient with postoperative Irvine-Gass syndrome who had preoperative CME that could not be visualized, so I guess assumed to be present. How would you proceed? So, here is a patient following cataract surgery with clinically significant macular edema and pseudophakic macular edema. Gary, do you want to answer that?

Abrams: Can I assume the patient also has diabetes?

Fine: Yes.

Abrams: I treat these patients initially the way I usually treat the patients with Irvine-Gass syndrome. I will usually start them out with fairly intensive topical steroids six or eight times a day, as well as topical nonsteroidal anti-inflammatory agents four times a day, trying to reduce the inflammation as much as possible. This will sometimes help to some degree, but in the diabetic it is often very disappointing. If they are not showing resolution of edema in a relatively short period of time – and that is usually in four to six weeks – I will go ahead and do a grid treatment in these patients. These patients do not respond as well as the usual diabetic with macular edema. They are much more resistant. They can get a severe exudative response with massive exudate throughout. One disturbing observation is diffuse leakage from the capillaries in the posterior pole. Following grid treatment, the fluid may go away, but they may precipitate exudate in the fovea as the edema resolves. Exudate will gradually resolve, but the long-term visual result is often not good, as one can imagine. So there are seldom good answers for these patients. You know, we are going to have to use all of the tools that we have to try to do the best that we can, and I think we can temper the degree of visual loss to some extent, but these eyes do not have a good prognosis when they have got extensive Irvine-Gass syndrome superimposed on diabetic macular edema.

Fine: I would like to ask Alan Bird, who is sitting at the back of the room, if there is a role for Diamox in the management of diabetics with pseudophakic macular edema.

Alan C. Bird: (from back of room) I do not know. I have never tried to. We usually treat in the standard fashion with laser.

Fine: I think Dr. Michael Novak from Cleveland had a brief report at a meeting a couple of weeks ago about using Diamox in a number of patients with diabetic macular edema who were recalcitrant to photocoagulation therapy. I did not hear the presentation. I do not know if you did, Dinny.

Davis: No.

Fine: I do not know if these were pseudophakics or not, but what I heard was that the results were not terribly encouraging. Dr. Franklin, you have had some experience recently concerning the interaction between lens implant surgery and the subsequent course of macular edema. Would you want to make any comments?

Rudolph M. Franklin: With Natalie Baziuk, one of our fellows, we did a retrospective study. We looked at all diabetics who had had cataract extractions over a seven-year period. We selected out only those patients who had uneventful cataract extractions with PCIOLs, and we looked at the visual acuities. We ended up with about 20 patients. The visual acuities were worse than 20/40 in almost 60% of patients, and the reason the vision was down was from macular edema. And it is the same kind of macular edema that Gary is talking about. It was more of an Irvine-Gass type diffuse leakage. You could almost always find some component of diabetic focal leaks, but for the most part it was just diffuse capillary ooze. So, I guess the take home message from our small study is that diabetics, if they have any pre-existing retinopathy, may well have a bad, at least not a good, visual outcome from macular edema, which is very difficult to treat, as we have already heard.

Fine: Rudy, thank you. Don, let me turn the session back over to you. Any announcements? Well, I would like to thank the audience and the panelists for their participation.

III

IDIOPATHIC MACULAR HOLES

IDIOPATHIC SENILE MACULAR HOLE

J. Donald M. Gass

Bascom Palmer Eye Institute, University of Miami School of Medicine, Miami, Florida

Definition

Spontaneous development of a full-thickness macular hole in a normal size eye unassociated with evidence of antero-posterior vitreomacular traction or contusion injury.

Clinical setting

1. Healthy patient usually over 50 years of age (mean 65 years)
2. Female to male ratio 2:1
3. Blurred vision, metamorphopsia, often discovered while covering one eye
4. Visual acuity 20/40 to 5/200 (mean 20/200)

Clinico-pathological anatomy

1. 400-500 μm diameter hole
2. 300-500 μm rim of retinal detachment
3. Receptor cell atrophy
4. Cystoid spaces
5. Yellow drusen-like deposits RPE
6. Epiretinal astrocytic membrane

Normal vitreoretinal anatomy

Firm attachment vitreous cortex to retina

1. Vitreous base
   a. strong attachment
   b. separates only by severe trauma
2. Along major retinal blood vessels
3. Margin optic disc
   a. moderate attachment
   b. usually separates with superior separation of vitreous
   c. free floating vitreous condensation ring or opacity in front of optic disc

Address for correspondence: J. Donald M. Gass, M.D., Bascom Palmer Eye Institute, University of Miami School of Medicine, Miami, Florida 33136

Retina and Vitreous, pp. 127-133
Proceedings of the Symposium on Retina and Vitreous,
organized by the New Orleans Academy of Ophthalmology
New Orleans, LA, USA, March 12-15, 1992
edited by Rudolph M. Franklin

4. Margin of fovea
   a. usually separates with superior separation of vitreous
   b. usually leaves no condensation ring on posterior hyaloid
   c. if condensation ring present, indicates tear (hole) in posterior hyaloid and hyaloid probably still attached to foveal retina

Premacular bursa

1. Optically empty mobile space in front of macula
2. Filled with liquid vitreous and lined posteriorly by vitreous cortex
3. Its anterior interface of condensed vitreous mistaken for separated posterior hyaloid

Pathogenesis & stages of development

Spontaneous contraction prefoveolar vitreous cortex

1. Anterior displacement (detachment) of foveolar retina = Stage 1A impending macular hole
   a. loss foveal depression
   b. yellow spot
   c. no vitreofoveal separation
   d. usually focal mild hyperfluorescence
2. Further cortical contraction, anterior displacement of foveal retina and tangential traction perifoveal retina = Stage 1B impending macular hole
   a. loss of foveal depression
   b. yellow ring
   c. radiating tractional lines in perifoveal retina
   d. no vitreofoveal separation
   e. visual acuity 20/25 to 20/70
   f. slit-beam sign negative
   g. usually mild focal hyperfluorescence
3. Further tangential traction = Stage 2 full-thickness macular hole (few days to few months)
   a. usually at edge of foveolar area
      - hole enlarges can-opener fashion
      - produces round hole with operculum
   b. less frequently, hole begins centrally
      - hole enlarges concentrically
      - produces hole without operculum
   c. visual acuity 20/30 to 20/200
   d. rim of subretinal fluid
   e. yellow drusen-like deposits
   f. slit-beam sign +/-
   g. focal moderate or marked hyperfluorescence

Retinal tissue contraction

Retinal tissue contraction causes concentric enlargement of Stage 2 hole to form fully developed 400-500 μm Stage 3 hole with or without operculum (2 to 6 months+).
1. Visual acuity 20/40 to 5/200
2. Rim of subretinal fluid

3. Yellow drusen-like deposits
4. Perifoveolar cysts
5. Positive slit-beam sign

Vitreomacular separation

1. Early with anterior displacement of operculum
2. Late complete vitreous separation from macula and optic disc = Stage 4 hole (40% or less)

Natural course

Stage 1 impending hole

1. Approximately 50% progress to full thickness holes
2. Approximately 50% spontaneously abort after spontaneous vitreofoveal separation
   a. improvement of visual acuity to near normal
   b. biomicroscopic return of foveal depression
   c. disappearance of yellow spot or ring
   d. one of the following:
      - pseudo-operculum
        - may cast yellow shadow
        - must distinguish from prominent foveal reflex
          - movement of latter with change in slit-beam position
          - ultrasound B-scan
        - usually no fluorescence
      - inner lamellar hole(s)
        - round, oval, sharply circumscribed reddish inner retinal defect, often with scalloped borders
        - no rim of detachment
        - usually operculum
        - negative slit-beam sign
        - visual acuity usually 20/30>
        - usually no fluorescence
      - stellate epiretinal opacity with radiating retinal folds
        - no operculum
        - negative slit-beam sign
        - visual acuity usually 20/30>
      - normal macula with no visible sign of vitreofoveal separation (vitreofoveal separation present but not visible)

Stage 2 hole

1. Most progress to Stage 3 two to six months
2. Few may remain <400 μm diameter permanently

Stage 3 hole

1. 40% or less progress to Stage 4
2. Visual acuity remains relatively stable 80% cases
3. RPE depigmentation in area of detachment frequent after one year

4. Pigmented demarcation may develop as soon as 6 months
5. Many develop epiretinal membranes
   a. may distort the hole
   b. may partly or completely bridge and close the hole
6. Spontaneous reattachment of retina occasionally occurs
   a. simulates inner lamellar hole
   b. visual acuity may be as good as 20/25
   c. slit-beam sign positive
   d. moderate to marked hyperfluorescence
   e. may develop redetachment and visual loss

Fellow eye

1. Vitreofoveal separation: NO RISK OF MACULAR HOLE
2. No vitreofoveal separation: <15% RISK OF MACULAR HOLE
3. Epiretinal membrane covering foveolar area, often with yellow spot: <1% RISK OF MACULAR HOLE
4. Criteria for vitreofoveal separation
   a. free floating optic nerve vitreous condensation ring
   b. vitreous interface anterior to macula attached to margin of optic disc
   c. pseudo-operculum
   d. inner lamellar macular hole
5. Stellate prefoveolar opacity with radiating retinal folds: NO RISK OF MACULAR HOLE
6. YELLOW SPOT OR RING WITH OTHER BIOMICROSCOPIC SIGNS OF STAGE 1 IMPENDING HOLE ARE THE ONLY CHANGES IN THE MACULA INDICATING FELLOW EYE AT HIGH RISK OF HOLE FORMATION

Lesions mistaken for stages of macular hole

Stage 1 impending hole

1. Yellow spot or ring lesions
   a. yellow spot beneath epiretinal membrane
      - crinkling of inner retina overlying and surrounding the yellow spot
      - usually posterior vitreous separation
      - yellow spot caused by underlying foveolar detachment
   b. drusen, RPE detachment, or focal area RFE depigmentation
      - no or minimal loss foveal depression
   c. idiopathic central serous retinopathy
      - loss of foveal depression
      - late fluorescein staining
      - usually male
   d. pseudo-operculum & yellow shadow
      - yellow shadow moves on RPE opposite direction of slit-beam source
      - yellow shadow disappears with diffuse illumination
   e. cystoid macular edema
      - multiple cysts
      - characteristic fluorescein staining pattern
   f. pattern dystrophy
      - usually similar lesion other eye

g. acquired juxtafoveal retinal telangiectasis
    - no loss foveal depression

h. Stargardt's disease
    - no loss foveal depression

i. solar maculopathy
    - no loss foveal depression
    - "silent" choroid

2. Yellow ring lesion
    a. pattern dystrophy
    b. Stage 2 hole
        - small hole retina usually near edge of foveola
        - greater focal hyperfluorescence in the area of the hole
        - slit-beam sign +/- positive
3. Other lesions
    a. inner lamellar hole
    b. pseudo-operculum
    c. epiretinal membrane
    d. stellate epiretinal opacity with radiating retinal folds
    e. perifoveal vitreous condensation ring

Stage 2 hole

1. Stage 1B hole
    a. no hole within yellow ring
    b. no focal area of exaggerated hyperfluorescence
    c. no rim of detachment
    d. slit-beam sign negative
2. Pseudomacular hole (hole in epiretinal membrane)
    a. crinkling inner retinal surface around hole
    b. visual acuity usually 20\30+

Stages 3 and 4 holes

1. Pseudomacular hole caused by hole in epiretinal membrane
    a. attached epiretinal membrane
    b. partly detached membrane
    c. detached membrane
2. Stage 1B hole
3. Inner lamellar hole
4. CME with large central cyst
5. Foveolar atrophy

"Disappearing" macular holes

1. Spontaneous peeling of epiretinal membrane (pseudomacular hole)
2. Spontaneous abortion Stage lB hole
3. Closure macular hole by overgrowth and contraction of epiretinal membrane
4. Spontaneous retinal reattachment around Stage 3 or 4 hole
5. Spontaneous disappearance CME with large central cyst

Surgical treatment Stage 1 impending macular hole

1. Pars plana vitrectomy and cortical peeling
2. Two uncontrolled feasibility studies suggest surgery reduces chances of hole from 50 to approximately 30%
3. Controlled trial underway

Surgical treatment Stages 2, 3 and 4 macular holes

Goal

Visual improvement by reattachment of retina around hole

Methods

1. Photocoagulation
2. Vitrectomy, cortical peeling, intravitreal gas, and face-down positioning (Kelly *et al.*, Poliner *et al.*)
3. + Tissue growth factor-beta (Glaser *et al.*)

Results (uncontrolled feasibility studies)

1. Visual results are better with vitrectomy techniques than with photocoagulation but complications are higher
2. All vitrectomy methods achieve 20/100 or better 40% of patients
3. Retinal reattachment rate higher with TGF-beta but patients achieving 20/40 acuity or better less than without (7% Glaser *et al. versus* 19% Kelly *et al.*)
4. Complications
   a. risk of cataract 50-90%
   b. risk loss of acuity from other causes 15-20%

Future needs

1. Controlled clinical trial
   a. randomize unilateral macular holes or
   b. confine study to second-eye cases only
2. Rigid determination pre- and postoperative visual acuities
3. Include only unequivocal full-thickness macular holes and eyes with 20/100 or less acuity, symptomatic for no longer than one year

References

1. Gass JDM: Idiopathic senile macular hole: its early stages and pathogenesis. Arch Ophthalmol 106:629, 1988
2. Johnson RN, Gass JDM: Idiopathic macular holes: observations, stages of formation, and implications for surgical intervention. Ophthalmology 95:917, 1988
3. Smiddy WE, Michaels RG, Glaser BM et al: Vitrectomy for impending idiopathic macular holes. Am J Ophthalmol 105:371, 1988
4. Jost BF, Hutton WL, Fuller DG et al: Vitrectomy in eyes at risk for macular hole formation. Ophthalmology 97:843, 1990

5. Smiddy WE, Michaels RG, de Bustros S et al: Histopathology of tissue removed during vitrectomy for impending idiopathic macular holes. Am J Ophthalmol 108:360, 1989
6. Kelly NE, Wendel RT: Vitreous surgery for idiopathic macular holes. Am J Ophthalmol 108:360, 1989
7. Glaser BM, Sjaarda RN, Kupperman BD et al: Transforming growth factor-beta in the treatment of full thickness macular holes. Presented Am Acad Ophthalmol, October 1991
8. Poliner LS, Tornambe PE, Poway CE: Retinal pigmentepitheliopathy following macular hole surgery. Presented Am Acad Ophthalmol, October 1991

IDIOPATHIC MACULAR HOLES AND PRECURSOR LESIONS

David R. Guyer and W. Richard Green

Eye Pathology Laboratory, Wilmer Ophthalmological Institute, The Johns Hopkins Medical Institution, Baltimore, MD, USA

Abstract

Idiopathic macular hole and its precursor lesions represent a complex and controversial group of conditions. The authors review the clinical appearance, differential diagnosis, theories of pathogenesis, natural history, and histopathology of this disorder. In addition they consider the management issues, including the controversial role of surgical intervention for macular holes and pre-macular hole lesions.

Introduction

Until the past several years, idiopathic macular hole and its precursors were not among the most fascinating subjects in retinal disease. However, the emergence of a classification that incorporates new ideas on pathogenesis[1,2] and the recognition that vitreous surgery might be beneficial for some patients[3-6] has generated a renewed interest in idiopathic macular hole and its precursor lesions.

Previous studies noted that no treatment could improve visual acuity in patients with idiopathic macular holes. Attention then focused on the identification of risk factors for macular hole formation in the fellow eye. Estimates for second eye involvement range from 3% to 89%[7-21]. Morgan and Schatz[12], for example, reported that if there were retinal pigment epithelium transmission defects in the fellow macula, the risk of hole formation was 80%. McDonnell and co-workers[9] reported that if the fellow eye had a macular cyst with 20/40 acuity or better, the two year risk of hole formation was 23%; whereas if the fellow eye had a macular cyst with acuity of 20/50 or worse, the risk was 89%.

Based in part on the estimated high risk of macular hole formation in the second eye of selected patients and in part on their surgical intuition, several ophthalmologists performed experimental vitreous surgery to reduce the risk of hole formation in second eyes that they believed to be at high risk[4,5]. In addition, recent reports[3-6] suggest a possible role for vitrectomy for full-thickness macular holes. However, several natural history studies have shown that some full-thickness macular holes and pre-macular hole lesions may spontaneously appear to resolve with time, often with improvement in vision[1,2,21]. Therefore, controlled studies are necessary to determine if surgical intervention is indicated for these patients.

In 1970 Aaberg[19] provided a comprehensive review of the clinical features of macular holes. Since then, recent findings have created much controversy concerning the correct

Address for correspondence: W. Richard Green, MD, Eye Pathology Laboratory, The Johns Hopkins Hospital, 600 N. Wolfe Street, Baltimore, MD 21287-9248, USA

Retina and Vitreous, pp. 135-162
Proceedings of the Symposium on Retina and Vitreous,
organized by the New Orleans Academy of Ophthalmology
New Orleans, LA, USA, March 12-15, 1992
edited by Rudolph M. Franklin

diagnosis and management of such patients. The terminology has also become confusing. Various lesions have been described, such as macular holes, lamellar holes, impending macular holes, macular cysts, stage 1 lesions, stage 2 lesions, resolved lesions, and involutional macular thinning. How do these lesions clinically differ from one another and what is the prognosis of each? Is surgical intervention indicated for any of these lesion? We examine this controversial area, with emphasis on recent observations and descriptions.

Clinical appearance and definitions[1,2,21]

Stage 3: full-thickness macular hole (Fig. 1)

This lesion is the classic macular hole. Biomicroscopic examination reveals a foveal area devoid of retinal tissue, approximately one-third of a disc diameter in size, which often is surrounded by a halo of detached retina with subretinal fluid present. Cystoid macular edema is often present (Figs. 2 and 3). An operculum is sometimes present (Fig. 4), and occasionally yellow deposits are seen at the level of the retinal pigment epithelium. These patients note total interruption of a fine slit beam focused over the hole (positive Watzke's sign). A stage 4 lesion is a full-thickness macular hole as described above associated with a posterior vitreous detachment.

Stage 2: full-thickness macular hole

This lesion is an early hole. The hole can be located eccentrically or centrally. There is less surrounding retinal detachment and cystoid macular edema than observed with a stage 3 lesion.

Stage 1: pre-macular hole lesions

Much confusion exists in the literature concerning these lesions. The terms macular cyst, stage 1 lesion, impending macular hole, and involutional macular thinning all have been used to describe the pre-macular hole lesion[1,2,9,11,12,19,21]. We believe that macular cysts, impending macular holes, and stage 1 lesions are all the same precursor lesion. These pre-macular hole lesions may be of three types[1,2,21]: a yellow-dot lesion (stage 1A), a yellow halo lesion (stage 1B) (Fig. 5), or a purely cystic-appearing lesion without yellow dots or halos. In all cases, biomicroscopic examination reveals a decreased or absent foveal depression without a macular hole. The yellow spot is usually 100-200 μm in diameter and the yellow ring is usually 200-350 μm in diameter[1,2].

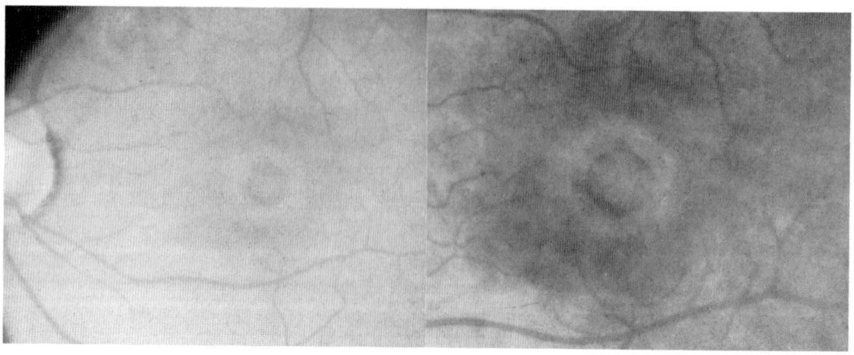

Fig. 1. Macular hole in left eye of a 63-year-old woman.

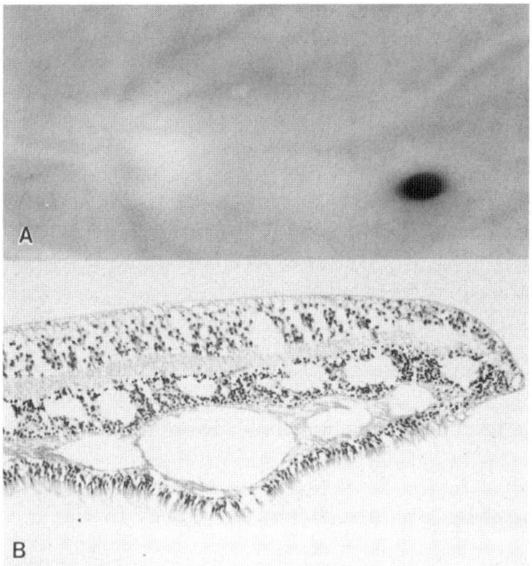

Fig. 2. Gross (A) and microscopic (B) appearance of idiopathic macular hole with rounded margins and moderate cystoid macular edema involving the outer plexiform and inner nuclear layers. Only minimal atrophy of the photoreceptor cells is present (hematoxylin and eosin: B, ×110). (From: Guyer DR, Green WR, De Bustros S, Fine SL: Histopathologic features of idopathic macular holes and cysts. Ophthalmology 97:1045-1051, 1990. Published courtesy of *Ophthalmology*.)

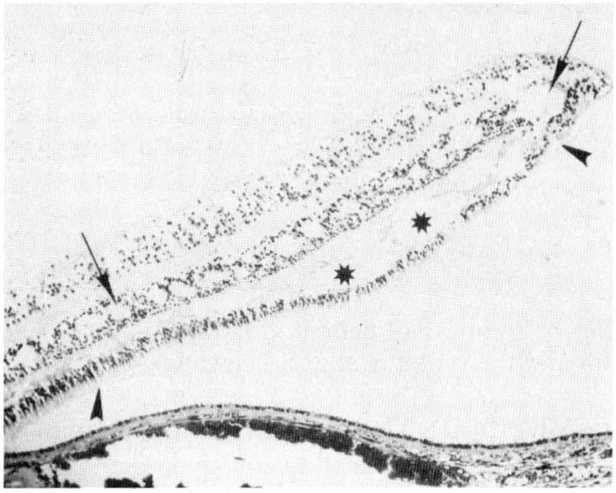

Fig. 3. One margin of an idiopathic macular hole with cystic edema in the inner nuclear layer (arrows) and to a lesser extent the outer plexiform layer (asterisks). Thinning of photoreceptor cell layer (between arrowheads) marks an area of detachment, although no demarcation adhesion is present (hematoxylin eosin, ×100). (From: Frangieh GT, Green WR, Engel HM: A histopathologic study of macular cysts and holes. Retina 1:311-336, 1981. Published courtesy of *Retina*.)

Occasionally, retinal striae can be observed radiating from the yellow ring. The center of the ring may appear reddish. Patients with these lesions note either widening or narrowing of the slit beam focused on the fovea, but no interruption of the slit beam (negative Watzke's sign)[21].

The difficulty in diagnosing pre-macular hole lesions has been highlighted by Gass and Joondeph[22]. Of 18 patients referred with the diagnosis of impending stage 1 macular holes, only one actually had a stage 1 lesion. The remaining patients had an aborted stage of macular hole formation (eight), stage 2 holes (four), stage 3 hole (one), and unrelated

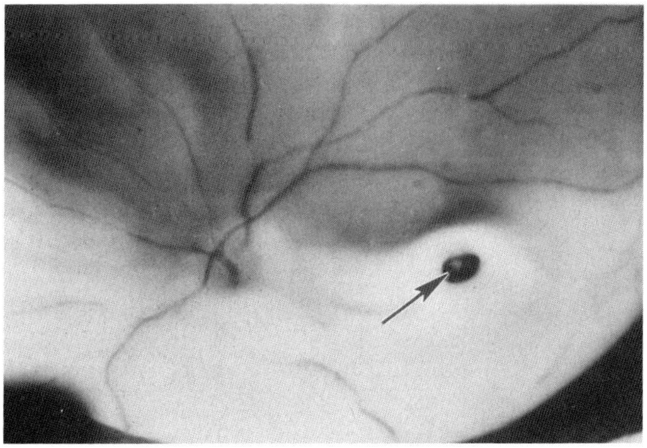

Fig. 4. Idiopathic macular hole with an operculum (arrow).

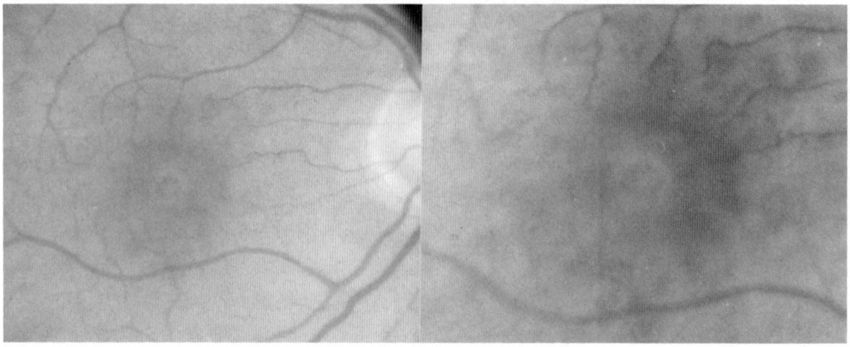

Fig. 5. Right eye of patient illustrated in Fig. 1 with an impending macular hole. There is a ring opacity and the center is slightly elevated.

lesions (four). The differentiating features of these lesions are discussed below in the section on differential diagnosis.

Gass[23] stresses that the diagnosis of impending macular hole be made only when the three following biomicroscopic features are present: loss of foveal depression, presence of a yellow spot or ring in the center of the fovea, and absence of posterior vitreous detachment.

Resolved lesions

Partial resolution of a macular cyst or hole was defined as improvement in the clinical appearance of the macula, often to a flat reddish-hue lesion without obvious cystic char-

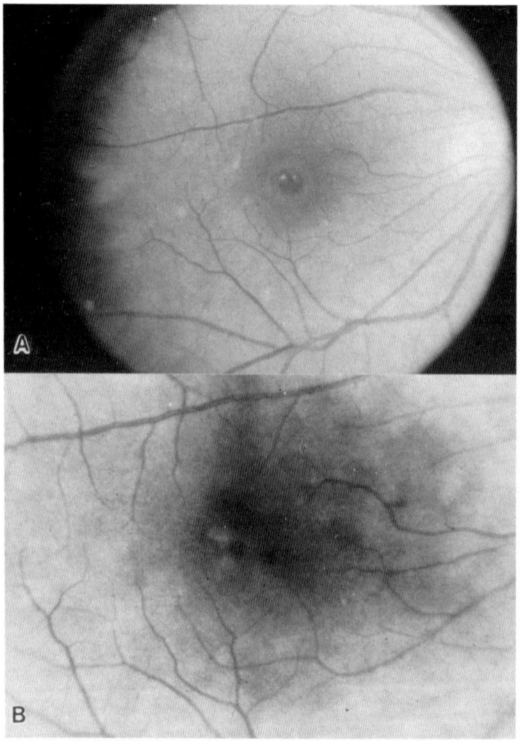

Fig. 6. Disappearance of macular hole. A. Initial appearance of macular hole of a 67-year-old woman with 20/80 vision. After 20 months (B) the hole is not apparent and vision improved to 20/40.

acteristics, subretinal fluid, or areas devoid of retinal tissue (Fig. 6)[21]. In cases with spontaneous vitreofoveal separation during stage 1, Gass[1] and Johnson and Gass[2] noted that a vitreofoveal opacity or pseudo-operculum is frequently present in front of the retina. Those authors[1,2] also observed a lamellar dehiscence of the inner retina with operculum formation in some cases. This dehiscence may appear as a very small "red foveolar facet". Some of his cases progressed to large red inner lamellar holes.

Gass (personal communication, 1989) believes that the flat reddish-hue lesion described in Guyer *et al.*'s series[21] may be a lamellar macular hole. In addition, the involutional macular thinning lesion of Morgan and Schatz[12] may be identical to the resolved flat reddish-hue lesion of Guyer *et al.*[21].

Lamellar macular holes

This lesion represents a partial-thickness macular hole. Inner lamellar holes are characterized by depression of the fovea, vitreofoveal separation with or without operculum formation, and one or more "sharply circumscribed round, oval, or petal-shaped, red depression in the inner retinal surface"[22]. These patients do not see interruption of a fine slit beam focused over the hole.

Differential diagnosis

Epiretinal membrane with a pseudo-hole

An epiretinal membrane with a hole can mimic a full-thickness macular hole. In the former the vision is usually much better than in the latter. Unlike a true macular hole, a pseudo-hole will not have a surrounding halo of fluid, an operculum, or yellow deposits at the level of the retinal pigment epithelium. A posterior vitreous detachment is present with macular epiretinal membranes.

Foveal detachment secondary to central serous chorioretinopathy

A yellow spot in the fovea can be noted in the early stages of central serous chorioretinopathy and can mimic a pre-macular hole lesion. The findings with fluorescein angiography are characteristic and allow these conditions to be easily distinguished. In addition, idiopathic macular holes are most common in elderly females, and central serous chorioretinopathy is typically seen in young to middle-aged males.

Solar retinopathy

The yellow lesion seen early in patients with solar retinopathy may be similar to the stage 1 pre-macular hole lesion. A history of sun-gazing is crucial in the differentiation of these two conditions. In addition, macular holes occur more commonly in elderly females, while solar retinopathy often occurs in younger males.

Cystoid macular edema

Cystoid macular edema, often associated with aphakia or pseudophakia, can mimic the yellow spot of a pre-macular hole lesion[22]. Extracellular fluid can apparently cause compression of xanthophyll and produce the yellow spot[14,22]. An epiretinal membrane is sometimes appreciated. A fluorescein angiogram and history of cataract extraction are useful in diagnosing the correct condition.

Central druse or retinal pigment epithelium depigmentation

Gass and Joondeph[22] described the case of a large central druse or retinal pigment epithelium depigmentation which was referred with a diagnosis of impending macular hole. Such patients do not have loss of the foveal depression sign (foveal reflex). However, if this condition is associated with a small amount of subretinal fluid, then it can be indistinguishable from a pre-macular hole lesion.

Central fibrocellular epiretinal membrane with a macular detachment

Gass and Joondeph[22] also described a patient with a central fibrocellular epiretinal membrane with macular detachment which was difficult to distinguish from a pre-macular hole lesion.

Aborted attempts at macular hole formation

Gass and Joondeph[22] described eight patients in whom aborted attempts at macular hole formation mimicked a pre-macular hole lesion. The cortical vitreous stayed attached to the fovea and formed a stellate, yellow plaque with radiating retinal folds in these patients. No hole was present.

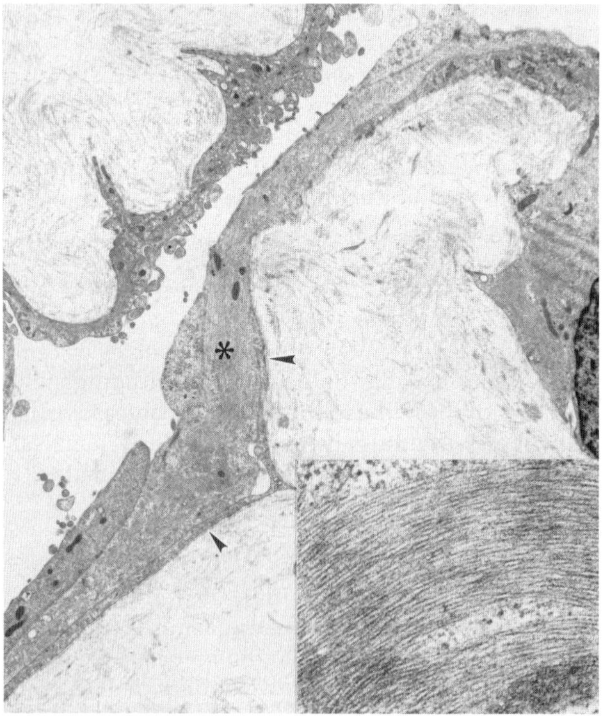

Fig. 7. Electron microscopic appearance specimen removed during vitrectomy for vitreomacular traction syndrome. The typical histopathologic features include the presence of fibrous astrocytes, which are identified by bundles of 10-nm cytoplasmic filaments (asterisk and inset) and basement membrane (arrowheads) (×5400; inset, ×52,000). (From: Smiddy WE, Michels RG, Green WR: Morphology, pathology, and surgery of idiopathic vitreoretinal macular disorders. Retina 10:288-296, 1990. Published courtesy of *Retina*.)

The vitreomacular traction syndrome

This condition is caused by vitreous traction on the macula due to an incomplete vitreous detachment[24-27], and can mimic an impending macular hole. The status of the vitreous is crucial in differentiating these conditions. This differential is extremely important as the vitreomacular traction syndrome can often be relieved by vitrectomy with removal of the epiretinal membrane and vitreous over the macula. In an electron microscopic study of specimens removed at the time of vitrectomy for vitreomacular traction syndrome, Smiddy *et al.*[24] found fibrous astrocytes to be the predominant cell type in all cases (Fig. 7).

Historical review and early theories on pathogenesis

Knapp[28] described the first case of a macular hole in 1869. The patient had a history of severe trauma and the initial diagnosis was that of a macular hemorrhage[19]. The first description of an idiopathic macular hole was by Noyes in 1871[29]. Ogilvie[30] coined the term "macular hole" in 1900.

The history of macular holes can be divided into three periods, each of which had its own favored pathogenesis for the condition. The first theory emphasized trauma as the only or most common mechanism for macular hole formation[28-32]. It was suggested that blunt trauma[18] could lead to an immediate macular hole or that the lesion could form later after breakdown of traumatic cystic changes[33-37]. Lister[38] stated that trauma led to the formation of cysts, which later ruptured and became a macular hole.

Clearly, these authors were not incorrect, since trauma can cause a macular hole. However, this mechanism accounts for only a small proportion of cases. Reese *et al.*[39] found that only 5% of macular holes were related to trauma, Aaberg *et al.*[16] reported 9% in their series, and McDonnell *et al.*[9] noted 15% due to accidental or surgical trauma. The most common type of macular hole is the idiopathic macular hole (83% of cases in the McDonnell *et al.* series[9]), which is seen most commonly in elderly females. It is this type of macular hole that has become the center of recent controversy, and which is the main subject of this review.

The second theory suggested that cystic degeneration was the main factor responsible for macular hole formation. In 1900, Kuhnt[40] suggested that macular holes were caused by a degenerated fovea and not secondary to trauma. He termed this condition "retinitis atrophicans sive rarificans centralis". Tower[41] also believed that macular cystic degeneration predisposed to hole formation. Coats[42] and Kuhnt[40] suggested that vasculature changes due to aging led to atrophy and then to macular hole formation.

Proponents of the third theory, the vitreous theory, believed that partial posterior vitreous detachment produced traction, which caused a macular cyst to form and then to rupture and form a macular hole. In 1924, Lister[38] noted the importance of the vitreous in this disease. Reese *et al.*[39] studied 43 phakic and eight aphakic eyes with macular holes and found that 15 (35%) and eight (100%) of the eyes respectively showed vitreoretinal traction. Yoshioka[43] found vitreoretinal adhesions and posterior vitreous detachments in five cases. Jaffe[44] reported 14 cases with vitreoretinal adherence, attachment, or traction. In 1970, Aaberg *et al.*[16] found posterior vitreous detachments in 84% and opercula in 26% of 90 eyes of 78 patients. A high incidence of posterior vitreous detachment was also reported in other series. For example, James and Feman[8] found a posterior vitreous detachment in all 24 of their with macular hole cases, and McDonnell *et al.*[9] reported that all eyes with macular holes had posterior vitreous detachment.

Interestingly, both the last two series[8,9] reported an increased incidence of systemic estrogen use or a history of hysterectomy in their patients. However, suitable matched control groups were not used. Nevertheless, McDonnell and associates[9] speculated that systemic estrogen fluctuations may promote liquefaction and destabilization of the vitreous and lead to vitreous traction, posterior vitreous detachment, and the formation of macular holes.

McDonnell *et al.*[9] added further support to the vitreous theory by noting that a posterior vitreous detachment occurred whenever any of their pre-macular hole lesions (in their terminology, "macular cysts") progressed to a macular hole. Avila and co-workers[10] suggested that vitreous traction extending from the vitreous base was crucial in the pathogenesis of this condition. These authors used a high-resolution precorneal lens and stated that posterior vitreous detachments were not present in 53% of cases.

Using laser biomicroscopy in the study of four cases, Ogura *et al.*[45] observed that an operculum may be supported by partially detached posterior vitreous and that macular holes are the result of tangential traction followed by axial traction caused by a contracted and detached cortical vitreous gel.

Trempe *et al.*[20], in 1986, reported on their series of patients using the El Bayadi-Kajiura preset lens to study the vitreous. These authors found that a posterior vitreous detachment was present in 39% and an operculum in 60% of cases. They also reported that eight of 28 fellow eyes without posterior vitreous detachments eventually progressed to a macular hole, while none of 21 fellow eyes with a posterior vitreous detachment developed a macular hole. This finding suggested that a complete posterior vitreous detachment may protect the fellow eye from macular hole formation. The strength of this study was that it used the El Bayadi-Kajiura lens, which enables a more detailed slit-lamp biomicroscopic study of the vitreous.

Recent surgical experience[4], however, has shown that it is difficult to determine reliably the status of the vitreoretinal relationship by slit-lamp biomicroscopy. In three of 15 patients, Smiddy *et al.*[4] observed a thin layer of cortical vitreous was noted on the retina intraoperatively, despite the simultaneous presence of a clinical apparent posterior vitreous detachment. In light microscopic evaluation of vitreous specimens in 29 cases of impending macular hole, Smiddy *et al.*[4] observed vitreous strands in all 29 specimens, fibrocellular membrane fragments in three, and fragments of internal limiting membrane in four. Seven of these specimens studied by electron microscopy disclosed native collagen in all seven (Fig. 8) and a fragment of internal limiting membrane with fibrous astrocytes in one specimen (Fig. 9)[46]. The most accurate way to determine whether a posterior vitreous detachment is present may be by endo-illumination during vitrectomy. Gass[1] and Johnson and Gass[2] have more recently suggested that posterior vitreous detachment is not as common or important in the pathogenesis of idiopathic macular holes as previously believed.

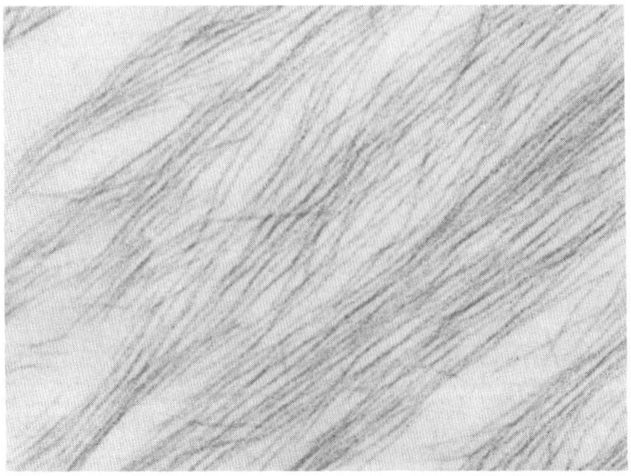

Fig. 8. Ultrastructural appearance of native cortical vitreous with collagen fibrils measuring about 12 nm in diameter removed from a patient with impending macular hole (×60,000).

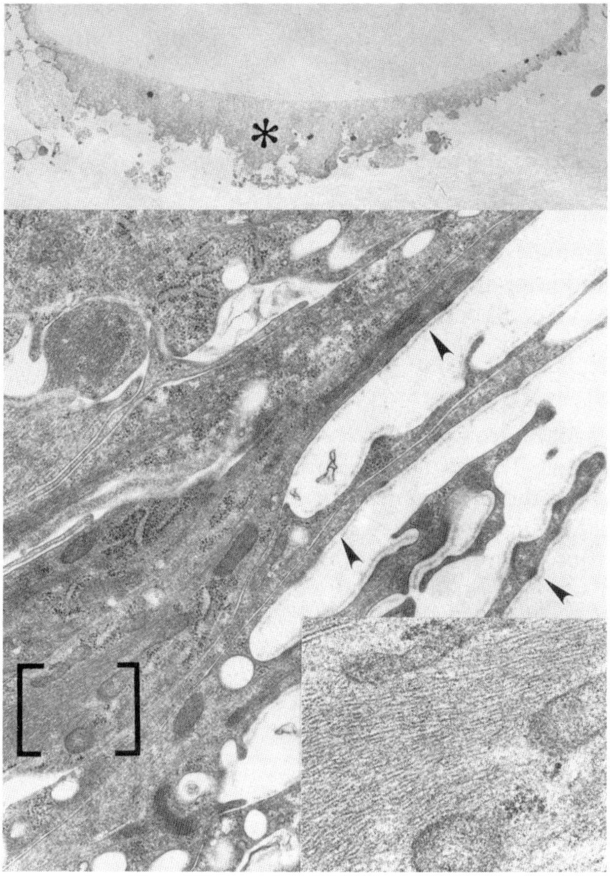

Fig. 9. Specimen from a patient with an impending macular hole contains a fragment of internal limiting membrane (asterisk, upper), numerous fibrous astrocytes (lower) as characterized by the presence of 10-nm cytoplasmic filaments (brackets and inset) and basement membrane formation (arrowheads) (upper, ×5400; lower, ×20,000; inset, ×60,000). (From: Smiddy WE, Michels RG, De Bustros S, De la Cruz Z, Green WR: Histopathology of tissue removed during vitrectomy for impending idiopathic macular holes. Am J Ophthalmol 108:360-364, 1989. Published with permission from *The American Journal of Ophthalmology*. Copyright by The Ophthalmic Publishing Company.)

In 1986, Morgan and Schatz[12] proposed a new pre-macular hole lesion termed involutional macular thinning and a new theory of pathogenesis. Involutional macular thinning is similar to the concepts of Kuhnt[40] and Coats[42]. Reduction of photoreceptor cells in the macular area of aged persons has also been described by Kornzweig *et al.*[47]. In the first of four steps in their theory, Morgan and Schatz[12] postulate that choroidal vascular changes lead to ischemia of the macula and retinal pigment epithelium. Consistent with this vascular hypothesis was the finding that 80% of their patients with pre-macular hole lesions had cardiovascular disease. The ischemia then leads to the formation of cystic changes (Step 2). In Step 3, atrophic changes occur in the macular and/or retinal pigment epithelium. Finally, vitreous traction on a thinned macula leads to macular hole formation (Step 4). This theory is interesting, but changes in the choroid have not been appreciated in histopathologic studies of idiopathic macular holes[48,49].

Morgan and Schatz's studies[11,12] supported earlier findings that vitreous traction is important in the pathogenesis of macular holes. Only two of 30 (7%) eyes which initially had a posterior vitreous detachment progressed to a macular hole at follow-up, while 15 of 34 (44%) without a posterior vitreous detachment initially developed a hole. Furthermore, ten of 12 (83%) of the eyes that developed a posterior vitreous detachment at follow-up also progressed to a macular hole.

Current concept of pathogenesis and classification

While anterior-posterior vitreous traction, with partial posterior vitreous detachment can cause a macular hole, recent findings suggest that this mechanism is not an important cause of most cases of idiopathic macular holes[1,2,14]. Two recent reports by Gass[1] and by Johnson and Gass[2], have changed our concepts about macular holes. Their studies have suggested a new classification and pathogenesis for this disease. These clinical studies[1,2] suggest that the vitreous appears to move freely without anterior-posterior vitreous traction. They noted that the fovea was elevated to the level of the parafoveal retina, there was often vitreous separation at the fovea but usually no posterior vitreous detachment and traction retinal tears. These findings mitigate against anterior-posterior vitreous traction being important in the pathogenesis of macular holes. Several contradictory studies may have been biased since they were retrospective in nature with reports by multiple examiners. In addition, there was no standardized definition for a posterior vitreous detachment, and in some cases, an optically empty posterior vitreous cavity representing a cystic area of liquefaction of the vitreous may have been misdiagnosed as a vitreous detachment[2]. This vitreous is often firmly attached to the macular area. An electron microscopy study by Foos[50] showed a firm vitreofoveal attachment in the posterior pole. Kishi *et al.*[51] also observed a firm vitreofoveal adhesion in 44% of autopsy eyes with partial posterior vitreous detachments.

Gass suggests that focal shrinkage of the foveal vitreous cortex is responsible for macular hole formation[1,2]. Initially, traction occurs which detaches the retina. Then, tangential traction of the foveal vitreous cortex causes the macular hole to occur. This hypothesis is supported by Smiddy *et al.*[4] who intraoperatively observed a layer of thin cortical vitreous on the retina in three eyes in which a posterior vitreous detachment had been diagnosed clinically. A recent histopathological study has confirmed the vitreous nature of this layer[46]. Two possible causes of this vitreous traction include hormonal changes and an abnormal vitreous adherence to the fovea[1,2,14,20]. The hormonal theory is supported by the findings that this condition usually occurs in elderly females and the association with hysterectomy and estrogen usage[9]. The latter hypothesis is supported by autopsy studies showing a firm vitreoretinal adhesion at the fovea.

The new classification system described by Gass[1,2] consists of four stages. In stage 1 (in other series, termed a macular cyst[9] or impending macular hole[4]) a foveal detachment occurs. In this stage there is an absent or decreased foveal depression and the visual acuity is usually between 20/25 and 20/70. A foveal yellow spot, 100-200 μm in diameter (stage 1A) or a yellow ring, 200-350 μm in diameter, with surrounding retinal striae (stage 1B) may also be observed. The latter lesion may have a red center. The yellow material noted probably represents xanthophyll, which is more easily observed with a foveal detachment, and is redistributed into a ring when a 1A lesion progresses to a 1B lesion. Fluorescein angiography may be normal or show early faint hyperfluorescence during this phase. Detection of this lesion may be difficult as only 55% of the patients in the series by Johnson and Gass[2] showed decreased visual acuity or an Amsler grid abnormality.

Early macular hole formation occurs in stage 2. The yellow ring (stage 1B) enlarges over weeks to months with formation of a full-thickness macular hole. The hole may start eccentrically at one edge of the lesion and enlarges with time. Yellow deposits at the level of the retinal pigment epithelium are variably observed. Fluorescein angiography may show early focal hyperfluorescence in the area of the hole, and cannot reliably differen-

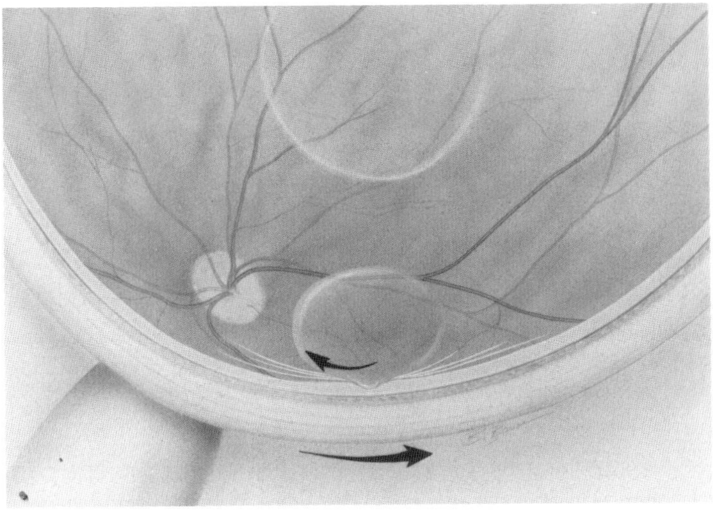

Fig. 10. Schematic representation of premacular bursa with fluid vitreous and how movement of the eye may create counter currents of the fluid vitreous which may create tension of the remaining formed vitreous. This in turn creates traction on the remaining cortical vitreous where it is thinnest – at the fovea.

tiate a stage 1 lesion from a stage 2 macular hole.

A stage 3 lesion is a full-thickness macular hole with vitreofoveal detachment. This lesion usually develops by three to six months, and the visual acuity is usually 20/70 to 20/400. The macular hole diameter is approximately 500 μm and an operculum may be observed. Gass[1,2] reports that, with time, one also may note drusen, epiretinal membranes, atrophy of the retinal pigment epithelium, and occasionally a posterior vitreous detachment.

A full-thickness macular hole with a posterior vitreous detachment is termed a stage 4 lesion.

These two reports from Miami[1,2] have added greatly to our current understanding of

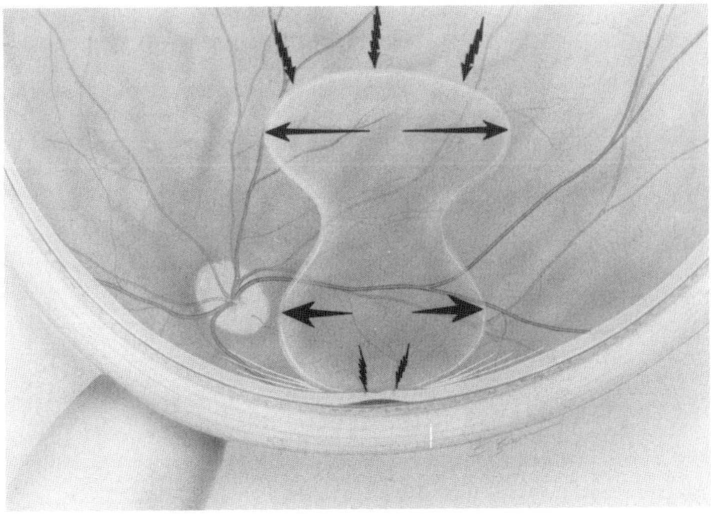

Fig. 11. Schematic representation illustrates enlargement of the premacular bursa with communication of the central area of vitreous degeneration. Fluid currents create tangential traction with elevation of foveal area (impending macular hole).

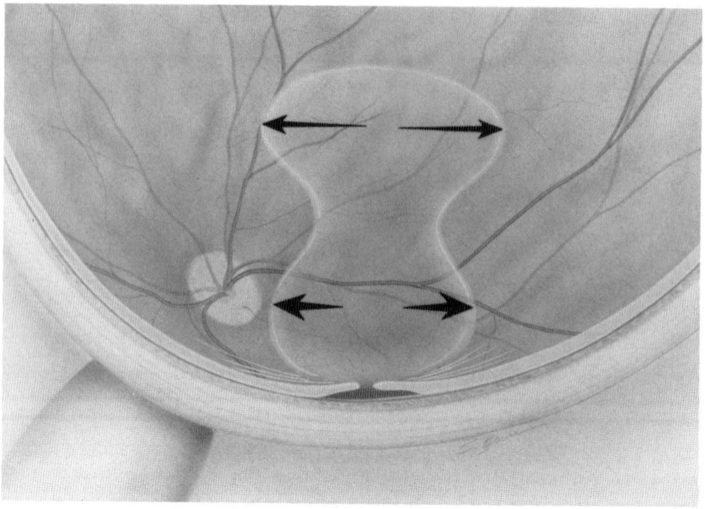

Fig. 12. Schematic illustration of tangential traction with macular hole and small area of surrounding detachment.

this complicated disease. However, one study[1] is based on observations of only 15 patients and a randomly selected group of 34 patients that were used to study vitreoretinal relationships. The second paper[2], however, reports on 158 eyes and notes similar findings. While the second study is a retrospective study, the percentage of patients with follow-up is excellent. In addition, Guyer *et al.*[21] have noted the presence of stage 1A and 1B lesions as described above, but also mention a third stage 1 lesion (1C lesion) cystic-appearing lesion without yellow spots or rings.

We believe that the tangential traction on the macula occurs by three possible mechanisms, fluid movements[52], cellular remodelling of cortical vitreous, and contraction of a cellular membrane on the inner surface of the cortical vitreous. Normally there is a premacular bursa – an area of fluid vitreous (Fig. 9). The bursa may enlarge with age and communicate with the larger central area of liquefaction. The posterior cortical vitreous

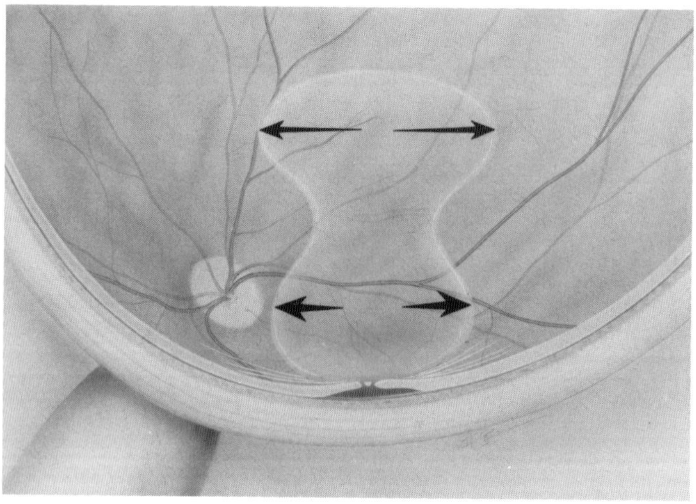

Fig. 13. Schematic illustration of tangential traction with macular hole and detachment and residual macular tissue attached to a thin bridge of cortical vitreous.

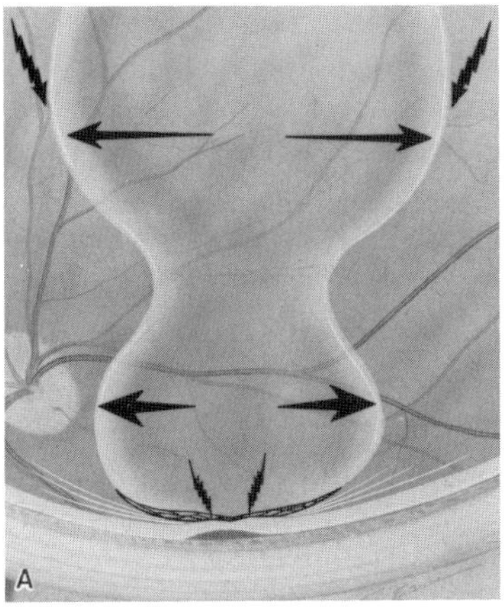

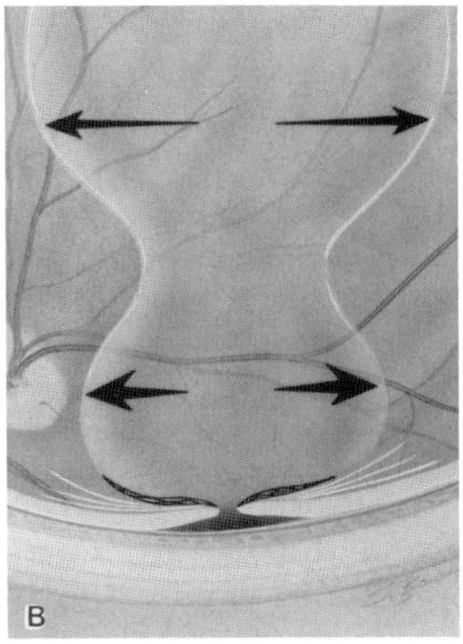

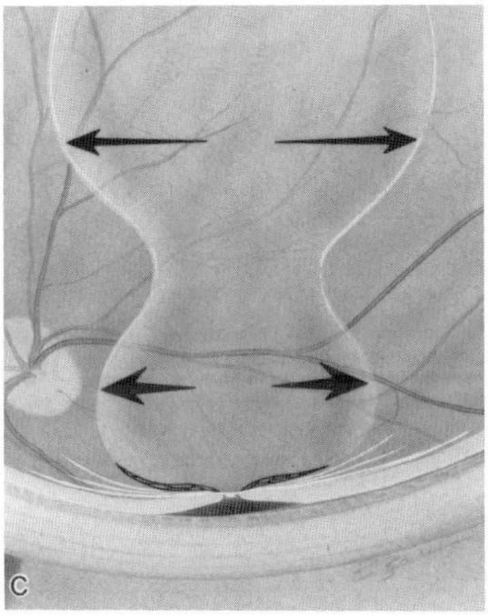

Fig. 14. Schematic representation fluid current-induced tangential traction with a cellular membrane on the inner surface of the thin tapered layer of cortical vitreous with impending macular hole (A), macular hole and detachment (B), and macular hole with operculum and detachment (C).

tapers to a thin layer over the foveal area. With movement of the eye there is a counter movement of the fluid vitreous in the pre-macular bursa (Fig. 9). This counter movement creates tension against the remaining cortical vitreous and the tension is greatest where the cortical vitreous is thinnest – at the fovea. This first leads to a localized foveal detachment (Fig. 10) and then hole formation (Fig. 11). A portion of foveal retina may remain attached to the thin cortical vitreous layer (Fig. 12).

Cellular proliferation in and on the inner surface of the thin cortical vitreous layer may also contribute to traction. Cells within the cortical vitreous may gather and realign cortical vitreous fibers. Proliferation of cells on the inner surface of the cortical vitreous may contract and the contracted state may be perpetuated by new collagen production. These forces may contribute to tangential traction on the fovea (Fig. 13).

Cellular proliferation, however, is more apt to be seen with pre-macular hole lesions and macular holes of longer duration. In a histopathology study of the surgical specimens from 29 eyes operated for impending idiopathic macular holes, Smiddy and co-workers[4] observed fibrocellular membrane fragments in only three (10%) of 29 specimens (Fig. 14). In a study of the specimen of cortical vitreous removed from two patients with pre-macular lesions, Campochiaro and coworkers[53] observed gial and retinal pigment epithelium using an immunocytochemical technique. Of these three mechanisms, fluid currents appears to be the most important.

Natural history

Pre-macular hole lesions

The visual prognosis of patients with pre-macular hole lesions (macular cysts, stage 1 lesions, or impending macular holes) is controversial in the literature. In the McDonnell *et al.* series[9], 50% of the macular cysts progressed to a macular hole. If the vision was 20/40 or better, then the two-year risk of macular hole formation was 23%. If the patient had 20/50 or worse vision, then 89% of the macular cysts progressed to a macular hole. This report suggested that a patient with a macular cyst and 20/50 or worse vision was at high risk to develop a macular hole. However, there are some problems with this study. First, it is a retrospective study with many patients lost to follow-up examination. Second, the findings are different from those of the study of Guyer *et al.*[21] which consists of the same study population, in part, with a longer follow-up period and a larger sample size. With a larger sample size, the denominator of this same subgroup doubled, while the numerator did not increase. Thus, in the Guyer *et al.* study[21], only five of 19 (26%) such patients were found to have progressed to a macular hole. This observation emphasizes the hazard of drawing conclusions from studies of small numbers of patients.

In addition, in reviewing photographs taken at the time of presentation of patients in the series of McDonnell *et al.*[9] Guyer *et al.*[21], found that five of the cases were actually stage 2 lesions and that one case was a stage 3 macular hole. The misdiagnosis problem highlights the fact that the criteria for diagnosis of macular holes and cysts is clearer than in the earlier study. The reported high rate of progression from a macular cyst to macular hole in eyes with a macular cyst and 20/50 or worse vision is hardly surprising considering that some of the cysts in the earlier series were probably Stage 2 macular holes at initial presentation.

One study of the predictive value of the focal electroretinogram in fellow eyes of patients with macular holes suggests that this technique can predict which eyes will progress to macular hole formation[54].

Morgan and Schatz[12] described a pre-macular hole lesion, termed involutional macular thinning (IMT), which they believed to be at a high risk to progress to a macular hole. They describe IMT as thinned, mildly atrophic reddish lesion, occasionally associated with striae, yellow rings, and cystic changes. Twenty-seven percent of these lesions developed a macular hole, compared to 0% of normal fellow eyes. Other risk findings in their series of IMT were retinal pigment epithelium defects on fluorescein angiography (80% risk) and no posterior vitreous detachment (44% risk). Of seven eyes with IMT, retinal pigment epithelium defects, and no posterior vitreous detachment, six (86%) progressed to a macular hole. However, other authors have not been able to confirm these findings[1,2,21]. Gass states that he cannot understand why their pre-macular hole lesion (IMT) is depressed rather than elevated, as reported by other series, and that the IMT lesion is suggestive of a lamellar macular hole[1,2]. Similarly, Guyer and associates[21] did not detect the IMT lesion but described a flat reddish-hue lesion, which they believe represents a resolved macular hole or cyst. Gass (Personal communication, October 1989) believes that the resolved lesion of Guyer *et al.*[21] may also be a lamellar macular hole. Gass[1] and Johnson and Gass[2] further report that stage 1 lesions may spontaneously undergo posterior vitreous detachment with formation of lamellar macular holes or facets. Thus, both the IMT lesion of Morgan and Schatz[12] and the resolved reddish-hue lesion of Guyer *et al.*[21] *may* represent the same lesion, which may actually be a lamellar macular hole. This concept would unify the San Francisco, Miami, and Baltimore studies, but would suggest that the IMT lesion is a resolved macular hole and not a pre-macular hole condition.

Gass[1] reported that ten of 18 (56%) stage 1 lesions progressed to a full-thickness macular hole. However, he noted that eight of 18 (44%) underwent spontaneous posterior vitreous detachment without full-thickness macular hole formation. In the latter instance, foveal reattachment occurred and the yellow dot or ring disappeared. In all but one case, the follow-up vision was 20/30 or better. A pseudo-operculum, occasionally with lamellar holes or facets, was often noted. Of those who developed a lamellar hole, Gass[1] stated that he has not noted enlargement of the lesion or decreased vision during follow-up. In one patient who had serial fluorescein angiograms, disappearance of the initial hyperfluorescence was noted.

Johnson and Gass[2] studied 11 patients with stage 1 lesions. Of nine patients with available follow-up information, six (67%) progressed to a macular hole. In addition, ten of 60 (16%) fellow eyes of patients with a macular hole had a prefoveal opacity and a lamellar hole. They suggested that those findings may represent a 16% frequency of unobserved resolution of stage 1 lesions. Wiznia[55] has reported three additional cases of reversibility of the early stages of this condition. Recently, Akiba and co-workers[56] reported that none of 28 patients with "early stage idiopathic macular hole" and vitreofoveal separation progressed to a full-thickness macular hole, while 10 of 27 (37%) patients without vitreofoveal separation progressed to a full-thickness macular hole.

The Miami series[1,2] are important because they describe the variable natural history of the pre-macular hole lesion. However, because of the lack of the follow-up information and a very small sample size, the actual percentage of pre-macular hole lesions that progress to a macular hole or that resolve, cannot be determined from those study.

Guyer *et al.*[21] reported that only two of 19 (10.5%) pre-macular hole lesions in their series progressed to a full-thickness macular hole, while 15 of 19 (79%) resolved to a flat reddish-hue lesion. Again, this retrospective study suffers from a small sample size and the loss of follow-up of many patients.

The best current information suggests that pre-macular hole lesions progress to a macular hole from 10.5% to 67% of the time. Both estimates are from retrospective studies, with significant biases. In the preceding presentation (pp. 127-133), Gass estimated that 50% of premacular lesions progress to hole formation. Nevertheless, in some cases, premacular hole lesions can resolve. A multi-centered prospective natural history study with strict criteria for lesion classification is necessary to support the above findings and to determine precisely the percentage of pre-macular hole lesions that progress to a full-thickness macular hole.

Full-thickness macular holes

Until recently, the visual prognosis of eyes with full-thickness macular holes has not been controversial. These eyes usually retain peripheral vision and central vision usually stabilizes at or near 20/200[9]. Five to 12% of eyes of patients with macular holes have spontaneous improvement of vision[9,11,16,21]. Of the 40 eyes in the series of Aaberg *et al.*[16], ten had decreased vision (only one to less than 20/200), three showed improved vision of three or more lines, and 27 were unchanged. Morgan and Schatz[11] reported that 82% of their patients retained their vision, although 63% of holes and 67% of associated retinal detachments enlarged during follow-up. Lewis *et al.*[57] reported a patient with a full-thickness macular hole in which the hole disappeared secondary to apparent shrinkage of an epiretinal membrane. The visual acuity improved from 20/70-2 to 20/30-2+2. In addition, Bidwell *et al.*[58] reported two patients with macular holes which disappeared over a period of two and four years. In both cases, visual acuity improved to 20/20. In the first case, the authors speculated that changes induced by an epiretinal membrane may have been responsible, as in the patient reported by Lewis and co-workers[57]. An explanation for the improvement of the second case was not apparent.

Guyer *et al.*[21] observed that three of 66 (5%) stage 3 full-thickness macular holes underwent apparent spontaneous partial resolution with the development of a flat reddish-hue lesion. These authors speculated that spontaneous release of vitreous traction could decrease the tension on the edges of the hole with a corresponding reduction in hole diameter. Resolution of subretinal fluid and intraretinal edema and flattening of the macula could then follow. This resolved flat reddish-hue lesion could show improved visual acuity secondary to the decrease in subretinal and intraretinal fluid. While speculative, this hypothesis is supported by recent information from surgical[3,6], histopathological[48], and scanning laser ophthalmoscopy[59] studies. First, Kelly and Wendel[3] were able, by removal of the preparafoveal cortical vitreous and fluid-gas exchange, to reattach the retina around the macular hole in 30 (58%) of 52 patients. Vision improved in 22 (73%) of 30 patients with reattached maculas. The postoperative appearance in some cases appeared identical to the flat reddish-hue lesion described by Guyer *et al.*[21]. Therefore, the same lesion that results from spontaneous release of vitreous traction also is noted after surgical release of vitreous traction. Second, a recent histopathologic study[48] describes three cases of the probable histopathologic correlate of the flat reddish-hue lesion. In a study of 22 idiopathic macular holes, the retina was reattached to Bruch's membrane by either glial cells or retinal pigment epithelium in two eyes. A small macular hole was present, but intraretinal and subretinal fluid was absent. Glial cells and retinal pigment epithelium seal the margin of the hole to Bruch's membrane. Intraretinal and subretinal fluid may have been reabsorbed by the retinal pigment epithelium. Only a small central macular hole remained, which might be too small to be seen by biomicroscopy. Thus, in the clinically described resolved lesion, no signs of a persistent macular hole may be noted.

Experimental studies[60] and more recent clinical studies[6] suggest that transforming growth factor-beta may be efficacious in sealing macular holes.

Finally, scanning laser ophthalmoscope studies[57,61] of macular holes have shown that an absolute scotoma is present in the area of the hole, but that functional retina is present in the area of the subretinal fluid surrounding the hole. This study supports the suggestion that viable photoreceptors may be present in the areas of the subretinal fluid and cystoid macular edema. Indeed, a scanning laser ophthalmoscope analysis of resolved flat reddish-hue lesions also showed potentially functional retina present. Thus, spontaneous release of tangential vitreofoveal traction may lead to flattening of the macular with a reduction in intraretinal and subretinal fluid, which could allow potentially viable photoreceptors to function again. This hypothesis of spontaneous resolution of macular holes is intriguing and speculative.

A major complication of full-thickness macular holes is retinal detachment. This complication is rare unless the patient is highly myopic. Aaberg *et al.*[16] reported that retinal detachment occurred in six of 81 such eyes. Five of the six eyes were myopic (greater than six diopters) and the other patient had vitreous organization secondary to trauma. Yaoeda[15] found that a retinal detachment occurred in 16 of 17 eyes with macular holes and myopia of six diopters or greater. Mikuni *et al.*[62] noted that in ten of 15 eyes with a macular hole and a retinal detachment, myopia of greater than six diopters was present. Previous therapy involved creation of a macular buckle[63-65] alone or in combination with macular photocoagulation[65]. In 1982, Gonvers and Machemer[66] introduced the concept of tamponade with treatment which included vitrectomy, partial gas-fluid exchange and prone positioning. Since that initial report, numerous other investigations have reported variable success with tamponade and positioning[67-72] and tamponade with photocoagulation[73-75]. In eyes in which retinal detachment recurred, some eyes have been successfully treated with a combination of pars plana vitrectomy, fluid-gas exchange, removal of an epiretinal membrane and laser photocoagulation[76]. Eight of nine eyes with recurrent retinal detachment with proliferative vitreoretinopathy were successfully treated by repeat vitrectomy, removal of epiretinal and vitreous membranes and direct sealing of the macular hole by cyanoacrylate tissue adhesive[77].

Stage 2 lesions

Limited natural history is available for this group of eyes with early hole formation. In Guyer *et al.*'s series[21], six of nine (67%) such lesions progressed to a classic full-thickness stage 3 macular hole at follow-up examination.

Normal fellow eyes of patients with macular holes and/or cysts

To most physicians and patients, the most important question is what is likely to happen to the fellow eye? The risk of fellow eye involvement is reported in the literature as being from 3 to 22%[7-19,21]. Guyer *et al.*[21] have reported that only one of 80 (1.2%) initially normal fellow eyes progressed to a macular hole at follow-up examination. Progression to a macular cyst was reported in two of 80 (2.5%) eyes. Therefore, it appears that the fellow eye has an excellent prognosis, if it is initially normal. However, these are retrospective studies.

In a recent prospective study, Fisher and Slakter[78] followed 39 patients with unilateral macular holes for an average follow-up period of 32 months. Five (13%) developed macular holes in the fellow eyes. Ultrasonic findings of attached vitreous in both eyes at the initial visit was a risk factor for the development of a macular hole in the fellow eye.

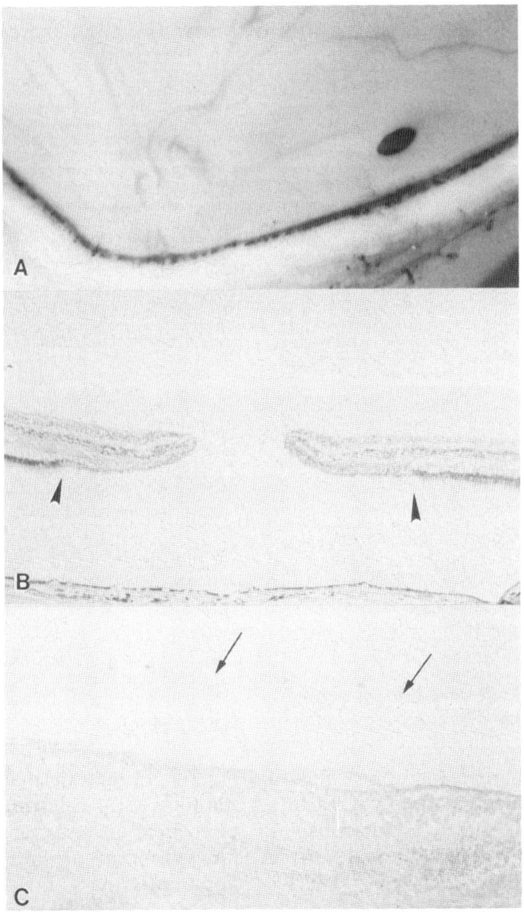

Fig. 15. Gross (A) and microscopic (B) appearance of an idiopathic macular hole with rounded margins and a 0.2 mm surrounding area of partial photoreceptor cell atrophy (between arrowheads). (C) A thin layer of cortical vitreous (arrows) remains attached to the macular retina. (Alcian blue: B, 34; C, ×340.)

Histopathology

Two large histopathologic series[48,49] have been reported on macular holes. Both these series are from the Eye Pathology Laboratory of the Wilmer Institute. In the most recent[48], cystoid macular edema (79%) and epiretinal membranes (68%) were noted frequently in 22 cases of idiopathic full-thickness macular holes. These findings suggest that these lesions may be potentially reversible. The degree of photoreceptor atrophy was variable (200 to 750 μm, mean 480 μm, from the edge of the hole margins). Therefore, some foveal photoreceptors may be functional in some cases. Further studies of these eyes revealed a thin, tapered layer of cortical vitreous is present over the macula (Figs. 15 to 17). It is postulated that fluid currents in the pre-macular bursa with eye movement lead to tangential traction on the foveal area (Figs. 10 to 13). With time, a fibroglial membrane may extend onto the inner surface of the thin, tapered layer of cortical vitreous (Fig. 14) and may contribute to tangential traction with full-thickness (Figs. 15 to 17) and lamellar (Fig. 18) macular hole formation.

An operculum was observed in only one of 22 eyes with idiopathic macular holes (Fig. 5). This configuration may simply represent a tag of residual tissue that remains adherent to the thin tapered layer of cortical vitreous (Figs. 13 and 14C). While anterior-posterior traction is possible, it apparently does not play a role in the formation of idiopathic macular holes. A major weakness with these histopathologic studies is that clinicopathologic correlation is not available, and so we do not know the time from the onset of the lesion

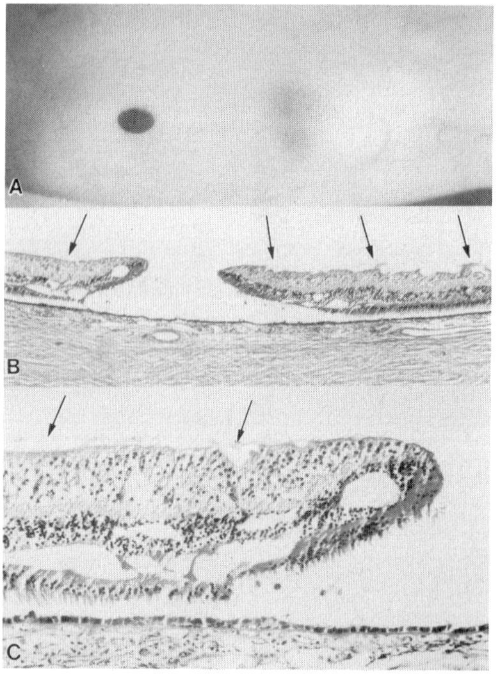

Fig. 16. Gross (A) and microscopic appearance (B and C) of an idiopathic macular hole with a thin, tapered layer of remaining cortical vitreous (arrows) with apparent tangential traction that elevates the retina at the margin of the hole. There is partial photoreceptor cell degeneration and a few cystic spaces are present in the adjacent area where the retina is detached (hematoxylin and eosin: B, ×34; C, ×340).

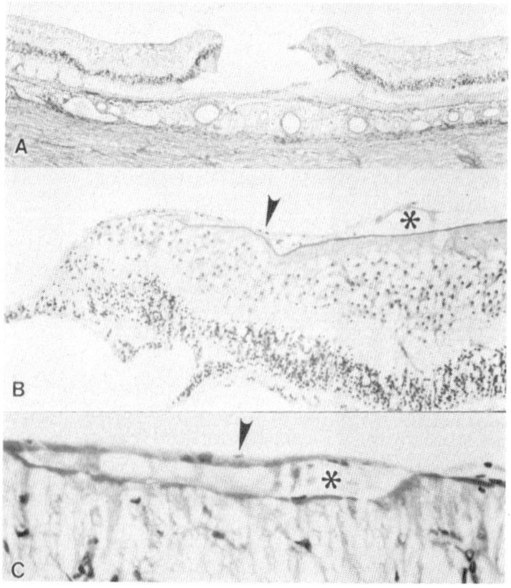

Fig. 17. Idiopathic macular hole with extensive photoreceptor cell atrophy. A thin tapered layer of cortical vitreous (asterisks) with a hypocellular membrane on its inner surface (arrowhead) apparently exerts tangential traction with elevation of the hole margins (periodic acid-Schiff: A, ×34; B, ×340, C, ×520).

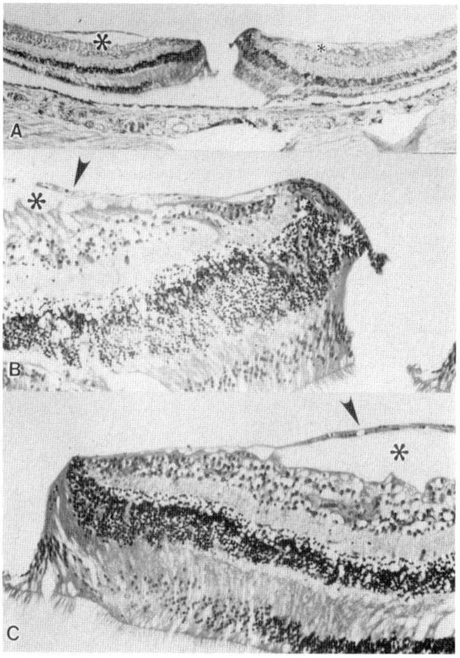

Fig. 18. A. Lamellar macular hole with apparent tangential traction of a thin tapered layer of cortical vitreous (asterisks) with a hypocellular membrane on its inner surface (arrowheads). The apparent traction has caused wrinkling of the internal limiting membrane and eversion of the margins of the hole (periodic acid-Schiff: A, ×30; B and C, ×340).

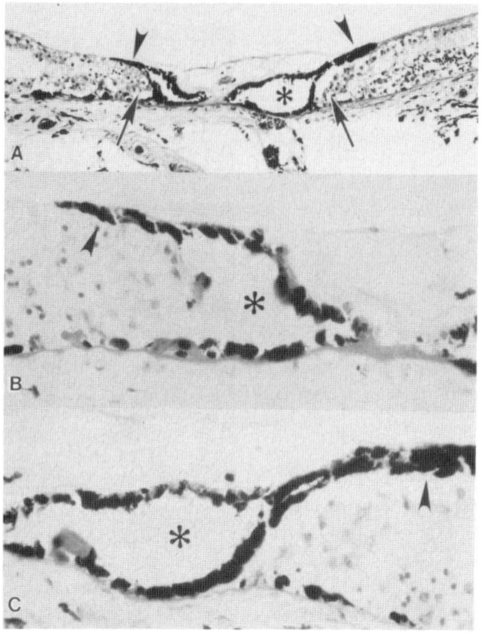

Fig. 19. A. Idiopathic macular hole (between arrows) is sealed by hyperplastic retinal pigment epithelium which forms a cyst-like structure (asterisks) and extends onto the inner surface of the retina (arrowheads) (periodic acid-Schiff: A, ×30; B and C, ×340).

to the death of the patient. We would expect that atrophy of the photoreceptors is related to the chronicity of the detachment, surrounding the macular hole.

In addition, two cases of the probable histopathologic correlate of the resolved lesion were described. In these cases, there was no surrounding retinal detachment present and the edges of the hole were re-apposed to Bruch's membrane. In one eye retina was adherent to Bruch's membrane with the margin sealed by hyperplastic retinal pigment epithelium (Fig. 19). In the other eye the margin of the hole was sealed by glial cell proliferation (Fig. 20).

Tangential traction by a thin epicortical vitreous membrane on the internal limiting membrane was observed in six of 12 eyes with lamellar (partial-thickness) macular holes. This mechanism is also important in the pathogenesis of lamellar macular holes. Epiretinal membranes in the macula most often occur with posterior vitreous detachment and do not commonly cause macular holes.

Macular cysts were found to be associated with cystoid macular edema in 67% of cases. Coalescence of edema spaces may play a role in cyst formation based on this study.

There are some weaknesses in these histopathologic studies. Artifactitious changes in the vitreous during gross examination and microscopic processing prohibit detailed study of the vitreous, which is essential in this condition. Clinicopathologic correlation is not available in most cases. Therefore, clinical verification and correlation of these lesions is not possible. In addition, the duration between onset of the lesion and the death of the patient is not known. Nevertheless, these studies provide some additional knowledge in

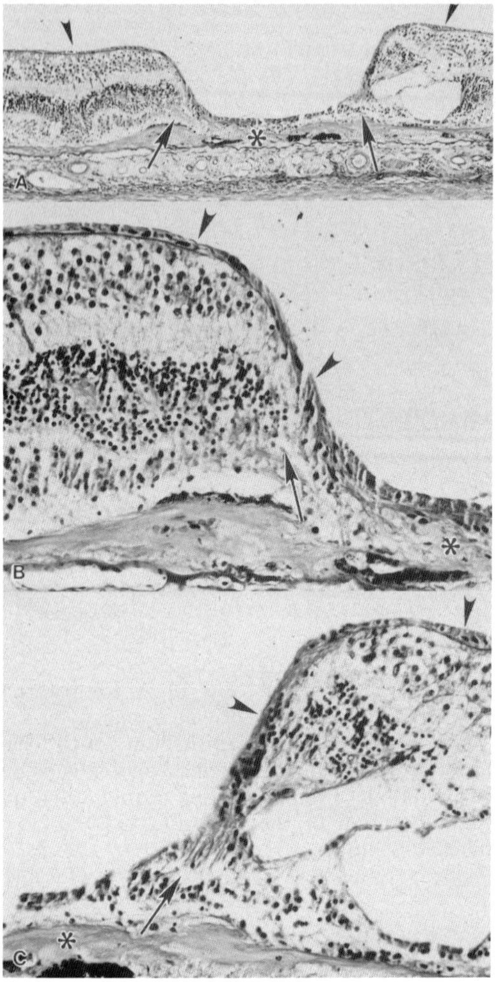

Fig. 20. A. Idiopathic macular hole (between arrows) in left eye of a 91-year-old woman. A fibroglial membrane is present on the inner surface of the retina (arrowheads), covers the margins of the hole and extends on the inner surface of a thin disciform scar (asterisk) in the area of the hole (periodic acid-Schiff; original magnification, ×70). Higher power view of temporal (B) and nasal (C) margins of macular hole (arrow) with a fibroglial membrane that covers the inner surface of the retina and margins of the hole (arrowheads) and the inner surface of a thin disciform scar (asterisk) (periodic acid-Schiff: B and C, ×220). (From: Guyer DR, Green WR, De Bustros S, Fine SL: Histopathologic features of idopathic macular holes and cysts. Ophthalmology 97:1045-1051, 1990. Published courtesy of *Ophthalmology*.)

understanding this condition. The observations of variable preservation of photoreceptor cells and cystoid macular edema in the adjacent retina further helps establish the rationale for surgery of macular holes.

Gass[79] reported the clinicopathologic features of a patient with bilateral lamellar macular holes associated with an epiretinal membrane and cystoid macular edema.

We have observed an additional possible mechanism of non-traumatic macular hole formation. This may be the same as the condition referred to as "involutional macular thinning". This type of macular hole occurs with age and, in some instances, is associated with diffuse drusen. With the development of diffuse drusen there is thinning of the outer nuclear layer (Fig. 21) and hole formation (Fig. 22).

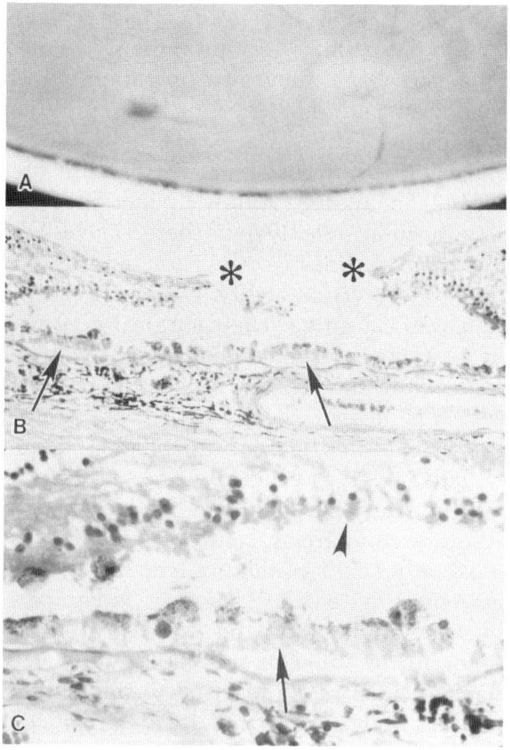

Fig. 21. A. Right eye of 94-year-old female with macular thinning associated with diffuse drusen. B. The foveal area is thin with only a few neural cells remaining. The tear in the foveal area (asterisks) is artifactitious as there is no rounding off and the margins are irregular. There is diffuse thickening of the inner aspect of Bruch's membrane (diffuse drusen) (arrows). The retinal pigment epithelium is partially atrophic (hematoxylin and eosin ×340). C. Higher power view of diffuse drusen (arrow) and rare cells of foveolar area (arrowhead) (hematoxylin and eosin ×520).

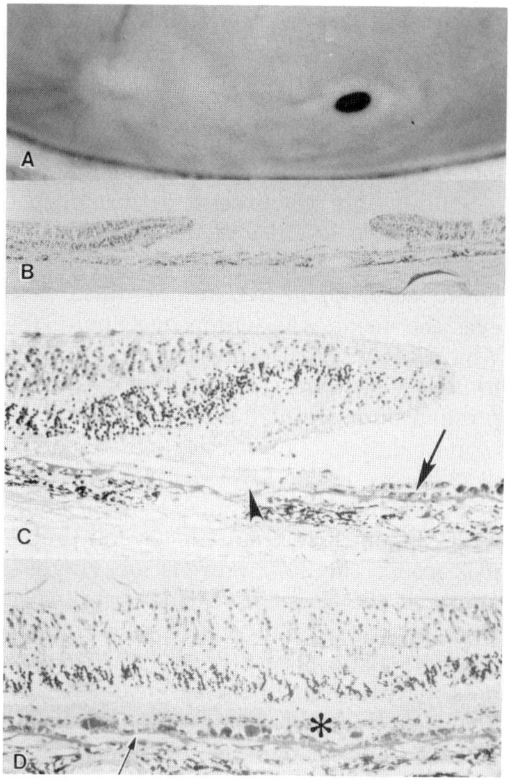

Fig. 22. A and B. Left eye of same patient illustrated in Fig. 21 has a macular hole associated with diffuse drusen. C. Margin of hole with diffuse drusen (arrow). In an area of areolar atrophy there is loss of the diffuse drusen, retinal pigment epithelium and photoreceptor cell layer (left of arrowhead). D. Parafoveal area with diffuse drusen (arrow) with partial atrophy of the photoreceptor cell layer (asterisks) and the retinal pigment epithelium (hematoxylin and eosin: B, ×34; C and D, ×340).

Management

Even more controversial than the pathogenesis and natural history of this disease is the appropriate management. Observation, laser photocoagulation, and vitrectomy all have been advocated.

Studies of vitrectomy for impending macular hole

Three uncontrolled studies[4,5,27] and one case report[80] have suggested the possible role of vitrectomy for impending macular holes. Margherio and associates[27] reported that 96% of 106 "carefully selected patients" had improved or stable vision after vitrectomy for impending macular holes. In this series, the authors attempted surgery when the vision was 20/50 or worse. Two retinal detachments and accelerated cataract formation in 16% of the eyes were reported. This study lacks a concurrent control group, and thus, conclusions on the benefits of surgery cannot be assessed. In addition, the patients in this series appear to be different from the typical patient with a pre-macular hole lesion. These patients often had macular epiretinal membranes, which are not usually very prominent or noted in patients with pre-macular hole lesions. This may be a subgroup of patients with epiretinal membranes and secondary cystic changes, and thus, peeling the epiretinal membrane may relieve traction and cause reabsorption of the cysts.

Smiddy and co-workers[4] performed pars plana vitrectomy in 15 patients with a pre-macular hole lesion and decreased vision. During an average follow-up period of 26 months, 12 of 15 (80%) eyes did not progress to a macular hole. Five of these 12 eyes had improved vision of two or more lines, three eyes had two lines worse vision, and in four eyes the vision was within one line of the preoperative visual acuity. Of the three eyes which lost vision, progressive cataract formation was causative. Their surgical goal was to release posterior vitreomacular adhesions. If a posterior vitreous detachment was not present, they peeled the posterior cortical vitreous from the retina with suction or a vitreoretinal pick. If a posterior vitreous detachment was present, they removed fine strands of cortical vitreous from the macula by using a vitreoretinal pick or tapered-tip suction needle. While these results show that only 20% of these eyes progressed to a full-thickness macular hole, there are several problems in the study. First, their series lacks a control group. The 20% figure is meaningless without a comparison control group. For example, in the Guyer *et al.*[21] natural history series, only 10.5% of the pre-macular hole lesions progressed to a full-thickness macular hole over five years. Therefore, in comparison to the natural history study, twice as many eyes may have progressed to a full-thickness macular hole in the surgical series. However, in the Johnson and Gass[2] study, 67% of pre-macular hole lesions progressed to a macular hole. In comparison to this natural history study, the surgical results appear three times better. Nevertheless, historical controls cannot be used to compare results. Without a concurrent control group, the series by Smiddy *et al.*[4] has a serious weakness and we cannot properly evaluate the role of surgery based on their study. An additional problem with this study is the small sample size with only 15 patients.

Jost and co-workers[5] performed vitrectomy on 15 eyes at risk for macular hole formation. In ten of 11 eyes with stage 1 lesions, macular holes did not occur. Two of four eyes with stage 2 lesions did not go on to macular hole formation. Macular holes developed by five weeks post-surgery in three of 15 cases (20%). This series is also uncontrolled and has a small sample size.

Finally, vitrectomy is not without complications. We may be subjecting eyes with relatively favorable natural history to surgical intervention and its possible complications. In the Smiddy *et al.*[4] series, no direct macular damage was noted intraoperatively, in the cases that developed a hole, but as these authors note, "whether the progression was inevitable and incidentally to the surgery or hastened by the operative procedure is not apparent". One peripheral retinal tear and progressive cataract formation in five of 14 (36%) of phakic patients were also reported. Although not reported in their series, retinal detachment and postoperative endophthalmitis are also potentially feared complications of such surgery.

Thus, while the surgical results of Smiddy *et al.*[4] and Jost and co-workers[5] are encouraging, we cannot presently recommend surgical intervention for pre-macular hole lesions because of the lack of control groups in their series and because of the potentially serious complications of vitrectomy. A prospective multi-centered randomized control study to determine if surgical intervention is warranted in these patients is presently underway. The study, *vitrectomy for impending macular hole*[81], is chaired by Dr. Serge de Bustros (Chicago, Illinois). Hopefully, in the near future, this study will provide us with the answer to the question of whether surgical intervention is indicated for patients with pre-macular hole lesions.

Treatment of full-thickness macular holes

Early suggestions concerning therapy for macular holes focused on psychosomatic and vasodilator treatment. Tower[41] advocated anti-anxiety and psychiatric therapy to alleviate circulatory problems responsible for the condition. He also suggested vasodilator therapy and specific treatments for systemic diseases. In addition, Gifford[81] suggested the use of vitamins, minerals, hormones, sedation, and abstinence from tobacco to relieve ocular angiospasm. All of those treatments have been abandoned. Today, the issues of treatment of macular holes centers on prevention, repair of retinal detachments secondary to macular holes, and the potential role of surgical intervention to promote resolution of the surrounding cuff of subretinal fluid.

In the pathogenesis section, we discussed how the spontaneous release of vitreofoveal traction could allow flattening of the retina adjacent to a macular hole. This flattening could lead to reabsorption of subretinal and intraretinal fluid and potentially improve vision. Histopathologic studies[48,49] of resolved macular hole and scanning laser ophthalmoscope analysis[57] support the concept that decreasing subretinal and intraretinal fluid could lead to improved vision. Preservation of photoreceptors was noted in the detached retina surrounding the macular hole[48].

Several studies have explored the possibility of causing reabsorption of this cuff of fluid. Schocket and associates[83] used argon or krypton laser photocoagulation at the rim of the hole to attempt to cause resolution of the surrounding halo of subretinal fluid. These authors treated 18 eyes with vision of 20/200 or less. The rim of the hole was not treated nasally 45 degrees above and below the raphe in 13 eyes. The entire circumference (360 degrees) of the rim was treated in five eyes. A 50-100 µm untreated space was left between applications. The mean follow-up period was 24.8 months. They reported that ten eyes (55.6%) showed visual improvement of three to eight lines, five eyes (27.8%) were stable, and three eyes (16.6%) lost three to five lines of vision. The major flaw in this study is the lack of a control group. While the results are encouraging, conclusions regarding such therapy cannot be made without an adequate prospective controlled randomized clinical trial.

In addition, it is potentially dangerous to treat these areas with laser photocoagulation since scanning laser ophthalmoscopy information[59] suggests that potentially viable photoreceptors may be present near or at the treated regions. One may be destroying the same photoreceptors that one is trying to save. Further study with pre- and postoperative scanning laser ophthalmoscopy and appropriate control groups are necessary to evaluate this potentially useful surgical intervention.

Kelly and Wendel[3] performed vitrectomies on 52 patients with full-thickness macular holes with surrounding areas of retinal detachment and were able to successfully reattach 30 (58%) of these patients. Improvement of vision was noted in 22 (73%) of the 30 successfully reattached patients. The overall success rate for improved vision was 42% and complications of surgery occurred in 15% of patients. They performed a pars plana vitrectomy with removal of the pre-foveal cortical vitreous, epiretinal membrane removal and a total gas-fluid exchange. In one of the successfully operated cases, the postoperative vision was 20/40, and there were no obvious clinical signs of a macular hole. A flat reddish-hue lesion, which was strikingly similar to the lesion described in the natural history study by Guyer *et al.*[21] was observed.

These cases suggest that full-thickness macular holes can appear partially to resolve if traction is relieved and if the surrounding retina reattaches. Since the natural history of full-thickness macular holes is so dismal compared to that of pre-macular hole lesions, it seems reasonable to consider surgical intervention in these patients. Cases of full-thickness macular holes that were acute in onset would be most desirable, as presumably more photoreceptors would be intact than in chronic cases.

Clinicopathologic studies[84] of the eyes obtained postmortem from one of the patients treated by pars plana vitrectomy and gas tamponade in the Kelley Wendel series[3] disclosed the macular hole was closed by glial cell proliferation in one eye and in the other eye the edges of the hole simply came together

Glaser and co-workers[6], in an uncontrolled small study, recently reported the use of transforming growth factor-beta in combination with total vitrectomy and fluid-air exchange in the treatment of full-thickness macular holes in 12 eyes. The edges of the hole flattened in seven of 12 eyes. Vision improved in five cases. This study lacks a control group, and therefore, valid conclusions concerning the results cannot be made. The potential role of transforming growth factor-beta is also uncertain. Until the results of a randomized trial are delineated the efficacy of surgery for macular holes has not been established. Some eyes will improve spontaneously according to natural history studies, and it is not yet clear whether the potential benefits of surgical intervention outweigh the potential risks[84]. In addition to the established risks of vitrectomy, retinal pigment epithelium changes may occur following surgery for macular holes[3,85].

Normal fellow eyes of patients with macular holes or cysts

These eyes do not require treatment, as they have an excellent visual prognosis based on studies described above.

Summary

Idiopathic macular hole and its precursor lesions are a complicated and controversial issue. We have attempted to alleviate some of the confusion associated with this disorder and have described what we perceive to be the present state of knowledge of this condition. In addition, we have suggested future avenues of research that need to be explored to learn more about this puzzling entity.

We first described the clinical appearance of the various lesions and provided photographic examples of each. Hopefully, the many terms used in the literature can become less confusing. Four types of macular holes exist: three are full-thickness holes (stages 2, 3 and 4), and one is a partial-thickness lamellar macular hole. Pre-macular hole lesions usually have yellow rings or dots, and have been termed macular cysts, impending macular holes, and stage 1 lesions. Finally, resolved lesions have been described, which may or may not be similar to lamellar macular holes.

The difficulty in diagnosis of these lesions has been highlighted recently in a report by Gass and Joondeph[22], who found that only one of 18 patients referred with the diagnosis of an impending macular hole actually had a stage 1 lesion. The differential diagnosis of this condition includes an epiretinal membrane with a pseudo-hole, foveal detachment secondary to central serous chorioretinopathy, solar retinopathy, cystoid macular edema, central druse or retinal pigment epithelium depigmentation, central fibrocellular epiretinal membrane with a macular detachment, aborted attempts at macular hole formation, and the vitreomacular traction syndrome.

Early theories of pathogenesis included traumatic and cystic theories. The vitreous theory followed. Recently, the concept of anterior-posterior vitreous traction being important in this condition has been abandoned in favor of the more common tangential traction and prefoveal cortical vitreous contraction theory of Gass[1,2]. Gass' new classification system was then described in this review article, with careful attention to the physical characteristics of each lesion.

We have applied the concept of fluid currents[52] in the pre-macular bursa as a possible mechanism of tangential traction. Two other features that may contribute to tangential traction are cortical vitreous remodeling and epicortical vitreous membrane contraction.

The controversial natural history of these lesions was next discussed. Retrospective studies suggest that pre-macular hole lesions progress to a macular hole anywhere from 10.5% to 67% of the time. Clearly, in some cases, these pre-macular hole lesions can resolve spontaneously. Biases from the retrospective nature of these studies do not enable us to know the actual rate of progression of these lesions. A prospective natural history study is needed to determine the actual percentage of cases that develop a macular hole. In addition, such a study is needed to verify the occurrence of and determine the frequency of cases of full-thickness macular holes that appear to partially resolve spontaneously.

A hypothesis concerning the spontaneous resolution of full-thickness macular holes has been proposed. Spontaneous release of vitreous traction can lead to re-apposition of the edges of the macular hole to Bruch's membrane-retinal pigment epithelium complex with resolution of the associated local retinal detachment. This reabsorption of the halo of subretinal fluid and intraretinal edema may lead to improved vision in some cases. Surgical[3,6], histopathological[48,49], and scanning laser ophthalmoscope[57] studies appear to support this hypothesis.

Normal fellow eyes of patients with macular holes and/or cysts appear to have an excellent prognosis. In one large series[21], only one of 80 (1.2%) of such eyes progressed to a macular hole.

Histopathologic studies[48,49] were considered next. Cystoid macular edema and epiretinal membranes are commonly noted in full-thickness macular holes. Thus, these lesions are potentially reversible. Histopathologic correlates of probable resolved lesions were described. Evidence of tangential traction by an epiretinal membrane on the internal limiting membrane was noted in many cases of lamellar or partial-thickness macular holes.

Finally, the management of these lesions was discussed. Several of these issues are not controversial. For example, the normal fellow eyes of patients with macular holes and cysts do not need to be treated due to their excellent natural history. Prophylactic treatment of macular holes with laser photocoagulation to prevent retinal detachments appears to be unnecessary. If a retinal detachment occurs secondary to a macular hole, prompt surgical intervention is required. The procedure of choice is vitreous surgery with or without laser photocoagulation. If these procedures fail, the use of tissue glue or the intravitreal injection of silicone oil can be attempted prior to scleral buckling of the posterior pole.

Two management issues remain controversial. The first is the potential role of vitreous surgery in patients with pre-macular hole lesions to prevent progression to macular holes. Pilot studies without control groups[4,5] have led to a multi-centered prospective randomized controlled clinical trial for this group of patients[81]. Until the results of this trial are reported, we cannot advocate vitrectomy for these patients. Some of these eyes will show spontaneous improvement according to retrospective natural history studies and the complications of vitreous surgery are not minimal.

The second controversial issue concerns surgical intervention for acute full-thickness macular holes (stages 2, 3 or 4). Both laser photocoagulation[83] and vitrectomy[3,6] have been advocated, but again, all of these studies have lacked adequate control groups. However, because this subgroup of patients has a dismal visual prognosis and due to the results of the above pilot studies, it is now reasonable to consider a multi-centered prospective randomized controlled clinical trial of surgical intervention with vitrectomy for patients with acute idiopathic macular holes. Hopefully, such a trial will begin in the near future. Future clinical studies are necessary to learn more about the natural history, pathogenesis, and management of idiopathic macular holes.

References

1. Gass JDM: Idiopathic senile macular hole: its early stages and pathogenesis. Arch Ophthalmol 106:629-639, 1988
2. Johnson RN, Gass JDM: Idiopathic macular holes: observations, stages of formation, and implications for surgical intervention. Ophthalmology 95:917-924, 1988
3. Kelly NE, Wendel RT: Vitreous surgery for idiopathic macular holes: results of a pilot study. Arch Ophthalmol 109:654-659, 1991
4. Smiddy WE, Michels RG, Glaser BM, De Bustros S: Vitrectomy for impending macular holes. Am J Ophthalmol 105:371-376, 1988
5. Jost BF, Hutton WL, Fullet, DG, Vaiser A, Snyder WB, Fish GE, Spencer R, Birch DG: Vitrectomy in eyes at risk for macular hole formation. Ophthalmology 97:843-847, 1990
6. Glaser BM, Sjaarda RN, Kuppermann BD, Pena RA, Michels RG: Transforming growth factor-beta in the treatment of full-thickness macular holes. Ophthalmology (Suppl) 98:145, 1991
7. Margherio RR, Schepens CL: Macular breaks. 1. Diagnosis, etiology, and observations. Am J Ophthalmol 74:219-232, 1972
8. James M, Feman SS: Macular holes. Graefe's Arch Clin Exp Ophthalmol 215:59-63, 1980
9. McDonnell PJ, Fine SL, Hillis AI: Clinical features of idiopathic macular cysts and holes. Am J Ophthalmol 93:777-786, 1982
10. Avila MP, Jalkh AE, Murakami K, Trempe CL, Stepens CL: Biomicroscopic study of the vitreous in macular breaks. Ophthalmology 90:1277-1283, 1983
11. Morgan CM, Schatz H: Idiopathic macular holes. Am J Ophthalmol 99:437-444, 1985

12. Morgan CM, Schatz H: Involutional macular thinning: a pre-macular hole condition. Ophthalmology 93:153-161, 1986
13. Bronstein MA, Trempe CL, Freeman HM: Fellow eyes of eyes with macular holes. Am J Ophthalmol 92:757-761, 1981
14. Gass JDM: Macular dysfunction caused by vitreous and vitreoretinal interface abnormalities. In: Stereoscopic Atlas of Macular Disease, 3rd edn, Vol 2, Ch 12, pp 671-726. St Louis: CV Mosby Co 1987
15. Yaoeda H: Clinical observation on macular hole. Acta Soc Ophthalmol Jpn 71:1723-1736, 1967
16. Aaberg TM, Blair CJ, Gass JDM: Macular holes. Am J Ophthalmol 69:555-562, 1970
17. Atmaca LS: Follow-up of macular holes. Ann Ophthalmol 16:1064-1065, 1986
18. Croll LF, Croll M: Hole in the macula. Am J Ophthalmol 33:248-253, 1950
19. Aaberg TM: Macular holes: a review. Surv Ophthalmol 15:139-162, 1970
20. Trempe CL, Weiter JR, Furukawa H: Fellow eyes in cases of macular hole. Arch Ophthalmol 104:93-95, 1986
21. Guyer DR, De Bustros S, Diener-West M, Fine SL: The natural history of idiopathic macular holes and cysts. Invest Ophthalmol Vis Sci (Suppl) 30:155, 1989
22. Gass JDM, Joondeph BC: Observations concerning patients with suspected impending macular holes. Am J Ophthalmol 109:638-646, 1990
23. Gass JDM: Risk of developing macular hole. Arch Ophthalmol 109:610-611, 1991
24. Smiddy WE, Green WR, Michels RG, De la Cruz Z: Ultrastructural studies of vitreomacular traction syndrome. Am J Ophthalmol 107:177-185, 1989
25. Smiddy WE, Michels RG, Green WR: Idiopathic macular disorders. Ophthalmology (Suppl) 96:94, 1989
26. Smiddy WE, Michels RG, Green WR: Morphology, pathology, and surgery of idiopathic vitreoretinal macular disorders. Retina 10:288-296, 1990
27. Margherio RR, Trese MT, Margherio AR, Cartright K: Surgical management of vitreomacular traction syndromes. Ophthalmology 96:1437-1445, 1989
28. Knapp H: Ueber isolierte Zerreissungen der Aderhaut in Folge von Traumen auf dem Augapfel. Arch Augenheilk 1:6-29, 1869
29. Noyes HD: Detachment of the retina, with laceration at the macula lutea. Trans Am Ophthalmol Soc 1:128-129, 1871
30. Ogilvie FM: On one of the results of concussion injuries of the eyes ("holes" at the macula). Trans Ophthalmol Soc UK 20:202-229, 1900
31. Collins ET: Unusual changes in the macular region (? the results of injury). Trans Ophthalmol Soc UK 20:196-197, 1900
32. Haab O: Die traumatische Durchlocherung der Macula lutea. Z Augenheilk 3:113-126, 1900
33. Alvarez-Luna PA: Edema de Belin y agupero de la macula. Arch Soc Oftal Hisp Am 7:221-225, 1947
34. Bonamour G: Le trou post-traumatique de la macula. Ann Ther Clin Ophtalmol 7:343, 1956
35. Fuchs E: Zur Veränderung der Macula lutea nach Contusion. Z Augenheilk 6:181-186, 1901
36. Zeeman WPC: Ueber Loch und Cystenbildung der Fovea centralis. Graefe's Arch Clin Exp Ophthalmol 80:259-269, 1912
37. Zentmayer W: Hole at the macula. Ophthalmic Rec 18:198-200, 1909
38. Lister W: Holes in the retina and their clinical significance. Br J Ophthalmol 8:1-20, 1924
39. Reese AB, Jones IS, Cooper WC: Macular changes secondary to vitreous traction. Am J Ophthalmol 64:544-549, 1967
40. Kuhnt H: Ueber eine eigenthümliche Veränderung der Netzhaut ad maculam (retinitis atrophicans sive rareficans centralis). Z Augenheilk 3:105-112, 1900
41. Tower P: Observations on hole in the macula. Ophthalmologica (Suppl) 40:1-60, 1954
42. Coats G: The pathology of macular holes. Roy Lond Ophthalmic Hosp Rep 17:69-96, 1907
43. Yoshioka H: Clinical studies on macular hole. III: On the pathogenesis of the senile macular hole. Acta Soc Ophthalmol Jpn 72:575-584, 1968
44. Jaffe NS: Vitreous traction at the posterior pole of the fundus due to alterations in the vitreous posterior. Trans Am Acad Ophthalmol Otolaryngol 71:642-652, 1967
45. Ogura Y, Shahidi M, Blair NP, Zeimer R: Improved visualization of macular hole lesions with laser biomicroscopy. Arch Ophthalmol 109:957-961, 1991
46. Smiddy WE, Michels RG, De Bustros S, De la Cruz Z, Green WR: Histopathology of tissue removed during vitrectomy for impending idiopathic macular holes. Am J Ophthalmol 108:360-364, 1989

47. Kornzweig AL, Feldstein M, Schneider JF: The pathogenesis of senile macular degeneration. Am J Ophthalmol 48:22-28, 1959
48. Guyer DR, Green WR, De Bustros S, Fine SL: Histopathologic features of idopathic macular holes and cysts. Ophthalmology 97:1045-1051, 1990
49. Frangieh GT, Green WR, Engel HM: A histopathologic study of macular cysts and holes. Retina 1:311-336, 1981
50. Foos RY: Vitreoretinal junction: topographical variations. Invest Ophthalmol 11:801-808, 1972
51. Kishi S, Demaria C, Shimizu K: Vitreous cortex remnants at the fovea after spontaneous vitreous detachment. Int Ophthalmol 9:253-260, 1986
52. Machemer R: The importance of fluid absorption, traction, intraocular currents, and chorioretinal scars in the therapy of rhegmatogenous retinal detachments. XLI Edward Jackson Memorial Lecture. Am J Ophthalmol 98:681-693, 1984
53. Campochiaro PA, Van Niel E, Vinores SA: Immunocytochemical labeling of cells in cortical vitreous from patients with premacular hole lesions. Arch Ophthalmol 110:371-377, 1992
54. Birch DG, Jost BF, Fish GE: The focal electroretinogram in fellow eyes of patients with idiopathic macular holes. Arch Ophthalmol 106:1558-1563, 1988
55. Wiznia PA: Reversibility of the early stages of idiopathic macular holes. Am J Ophthalmol 107:241-245, 1989
56. Akiba J, Yoshida A, Trempe CL: Risk of developing a macular hole. Arch Ophthalmol 108:1088-1090, 1990
57. Lewis H, Cowan GM, Straatsma BR: Apparent disappearance of a macular hole associated with development of an epiretinal membrane. Am J Ophthalmol 102:172-175, 1986
58. Bidwell AE, Jampol LM, Goldberg MF: Macular holes and excellent visual acuity. Arch Ophthalmol 106:1350-1351, 1988
59. Guyer DR, Sunness JS, Fine SL, De Bustros SN: Idiopathic macular holes and cysts: a scanning laser ophthalmoscope analysis. Ophthalmology (Suppl) 97:152, 1990
60. Smiddy WE, Glaser BM, Green WR, Conner JB Jr, Roberts AB, Lucas R, Sporn MD: Transforming growth factor beta: a biological chorioretinal glue. Arch Ophthalmol 107:577-580, 1989
61. Acosta F, Lashkari K, Reynaud X, Jalkh AE, Van de Velde F, Chedid N: Characterization of functional changes in macular holes and cysts. Ophthalmology 98:1820-1823, 1991
62. Mikuni M, Kobayashi S, Yaoeda H: Treatment of retinal detachment with macular hole. Fol Ophthalmol Jpn 18:659-668, 1967
63. Feman SS, Hepler RS, Straatsma BR: Rhegmatogenous retinal detachment due to macular hole: management with cryotherapy and a V-shaped sling. Arch Ophthalmol 91:371-372, 1974
64. Leaver PK, Cleary PE: Macular hole and retinal detachment. Trans Ophthalmol Soc UK 95:145-147, 1975
65. Alexandridis E, Kohl-Eisenhut H: Treatment of retinal detachment with macular hole. Graefe's Arch Clin Exp Ophthalmol 224:11-12, 1986
66. Gonvers M, Machemer R: A new approach to treating retinal detachment with macular hole. Am J Ophthalmol 94:468-472, 1982
67. Vallet M: Surgical treatment of retinal detachment from macular hole. Graefe's Arch Clin Exp Ophthalmol 224:238-239, 1986
68. Chignell AH, Billington B: The treatment of macular holes pars plana vitrectomy and internal aid/SF6 exchange. Graefe's Arch Clin Exp Ophthalmol 224:67-68, 1986
69. Blankenship GW, Ibanez-Langlois S: Treatment of myopic macular hole and detachment. Intravitreal gas exchange. Ophthalmology 94:333-336, 1987
70. Miyake Y: A simplified method of treating retinal detachment with macular hole. Am J Ophthalmol 97: 243-245, 1984
71. Miyake Y: A simplified method of treating retinal detachment with macular hole: long-term follow up. Arch Ophthalmol 104:1234-1236, 1986
72. Kariyama S, Matsumura M, Harada T, Ishigooka H, Ogino N: Surgical techniques and reattachment rate in retinal detachment due to macular hole. Arch Ophthalmol 108:1559-1561, 1990
73. Rashed O, Sheta S: Evaluation of the functional results after different techniques for treatment of retinal detachment due to macular holes. Graefe's Arch Clin Exp Ophthalmol 227:508-512, 1989
74. Harris MJ, De Bustros S, Michels RG: Treatment of retinal detachments due to macular holes. Retina 4:144-147, 1984
75. Schachat AP, De la Cruz Z, Green WR, Patz A: Macular hole and retinal detachment in Best's disease. Retina 5:22-25, 1985
76. Strirpe M, Michels RG: Retinal detachment in highly myopic eyes due to macular holes and epiretinal traction. Retina 10:113-115, 1990

77. Sheta SM, Hida T, McCuen BW II: Cyanoacrylate tissue adhesive in management recurrent retinal detachment causes by macular hole. Am J Ophthalmol 109:28-32, 1990
78. Fisher YL, Slakter JS: Ultrasound evaluation of the vitreoretinal interface in macular hole formation. Ophthalmology (Suppl) 98:146, 1991
79. Gass JDM: Lamellar macular hole: a complication of cystoid macular edema after cataract extraction. Ophthalmology 94:793-800, 1976
80. Mein CE, Flynn HW Jr: Recognition and removal of the posterior cortical vitreous during vitreoretinal surgery for impending macular hole. Am J Ophthalmol 111:611-613, 1991
81. De Bustros S: Early stages of macular holes: to treat or not to treat. Arch Ophthalmol 108:1085-1086, 1990
82. Gifford SR: An evaluation of ocular angiospasm. Trans Am Acad Ophthalmol Otolaryngol 48:19-30, 1943
83. Schocket SS, Lakhanpal V, Xiaoping M, Kelman S, Billings E: Laser treatment of macular holes. Ophthalmology 95:574-582, 1988
84. Funata M, Wendel RT, De la Cruz Z, Green WR: Clinicopathologic study of bilateral macular holes treated with pars plana vitrectomy and gas tamponade. Retina 4/12:289-298, 1992
85. Fine SL: Vitreous surgery for macular hole in perspective. Is there an indication? Arch Ophthalmol 109:635-636, 1991
86. Poliner LS, Tornambe PE: Retinal pigment epitheliopathy following macular hole surgery. Ophthalmology (Suppl) 98:146, 1991

VITRECTOMY SURGERY FOR IDIOPATHIC MACULAR HOLES

Everton L. Arrindell and Gary W. Abrams

Department of Ophthalmology, Medical College of Wisconsin, Milwaukee, WI, USA

Background

Idiopathic macular hole formation is a disorder occurring more frequently in healthy women beyond the fifth decade of life[1]. Full-thickness macular hole is often associated with patient complaints of metamorphopsia and decreased vision, with a decline in visual acuity to a median level of 20/200[1]. The incidence of bilateral macular hole formation ranges from 6%[2] to as high as 28%[3], but is generally thought to be in the range of 10%. A number of etiologic factors have been ascribed to idiopathic macular hole formation including cystic retinal degeneration[4-7], systemic vascular disease processes[2,4,5,8,9], retinal pigment epithelial disorders[5,9], hormonal changes and systemic estrogen therapy[2,10], and vitreous tractional forces[1,2,4,5,8,9].

Vitreoretinal tractional forces and abnormal vitreoretinal relationships have been implicated in a variety of other ocular macular disorders, including macular epiretinal membranes[11], tractional macular retinal detachments[2,12], aphakic cystoid macular edema[13] and central serous choroidopathy[14]. The role of the vitreous in the pathogenesis of idiopathic macular holes and cysts has long been the subject of intense interest and study[4,15]. More recently, a better understanding of the pathophysiology and the natural history of this disorder, coupled with advances in vitreoretinal surgery, has sparked interest regarding the role of surgical intervention for patients with full-thickness and impending macular holes. In invoking a surgical intervention for any ocular disorder, several important factors should be considered. Firstly, an understanding of the pathogenesis of the condition is important. What are the pathophysiologic or pathoanatomic changes associated with the condition? Secondly, the natural history of the condition should be contemplated. Obviously conditions with a favorable long-term anatomic and visual outcome might not warrant surgical intervention. Thirdly, does the proposed surgical procedure alter the existing pathoanatomic or pathophysiologic processes? Fourthly, does the surgical intervention alter the natural history with regard to outcome? Fifthly, do the risks of surgery outweigh the potential benefits? Finally, are there alternative treatment modalities which might provide an equivalent or better result at less risk to the patient? In past years, a variety of non-surgical treatments have been offered to patients with idiopathic macular holes[4], however, the results have been in general equivocal or disappointing in altering the natural history of the disease. More recent studies[16-19] suggest a role for vitreous surgery using modern vitreoretinal techniques. These clinical stu-

Supported in part by Core Grant EY01931-15 from the National Eye Institute/NIH, Bethesda, MD, and an unrestricted grant from Research to Prevent Blindness, Inc., New York, NY

Address for correspondence: Gary W. Abrams, MD, Eye Institute, 8700 W. Wisconsin Avenue, Milwaukee, WI 53226, USA

Retina and Vitreous, pp. 163-172
Proceedings of the Symposium on Retina and Vitreous,
organized by the New Orleans Academy of Ophthalmology
New Orleans, LA, USA, March 12-15, 1992
edited by Rudolph M. Franklin

dies, while providing encouraging results, are mostly non-randomized and lack standardized pre- and postoperative visual acuity assessment, thus making interpretation of results difficult.

In this report, the role of vitreous surgery for patients with macular holes and impending macular holes is examined. The surgical goals and results of early pilot studies are reviewed. The importance of obtaining standardized visual acuity measurements both pre- and postoperatively in patients with this localized macular pathology is emphasized.

Etiology, pathogenesis and stages of hole formation

A role for the vitreous in macular hole formation has long been postulated[15]. An ever-growing body of information lends support to this claim[1,15,21-23]. In 1909, Zentmayer[20] first described the presence of connective tissue proliferation at the edges of a macular hole. Others have documented the presence of these vitreomacular membranes in patients with macular holes[23,24]. More recently, additional support for the role of vitreomacular traction, either tangential[4,5,17,18,25,26], anteroposterior[4,5,9,18,21,22], or a combination[4,18] has been garnered. Tangential vitreomacular traction was detected at the time of surgery in 73% of eyes undergoing vitrectomy for vitreomacular traction syndrome[18]. Gass has postulated that focal shrinkage of the vitreous cortex in the foveal region with exertion of tangential vitreomacular traction is a pathogenic feature of macular hole formation[4,25].

Stages of hole formation

Until recently, much confusion existed in the ophthalmic literature regarding the classification or staging of macular holes. As Gass has pointed out, several clinical conditions including pseudoholes and inner lamellar holes may be confused with the early stages of idiopathic macular hole formation[27]. In 1988, based on his clinical observations and a review of patient records, he described the distinctive clinical features, and the evolution of the clinical stages of macular hole formation. The earliest stage, stage 1A, was characterized clinically by a yellowish spot measuring 250-300 μm with some loss of the normal foveal depression. In his series 55% of patients with this finding complained of metamorphopsia or decrease in vision. The enlargement of this yellow spot, appearance of a yellow halo, and additional loss of the foveal depression was classified as stage 1B. Stage 2 was marked by early central or eccentric hole formation associated with a grayish halo of marginal detachment of the sensory retina, and the absence of a posterior vitreous separation. Approximately 90% of these patients in Gass' series were symptomatic. Circumferential enlargement of the hole with a vitreofoveal separation, and frequent association of an overlying operculum was termed stage 3. Complete posterior vitreous separation in association with a full-thickness hole was designated as a stage 4 lesion.

In addition to these descriptive features several additional points regarding the presentation and natural history of this condition are noteworthy. First, 66% of patients with stage 1 lesions progressed to full-thickness macular hole formation over weeks to months[25]. Consequently, if a high risk group of patients with these characteristics could be reliably identified, they may benefit from interventional therapy. It has been suggested that patients with a full-thickness hole in one eye and a symptomatic stage 1 lesion in the fellow eye may be at high risk for progression to full-thickness hole formation[25]. Others have reported that patients with cystic retinal changes[2,3], retinal pigment epithelial abnormalities[3], and involutional macular thinning[5,6] may have upwards of a 50% risk of full-thickness macular hole formation. Another important point with potential implications for surgical intervention is that in Gass' series 68% of full-thickness macular holes had no posterior vitreous separation. The presence of a posterior vitreous separation is thought to be protective against subsequent macular hole formation[4,6]. In addition, 30% of these eyes had an associated epiretinal membrane. This latter figure is in agreement with a report by Morgan and Schatz who noted epiretinal membrane formation clinically in 25% of their patients with macular holes[9]. Histopathologic evidence has been garnered which supports the hypothesis of tangential retinal traction, and an incidence of epiretinal membrane formation of as high as 73% in eyes with macular holes[23].

Goals of surgery/surgical techniques

The strong evidence implicating vitreous tractional forces in the pathogenesis of macular hole formation has sparked interest in the potential role of vitreous microsurgical techniques in the management of this disorder. The central questions are:
1. does release of vitreous tractional forces in patients with stage 1 lesions abort progression to full-thickness macular hole formation? and
2. in patients with stage 3 or 4 lesions, does vitrectomy with release of vitreous traction and presumed closure of the retinal defect allow for resolution of the associated neurosensory detachment and improvement in the visual outcome of these patients?

The primary goal of vitreous surgery in this disorder is to relieve vitreomacular traction. In patients with stage 1 lesions, this might allow for foveal re-attachment. A number of surgical techniques used in the vitreous surgery of other tractional disorders might be employed. Surgical separation of the posterior hyaloid using a needle, a soft-tip extrusion device or a barbed microvitreoretinal blade may be carried out as described by Han *et al.*[28]. We have found the soft-tip extrusion method safe and effective in separation of the posterior hyaloid in patients with macular pathology (Fig. 1). In a series of 106 patients considered to be at risk for idiopathic macular hole formation, Margherio *et al.*[18] performed pars plana vitrectomy, and described a "can opener" technique using a bent 23-gauge needle first to circumcise the fovea of these patients. Dissection of membranes was

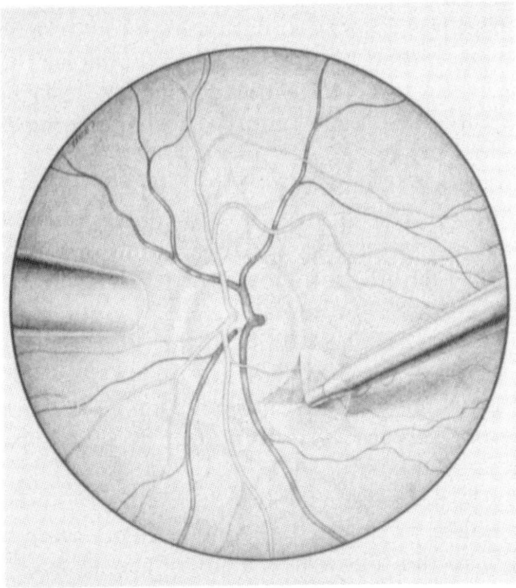

Fig. 1. Surgeon's view of left eye showing aspiration and elevation of posterior hyaloid at disc margin with tapered extrusion needle attached to linear suction. Papillomacular bundle, retinal vasculature, and disc itself are avoided with needle tip. (Reprinted with permission from Han DP, Abrams GW, Aaberg TM: Surgical excision of the attached posterior hyaloid. Arch Ophthalmol 106:998-1000, 1988.)

then carried out towards the fovea, with the membranes cut with intravitreal scissors close to the fovea. The authors proposed that such a technique would be less likely to promote macular hole formation than peeling of membranes over the fovea. Regardless of the technique used, the macular pathology should probably be addressed early in the surgical procedure to maximize the surgeon's visualization and minimize vitreous manipulation prior to separation of the posterior hyaloid. With these methodological approaches and careful attention to the vitreoretinal anatomy intraoperatively, successful separation of the posterior hyaloid and cortical vitreous remnants may be achieved using these techniques. Careful biomicroscopic examination of the patient within a 24-hour time period prior to surgery should be carried out to re-assess the vitreoretinal anatomy. This is particularly important in patients undergoing surgery for stage 1 lesions where spontaneous separation of the posterior vitreous may obviate the need for surgical intervention.

In patients with stage 3 or 4 lesions, the goals of surgery may be multiple. These lesions are characterized by a central, full-thickness retinal defect of approximately 485 μm with usually an associated neurosensory retinal detachment. In these patients, relief of vitreous traction, removal of any associated epiretinal membranes, and closure of the retinal defect by the use of intraoperative and postoperative tamponading agents may all be important. The removal of any associated epiretinal membranes may be important as persistent membranes may allow for continued traction, eversion of the edges of the macular hole, and persistence of the surrounding neurosensory detachment postoperatively. Others have suggested the intraoperative use of laser photocoagulation[29] or tissue adhesives[30] which have been used to treat macular holes associated with more extensive retinal detachments. However, at this time there is insufficient clinical data to support such recommendations for patients with idiopathic macular holes.

Results of surgery

High risk and impending macular holes

Previously described findings associated with a high risk of macular hole formation include cystic retinal changes, retinal pigment epithelial abnormalities, involutional macular thinning, and symptomatic stage 1 macular lesions as described by Gass. Electroretinographic abnormalities have also been reported to have some predictive value in eyes at risk for macular hole formation[31].

Several studies have reported the use of vitrectomy techniques to prevent macular hole formation in eyes thought to be at high risk[17-19]. In 1988, Smiddy *et al.*[17] reported on 15 high-risk patients undergoing vitrectomy for impending macular holes. Twelve of these patients had an idiopathic hole in the fellow eye with visual decrease in the range of 20/100 to 20/400. All eyes were symptomatic with preoperative vision in the involved eye ranging from 20/20 to 20/70. The details of the surgical procedures used were not reported, however, the authors reported that macular holes subsequently developed in only three eyes (20%) and visual acuity as measured on a Snellen acuity chart, was stable or improved in 12/15 eyes. Decreased vision in three eyes postoperatively was attributed to development of nuclear sclerosis.

A subsequent study by Jost *et al.*[19] in 1990 reported on 15 eyes undergoing vitrectomy for impending macular holes. In this series, nine patients were noted preoperatively to have a full-thickness hole in the fellow eye. Four of the 15 eyes undergoing vitrectomy for impending macular holes were noted to have small, full-thickness foveal defects (stage 2 lesions) intraoperatively. In none of the 15 eyes was there preoperative or intraoperative evidence of a posterior vitreous detachment. Eleven patients were noted to have tangential vitreoretinal traction, and three eyes were noted to have anteroposterior traction. With a median follow-up of 18 months, only one of 11 eyes with a stage 1 lesion progressed to full-thickness macular hole formation. Two of the four eyes operated on with stage 2 lesions progressed to stage 3 macular holes. All 12 eyes that did not progress to macular hole formation were reported to experience a significant improvement in vision, with 58% of eyes attaining a visual acuity of 20/25 or better. They also reported that postoperative foveal electroretinogram amplitudes were higher than preoperative measurements in five of six eyes tested. Apparent resolution of the foveal lesion with stabilization or improvement of vision may be noted in some patients following vitrectomy (Fig. 2).

Other studies have addressed the role of vitrectomy in eyes with various forms of vitreomacular traction. In a series of 106 symptomatic patients undergoing vitrectomy for premacular hole conditions and various forms of vitreomacular traction syndromes, a 2% incidence of macular hole formation was reported[18]. The status of fellow eyes in this series was not provided. The authors believed that macular hole formation in these two eyes

A

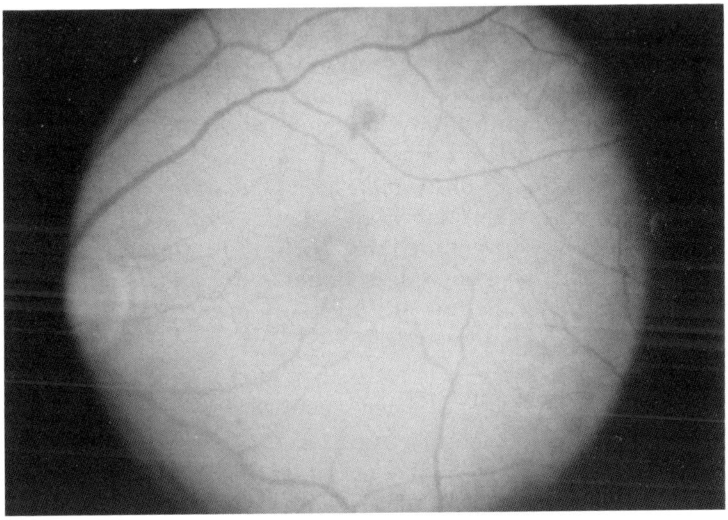

B

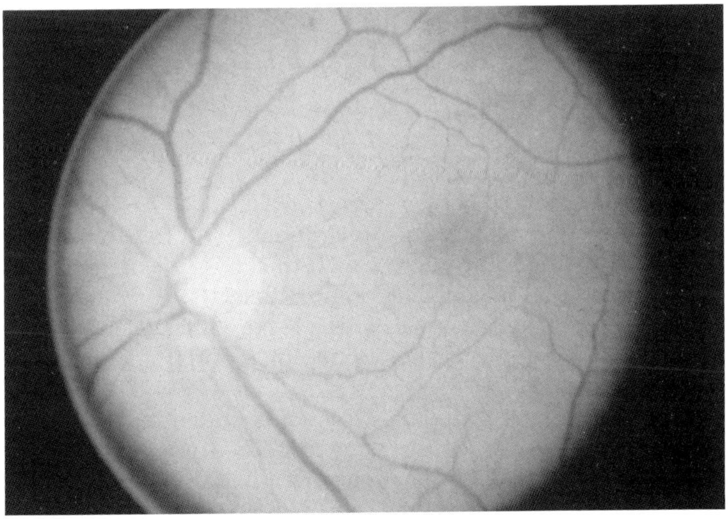

Fig. 2A. This 81-year-old woman with metamorphopsia and visual acuity of 20/25 underwent vitrectomy for stage 1B macular hole. *B.* Postoperatively the lesion has resolved, the patient is less symptomatic, and visual acuity remains 20/25. (Photograph courtesy of William F. Mieler, MD.)

might have been averted had their "can opener" surgical technique used in latter cases in this series been employed in the two earlier cases with subsequent macular hole formation. Visual acuity improved in 89% of patients, was unchanged in 7% and decreased in 4%. Acceleration of nuclear sclerosis developed in 16% over an average follow-up period of 35 months. Retinal detachments and macular epiretinal membranes occurred in 2% of patients postoperatively. Smiddy *et al.* also reported on a group of 15 patients undergoing vitrectomy for a vitreomacular traction syndrome characterized by cystic macular changes, a dumbbell-shaped area of vitreous attachment to the optic disc and macula, and partial posterior vitreous detachment. All patients had symptomatic decrease in vision, most often to the level of 20/200. Vitrectomy techniques used to relieve anteroposterior vitreous traction resulted in a stabilization of Snellen visual acuity in six eyes and improvement of visual acuity in ten eyes. Nuclear sclerosis developed in five of 15 eyes postoperatively. This subpopulation of patients is thought to represent a specific vitreomacular traction syndrome distinct from patients with stage 1 macular holes[24]. However, the natural history of this vitreomacular tractional syndrome is not fully known.

Although the results of these studies are encouraging, several significant weaknesses are evident. These studies all lack randomization with appropriate control groups. Additionally, in none of the above studies was a standardized visual acuity with refraction (as per the Macular Photocoagulation Study, or the Early Treatment Diabetic Retinopathy Study protocol) obtained. Interpretation of visual outcome is therefore difficult. Nonetheless, the anatomic results (absence of macular hole formation) cannot be disputed. However, it is still unclear exactly what percentage of eyes with stage 1 lesions go onto hole formation. These pilot studies have added useful clinical information regarding management of these patients, and have served as impetus for organization of a randomized clinical trial to further evaluate the role of vitrectomy in these patients. Such a study has already been proposed and is underway[32].

Table 1. Visual acuity and potential acuity meter readings with documented full-thickness macular holes

Patient	*Snellen visual acuity*	*MPS* visual acuity*	*Potential acuity meter*
1	20/400	20/63	20/80
2	20/200	20/80	20/200
3	20/100	20/63	20/70

*Macular Photocoagulation Study protocol. Note discrepancies between Snellen visual acuity and standardized visual acuity measurements using the MPS protocol

Results of vitrectomy for full-thickness macular holes

The role of vitrectomy in the management of patients with full-thickness macular holes has been the subject of much recent interest. Full-thickness macular holes (stages 3 or 4) are usually characterized by a full-thickness retinal defect, a surrounding cuff of subretinal fluid, and a permanent visual decrease to the level of 20/200. Although traditionally these eyes have been considered untreatable, recent reports have suggested vitrectomy might be beneficial[16,33,34].

In 1991, Kelly and Wendel[16] reported on 52 patients undergoing vitrectomy for stage 3 or 4 macular holes. Snellen visual acuities were measured preoperatively and postoperatively using the refraction provided by the referring physician. Intraoperatively, adherent cortical vitreous and epiretinal membranes were removed and a total fluid-gas exchange performed, leaving sulfur hexafluoride in the eyes. Patients were kept in a prone position postoperatively while the gas bubble tamponaded the macular hole. The authors reported an anatomic success (foveal re-attachment) in 30 (52%) patients. Of these patients, 73%

achieved an improvement in visual acuity of two lines or better. Overall, 42% of patients had an improvement in visual acuity postoperatively. No predictive factors for anatomic failure were identified in the 48% of patients who failed surgery. Other small series have reported improved anatomic success and visual improvement in patients undergoing vitrectomy for stage 3 and 4 macular holes. Glaser *et al.*[34] presented preliminary data on the intraoperative adjunctive use of transforming growth factor-β (TGF-β) in 12 eyes undergoing vitrectomy for full-thickness macular holes. This growth factor is thought to stimulate fibroglial proliferation with closure of the retinal defect. They reported foveal re-attachment in seven eyes, and an improvement in visual acuity in five eyes using these methods.

The mechanisms whereby vitrectomy surgery might improve visual acuity in patients with full-thickness macular holes are unknown. It has been postulated that closure of the retinal defect with resolution of the surrounding subretinal fluid might allow for some return of vision in the previously detached fovea[16]. Yet others believe that an eccentric location of the macular hole in some patients might explain the improvement in postoperative visual results[35]. Additionally, it has been suggested that the size of the macular hole may be much smaller than apparent preoperatively[33]. The presence of vitreous traction, associated epiretinal membranes[36], and subretinal fluid may exert forces which allow the retinal hole to gape more than the actual anatomic defect. With release of these forces the anatomic integrity of the retina may be restored with the presence of a much smaller defect. Although histologic studies demonstrate a full-thickness defect, the apparent postoperative disappearance of the retinal defect reported in some patients[36] might be explained by the above. However, we are not aware of published histopathologic studies of eyes previously undergoing vitrectomy for macular holes.

Randomized studies assessing the role of vitrectomy with or without surgical adhesives or biologically active adjuncts in eyes with stage 3 or 4 macular holes are lacking. Again, major pitfalls in all previous studies are the absence of randomization and the lack of standardized pre- and postoperative visual acuity assessment. Further to evaluate and demonstrate the importance of this point, we examined three patients with documented stage 3 or 4 macular holes. Visual acuities were obtained by a trained technician using standard Snellen acuity charts, visual acuity with refraction (and encouragement) as per the Macular Photocoagulation Study protocol, and the potential acuity meter (PAM). These findings illustrate the paramount importance of obtaining standardized visual acuity assessment in patients with macular pathology. Because of the wide disparity in visual acuities measured by the two techniques, there is a significant potential for bias towards better postoperative visual acuities in patients who "try harder" to see following surgery. This is particularly significant since the primary measure of surgical success is the patient's visual outcome.

Complications of surgery for macular holes

The natural history of a macular hole rarely leads to a visual acuity of worse than 20/400. The possibility of surgical complications with a worse visual result must be considered. We have observed phototoxic maculopathy in an eye undergoing surgery for an impending macular hole with diminution of visual acuity from 20/40 preoperatively to 20/200 postoperatively (Fig. 3). Postoperative macular pigment abnormalities possibly due to a phototoxic mechanism have been reported by others[16,37]. In addition, we are aware of two eyes which underwent surgery for stage 3 macular holes which developed postoperative retinal detachments, one with proliferative vitreoretinopathy, and one with a giant retinal tear. There is risk of intraoperative or postoperative progression of a stage 1 impending hole to a full-thickness hole[17].

A

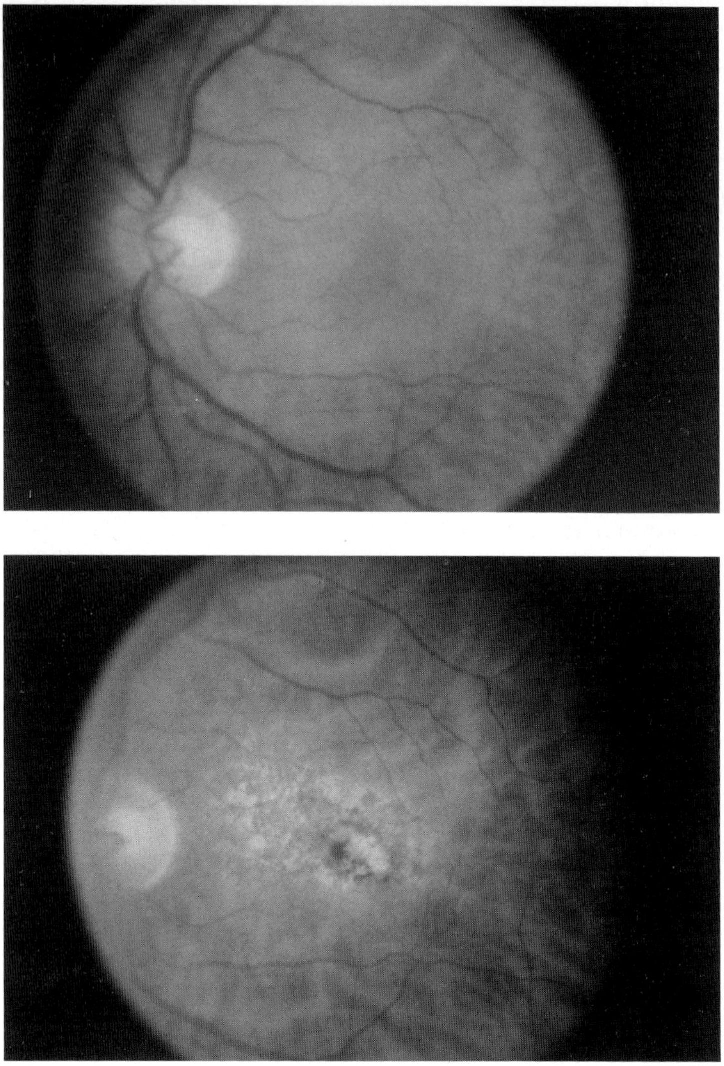

B

Fig. 3A. Stage 1B macular hole in a 60-year-old woman. visual acuity was 20/40. *B.* One month postoperatively, visual acuity was 20/200 with marked macular pigmentary abnormalities.

Summary and conclusions

In summary, our recent increased understanding of the pathogenesis, stages, and natural history of idiopathic macular holes have stimulated interest in the use of modern microsurgical techniques in an attempt to alter the natural history of this disease process. In patients with stage 1 lesions, or patients with retinal findings considered to be at risk for full-thickness macular hole, several early, non-randomized pilot studies have suggested that vitrectomy may be beneficial in reducing the risk of subsequent hole formation. By removing or relieving tractional forces, vitrectomy may allow for foveal re-attachment and stabilization or improvement in vision. However, the benefit of surgery over the natural history of these stage 1 lesions untreated is still not clear. Therefore, a randomized clinical trial of surgery for impending macular holes is currently underway.

In patients with full-thickness, stage 3 or 4 macular holes the role of vitrectomy is even less clearly delineated. Although vitrectomy techniques may be used for release of residual vitreous traction, removal of epiretinal membranes with perhaps closure of the retinal defect and resolution of the surrounding neurosensory detachment, the results on visual acuity are less clear. However, preliminary studies, despite their weaknesses, suggest that surgical intervention may be beneficial in some cases. Currently a prospective, randomized clinical trial is underway to assess the role of vitrectomy with retinal tamponade using intraocular gas on the anatomic and visual outcomes in these patients. The critical assessment of pre- and postoperative visual acuities using Snellen visual acuity, standardized refraction using the Macular Photocoagulation Study protocol, and the potential acuity meter which has been proposed for use in this study, will hopefully allow for more accurate interpretation of visual outcomes. These prospective studies should provide us with additional information regarding the natural history and management options in patients with this unfortunate condition.

References

1. Gass JDM: Stereoscopic Atlas of Macular Diseases: Diagnosis and Treatment, 3rd edn, pp 684-693. St Louis: CV Mosby Co 1987
2. McDonnell PJ, Fine SL, Hillis AI: Clinical features of idiopathic macular cysts and holes. Am J Ophthalmol 93:777-786, 1982
3. Bronstein MA, Trempe CL, Freeman HM: Fellow eyes with macular holes. Am J Ophthalmol 92:757-761, 1981
4. Aaberg TM: Macular holes: a review. Surv Ophthalmol 15:139-162, 1970
5. Morgan CM, Schatz H: Involutional macular thinning: a premacular hole condition. Ophthalmology 93:153-161, 1986
6. Trempe CL, Weiter JJ, Furukawa H: Fellow eyes in cases of macular hole: biomicroscopic study of the vitreous. Arch Ophthalmol 104:93-95, 1986
7. Frangieh GT, Green WR, Engel HM: A histopathologic study of macular cysts and holes. Retina 1:311-336, 1981
8. Margherio RR, Schepens CL: Macular breaks: I. Diagnosis, etiology, and observations. Am J Ophthalmol 74:219-232, 1972
9. Morgan CM, Schatz H: Idiopathic macular holes. Am J Ophthalmol 99:437-444, 1985
10. James M, Feman SS: Macular holes. Graefe's Arch Klin Exp Ophthalmol 215:59-63, 1980
11. Hirokawa H, Jalkh AE, Takahashi M et al: Role of the vitreous in idiopathic preretinal macular fibrosis. Am J Ophthalmol 101:166-169, 1986
12. Smiddy WE, Michels RG, Glaser BM, De Bustros S: Vitrectomy for macular traction caused by incomplete vitreous separation. Arch Ophthalmol 106:624-628, 1988
13. Tolentino FI, Schepens CL: Edema of the posterior pole after cataract extraction: a biomicroscopic study. Arch Ophthalmol 74:781-786, 1965
14. Jaffe NS: Vitreous traction at the posterior pole of the fundus due to alterations in the vitreous posterior. Trans Am Acad Ophthalmol Otolaryngol 71:642-652, 1967
15. Lister W: Holes in the retina and their clinical significance. Br J Ophthalmol 8:1-20, 1924
16. Kelly NE, Wendel RT: Vitreous surgery for idiopathic macular holes: results of a pilot study. Arch Ophthalmol 109:654-659, 1991
17. Smiddy WE, Michels RG, Glaser BM, De Bustros S: Vitrectomy for impending idiopathic macular holes. Am J Ophthalmol 105:371-376, 1988
18. Margherio RR, Trese MT, Margherio AR, Cartright K: Surgical management of vitreomacular traction syndromes. Ophthalmology 96:1437-1445, 1989
19. Jost BF, Hutton WL, Fuller DG et al: Vitrectomy in eyes at risk for macular hole formation. Ophthalmology 97:843-847, 1990
20. Zentmayer W: Hole at the macula. Ophthalmol Rec 18:198-200, 1909
21. Schepens CL: Fundus changes caused by alterations of the vitreous body. Am J Ophthalmol 39:631-633, 1955
22. Avila MP, Jalkh AE, Murakami K et al: Biomicroscopic study of the vitreous in macular breaks. Ophthalmology 90:1277-1283, 1983

23. Guyer DR, Green WR, De Bustros S, Fine SL: Histopathologic features of idiopathic macular holes and cysts. Ophthalmology 97:1045-1051, 1990
24. Smiddy WE, Michels RG, Green WR: Morphology, pathology, and surgery of idiopathic vitreoretinal disorders: a review. Retina 10:288-296, 1990
25. Gass JDM: Idiopathic senile macular hole: its early stages and pathogenesis. Arch Ophthalmol 106:629-639, 1988
26. Johnson RN, Gass JDM: Idiopathic macular holes: observation, stages of formation, and implications for surgical intervention. Ophthalmology 95:917-924, 1988
27. Gass JDM, Joondeph BC: Observations concerning patients with suspected impending macular holes. Am J Ophthalmol 109:638-646, 1990
28. Han DP, Abrams GW, Aaberg TM: Surgical excision of the attached posterior hyaloid. Arch Ophthalmol 106:998-1000, 1988
29. Schocket SS, Lakhanpal V, Xiaoping M, Kelman S, Billings E: Laser treatment of macular holes. Ophthalmology 95:574-582, 1988
30. Sheta SM, Hida T, McCuen BW: Cyanoacrylate tissue adhesive in the management of recurrent retinal detachment caused by macular holes. Am J Ophthalmol 109:28-32, 1990
31. Birch DG, Jost BF, Fish GE: The focal electroretinogram in fellow eyes of patients with idiopathic macular holes. Arch Ophthalmol 106:1558-1563, 1988
32. De Bustros S: Early stages of macular holes: to treat or not to treat. Arch Ophthalmol 108:1085, 1990
33. Geiger GL: Surgical management of macular holes. Media Guide to Special Problems in Ophthalmology 1:1-4, 1991
34. Glaser BM, Sjaarda RN, Kuppermann BD, Pena PA, Michels RG: Transforming growth factor-beta in the treatment of full thickness macular holes. Ophthalmology (Suppl) 98:145, 1991
35. Bidwell AE, Jampol LM, Goldberg MF: Macular holes and excellent visual acuity (Letter). Arch Ophthalmol 106:1350-1351, 1988
36. Lewis H, Cowan GM, Straatsma BR: Apparent disappearance of a macular hole associated with development of an epiretinal membrane. Am J Ophthalmol 102:172-175, 1986
37. Poliner LS, Tornambe PE: Retinal pigment epitheliopathy following macular hole surgery. Invest Ophthalmol Vis Sci (Suppl) 32:685, 1991

MACULAR HOLE SURGERY

Stuart L. Fine

Department of Ophthalmology, Scheie Eye Institute, Philadelphia, Pennsylvania, USA

Macular hole affects approximately 100,000 people in the United States over the age of 55. According to the Baltimore Eye Survey, the prevalence is 3.3 per 1000[1]. As a cause of vision loss in people over 55, macular hole compares in frequency with both diabetic retinopathy and glaucoma. Eighty percent of those affected are women, the average age is 70, and both Caucasians and African-Americans are affected. With such a high prevalence, there should be nearly incontrovertible data before making any therapeutic recommendations.

Several retrospective studies have shown that the majority of macular hole patients maintain acuity in the range of 20/80 to 20/200 and that fellow eyes are involved, on average, in only 10% of patients. In one report of patients with unilateral macular hole and a normal fellow eye, there was only a 1% risk of the second eye developing a hole over the next five years[2]. So, in most patients, macular hole is unilateral, and the visual acuity probably will remain good in the fellow eye.

Three years ago, Kelly presented the first results of vitreous surgery for macular hole[3]. Of 52 patients operated on, the hole was closed in 30. Forty-two of the patients experienced some improvement in vision, but only 20% improved to 20/40. In discussing that paper and in a subsequent editorial, the author stated that since macular hole was unilateral in approximately 90% of patients, perhaps only 2% of patients actually achieved a better quality of life in the operated eye[4].

There was new information about macular hole surgery presented at the 1992 annual meeting of the American Academy of Ophthalmology[5-7]. Each study had well-defined entrance criteria, employed a standardized operation performed by experienced surgeons, and had relatively complete follow-up information. However, there was only short-term follow-up and sparse data on complications.

In the years since the initial report by Kelly and Wendel, it appears that progress is being made. The following statements probably are true. Closed holes probably have better acuity, at least within the first six months after surgery[6,7]. Surgery probably does increase the likelihood of closure. Application of TGF-Beta 2 probably does increase the surgical success rate in operated eyes in which no epiretinal membrane dissection is performed; however, it may not be advantageous if all tangential traction can be removed surgically. And finally, the duration of symptoms may influence the final visual outcome. What we need, however, are standardized outcome measures and frequency of complica-

This discussion was presented in part at the Annual Meeting of the American Academy of Ophthalmology in Dallas, Texas on November 5, 1992. It is printed with permission of the American Academy of Ophthalmology. Portions of this discussion will appear in *Ophthalmology* in June, 1993

Address for correspondence: Stuart L. Fine, M.D., Department of Ophthalmology, University of Pennsylvania, Scheie Eye Institute, Myrin Circle, 51 North 39th Street, Philadelphia, PA 19104, USA

Retina and Vitreous, pp. 173-174
Proceedings of the Symposium on Retina and Vitreous,
organized by the New Orleans Academy of Ophthalmology
New Orleans, LA, USA, March 12-15, 1992
edited by Rudolph M. Franklin

tions at six month intervals for three to five years. What is the likelihood of a cataract developing one to two years after macular hole surgery which requires another operation? What is the visual outcome one year after the cataract surgery? If there were cystoid macular edema after IOL surgery, and if there were phototoxic pigment epitheliopathy during both procedures, will the combination reduce the acuity in two to three years even though the hole is closed? What is the frequency of retinal detachment, long term? What are the prognostic risk factors that determine visual outcome? These factors might include duration of symptoms, initial acuity, size of the hole, amount of subretinal fluid, stage of the hole, and fluorescein angiographic features. And finally, what is the likelihood of restoring, in the operated eye, vision which is sufficient for reading and driving in a monocular patient?

The majority of patients with macular hole have a normal fellow eye which will not be involved with significant pathology over the next five years. The average age of these patients is nearly 70. They may pay a significant price for partial restoration of vision for a generally monocular condition. The potential benefits after successful surgery are improved distance vision, reading vision, functional vision, and quality of life, but the costs are substantial: Seven to ten postoperative days in a face-down position, anxiety about the outcome, postoperative discomfort, anxiety about the risk of a second procedure, and up to US$ 20,000 in professional and hospital fees for two surgical procedures.

For all these reasons, the author believes that it is now appropriate to conduct a randomized trial to evaluate the role of vitreous surgery for macular holes. Only when such a trial is completed can we be comfortable recommending therapy with the same degree of confidence as is true for our patients with diabetic retinopathy, branch retinal vein occlusion, and other conditions for which randomized trials have been completed. Fortunately, one multi-center trial has been enrolling patients for more than one year, while another trial has completed the pilot phase and is awaiting funding. Thus, in time, we shall have the information we need to advise our patients properly. Until then, caution is advisable especially for the patient with unilateral macular hole and a normal fellow eye. And finally, consider this question: Would you recommend cataract surgery for a 70 year old with a good fellow eye if you expected an average visual improvement of two lines on the Snellen chart? Q. E. D.

References

1. Tielsch J: Data from fundus photograph grading of 2732 participants in the Baltimore Eye Survey. Personal communication, November 4, 1992
2. Guyer DR, DeBustros S, Diener-West M, Fine SL: Observations on patients with idiopathic macular holes and cysts. Arch Ophthalmol 110:1264-1268, September 1992
3. Kelly NE, Wendel RT: Vitreous surgery for idiopathic macular holes: results of a pilot study. Arch Ophthalmol 109:654-659, 1991
4. Fine SL: Editorial: Vitreous surgery for macular hole in perspective: is there an indication? Arch Ophthalmol 109:635-636, May 1991
5. Wendel RT, Patel AC, Kelly NE, Salzano TC: Macular hole surgery. Presented at the Annual Meeting of the American Academy of Ophthalmology, Dallas, Texas, November 5, 1992
6. Smiddy WE, Glaser BM, Thompson JD, Sjaarda RM, Flynn HW Jr, Hanham A, Murphy RP: Transforming growth factor-beta 2 significantly enhances the ability to flatten the rim of subretinal fluid surrounding macular holes: preliminary results of a multi-center prospective randomized study. Presented at the Annual Meeting of the American Academy of Ophthalmology, Dallas, Texas, November 5, 1992
7. Lansing MB, Glaser BM, Liss H, Hanham A, Thompson JT, Sjaarda RM, Gordon AJ: The effect of pars plana vitrectomy and transforming growth factor beta-2 without epiretinal membrane peeling on full thickness macular holes. Presented at the Annual Meeting of the American Academy of Ophthalmology, Dallas, Texas, November 5, 1992

IV

CHOROIDAL MELANOMA

MANAGEMENT OF PATIENTS WITH CHOROIDAL AND CILIARY BODY MELANOMAS

J. Donald M. Gass

Bascom Palmer Eye Institute, University of Miami School of Medicine, Miami, Florida, USA

Clinical history, external, biomicroscopic, and indirect ophthalmoscopic examinations are most important in determining whether a tumor is a malignant melanoma, a benign melanocytic tumor, or a mass simulating them. Special tests including fluorescein angiography and ultrasonography may provide helpful information in those cases where the diagnosis is uncertain. Radioactive phosphorous 32 has once again been largely abandoned because of the high incidence of false positive tests in those lesions that may simulate melanomas. Rarely it and other techniques, such as computerized tomography and magnetic resonance imaging, may provide some assistance in diagnosis, particularly in eyes with media that preclude visualization of the tumor. As a general rule, it is prudent to rely more heavily on your own observations than upon results of special investigations. Biopsy is rarely employed because:

1. the diagnosis is usually evident ophthalmoscopically and biomicroscopically;
2. a short period of observation of suspicious lesions permits evaluation of their growth potential;
3. difficulty of interpretation of needle biopsy particularly with regard to differentiation of benign from malignant melanocytic tumors; and
4. concern for extraocular spread of tumor during the course of biopsy.

This discussion will be limited primarily to the diagnosis and management of patients whose general medical work-up is negative for extraocular malignancy, and whose tumor is judged to be either a malignant melanoma or a melanocytic tumor of uncertain growth potential.

Symptoms and signs that indicate a likelihood of a malignant melanoma are: recent loss of vision and photopsia, a pigmented mass larger than 10 mm in diameter and 3 mm in height arising in the choroid, associated with derangement of the overlying retinal pigment epithelium, including clumping of orange pigment on its surface; extension of the tumor through Bruch's membrane in a mushroom configuration; exudative retinal detachment; fluorescein angiographic evidence of multiple pinpoint leaks on the tumor surface and evidence of intratumoral blood vessels near its inner surface; and low reflectivity ultrasonographically[1-3]. The more of these signs present, the higher the likelihood of a malignant melanoma. No one or a combination of several of these sign alone, however, is definite evidence of a malignant melanoma.

Signs that indicate low growth potential of a melanocytic tumor include: small diameter and low height; presence of multiple drusen on its surface or absence of overlying

Address for correspondence: J. Donald M. Gass, MD, Bascom Palmer Eye Institute, University of Miami School of Medicine, Miami, FL 33101, USA

Retina and Vitreous, pp. 177-179
Proceedings of the Symposium on Retina and Vitreous,
organized by the New Orleans Academy of Ophthalmology
New Orleans, LA, USA, March 12-15, 1992
edited by Rudolph M. Franklin

RPE changes, presence of adjacent zones of RPE atrophy and intraretinal migration of pigment surrounding the tumor, frequently at its inferior border; evidence of overlying subretinal neovascularization; and absence of exudative detachment of the retina. The presence of drusen on its surface is only significant if no drusen are present in the same area in the fellow eye. The presence of subretinal exudate is not necessarily of significance if other signs of low growth potential are present. Fluorescein angiography is helpful in the detection of subtle RPE changes caused by a large nevus. Ultrasonography is of minimal value in the differential diagnosis of small choroidal tumors.

Although the signs and symptoms outlined previously are helpful in predicting growth potential, there are important exceptions to the significance of individual signs. As in the case of cutaneous nevi, most melanocytic choroidal nevi are small but some may be similar in size to medium and large malignant melanomas[2]. In such cases, the absence of symptoms and the presence of other signs suggesting low growth potential should alert the clinician to this possibility. At the same time the presence of other signs ordinarily suggestive of high growth potential, such as a mushroom shape, may reflect only the end result of accelerated growth that occurred during the first decade of life and that terminated soon afterward, as is typical of nevi. Ultrasonographic and P^{32} findings in these large nevi may be identical to that of a malignant melanoma. Since the gross cytologic construction of a malignant melanoma and a large nevus is similar, it is unlikely that CT and MRI scans will prove helpful in the differential diagnosis.

In the management of patients with melanocytic lesions we should be mindful of the following:

1. melanomas display a wide range of growth rates and malignant potential;
2. each melanoma, however, has a marked tendency to grow at a constant rate;
3. there is in general a direct correlation between growth rate of melanomas and their malignant potential;
4. it is uncertain whether early treatment influences the risk of metastasis;
5. there is no evidence that observing tumors for evidence of growth potential poses a significant risk to the patient; and
6. the relative risks of metastasis for the various modes of treatment are unknown[3,4].

In the case of a patient with a small lesion and signs of low growth potential, photographic documentation of the tumor, reassurance of the patient, and follow-up are indicated. If this same patient has in addition a serous detachment of the macula, the follow-up should be more frequent. If the detachment persists for several months and the tumor shows no signs of growth, photocoagulation to the site of fluorescein angiographic leakage is helpful in restoring central acuity, while continuing to observe the patient[3,5]. I do not share the concern of Erie and co-workers that such treatment influences in any way the likelihood of the tumor growing or of added risk to the patient if such growth occurs[6]. I am concerned that failure to treat may result in permanent loss of central vision in these patients, some of whose tumors, in my experience, have failed to grow on follow-up.

Most patients with a small lesion showing more signs of growth potential and good visual function probably should also be followed for evidence of growth before recommending treatment. Ultrasonographic documentation of tumor height as well as stereoscopic fundus photographs are helpful in detection of growth.

I believe that patients with moderate and large tumors which are discovered on routine eye examination, which are not associated with exudative retinal detachment, and which show other signs of low growth potential, should also be followed for evidence of active growth before recommending treatment.

Patients whose tumors have demonstrated growth and those who present with medium-sized or large tumors with multiple other signs of high growth potential, are candidates for treatment. Many factors, including visual function of the affected and fellow eye, the patient's general health, and the size and location of the tumor will determine which treatment is best for the individual. Discussion of the treatment with the patient should include: our lack of knowledge concerning the relative safety of the various treatment options, the operative procedures and costs involved for each of the treatment options, their short- and long-term complications, and the frequency of follow-up required for each. During the course of a careful explanation of all the treatment options, the physician can usually sense, without having made any recommendations, whether the patient will choose enucleation *versus* one of the eye-preserving options.

References

1. Augsburger JJ, Schroeder RP, Territo C, Gamel JW, Shields JA: Clinical parameters predictive of enlargement of melanocytic choroidal lesions. Br J Ophthalmol 73:911-917, 1989
2. Gass JDM: Problems in the differential diagnosis of choroidal nevi and malignant melanomas. Trans Am Acad Ophthalmol 83:19, 1977
3. Gass JDM: Observation of suspected choroidal and ciliary body melanomas for evidence of growth prior to enucleation. Ophthalmology 87:523, 1980
4. Gass JDM: Comparison of uveal melanoma growth rates with mitotic index and mortality. Arch Ophthalmol 103:924, 1985
5. Folk JC, Weingeist TA, Coonan P, Blodi CF, Folberg R, Kimura AE: The treatment of serous macular detachment secondary to choroidal melanomas and nevi. Ophthalmology 96:547-551, 1989
6. Erie JC, Robertson DM, Mieler WM: Presumed small melanomas with serous macular detachments with and without surface laser photocoagulation treatment. Am J Ophthalmol 109:259-264, 1990

COMPLICATIONS OF ENUCLEATION SURGERY
COMS Report Number 2

Collaborative Ocular Melanoma Study Group*

Abstract

As of June 30, 1992, Collaborative Ocular Melanoma Study investigators had enucleated 981 eyes of patients with choroidal melanoma who had been enrolled in randomized clinical trials. This report summarizes the intraoperative and perioperative complications that had been observed. There were neither intraoperative or perioperative deaths nor cases of intraoperative rupture of the globe. Unanticipated extrascleral extension was found in 15 patients (1.5%). Potentially important anesthetic or cardiopulmonary problems occurred in nine patients (0.9%). Overall, the risk of any complication was quite low. Only 27 patients (2.8%) were reported to have had any complication.

Introduction

The Collaborative Ocular Melanoma Study (COMS) Group, consisting of ophthalmologists and other researchers in 43 clinical centers across North America, is investigating the relative benefits of radiation and enucleation for patients with choroidal melanoma in prospective randomized clinical trials. Relative survival benefit is being assessed for patients with medium sized tumors treated either with enucleation or radioactive ^{125}I plaque application. For patients with larger tumors, all eyes are enucleated, but half of the patients receive preoperative external beam radiation. As of June 30, 1992, 654 patients had been randomized in the medium tumor study of ^{125}I plaque *versus* enucleation and 687 patients had been randomized in the large tumor study comparing enucleation with and without preoperative external beam radiation. Combining the two trials, overall, approximately three out of four COMS patients have had an enucleation procedure.

Complications of enucleation surgery may be seen immediately (first 24 hours), early (first several weeks), or as late manifestations after surgery. Although these complications

Presented in part at the Annual Meeting of the American Academy of Ophthalmology, Anaheim, October, 1991

Support for COMS provided through cooperative agreements EYO6253, EYO6257, EYO6258, EYO6259, EYO6260, EYO6264, EYO6265, EYO6266, EYO6268, EYO6269, EYO627O, EYO6274, EYO6275, EYO6276, EYO6279, EYO628O, EYO6282, EYO6283, EYO6287, EYO6288, EYO6289, EYO6291, EYO6839, EYO6844, EYO6848, EYO6858, EYO6899, EYO6843 and EYO6284 with the National Eye Institute, National Institutes of Health

*Manuscript prepared for the Collaborative Ocular Melanoma Study (COMS) Group by Andrew P. Schachat, M.D., Jonathan J. Dutton, M.D., Barbara S. Hawkins, Ph.D., and Jeffrey A. Nerad, M.D.
A listing of the COMS Group at the end of this paper

Address for correspondence: Barbara S. Hawkins, COMS Coordinating Center, 9th Floor, 550 North Broadway, Baltimore, MD 21205, USA

Retina and Vitreous, pp. 181-190
Proceedings of the Symposium on Retina and Vitreous,
organized by the New Orleans Academy of Ophthalmology
New Orleans, LA, USA, March 12-15, 1992
edited by Rudolph M. Franklin

are well known and clearly described in the literature, their incidence has not been documented in a large series of patients. The most common medically significant early complications include systemic complications such as cardiovascular events and local surgical site problems such as rupture of the globe, infection, hemorrhage, and ocular implant extrusion. Later, cosmetic complications become more prominent. These may include enophthalmos, poor prosthetic motility, superior sulcus deformity, upper eyelid ptosis, loss of forniceal fixation, epithelial cysts, and late implant extrusion.

Little information exists in the literature regarding the operative complications of enucleation surgery. This report summarizes the experience of COMS investigators with immediate complications in a consecutive series of 981 enucleation surgeries performed for patients enrolled in COMS randomized trials during the first five years of the study. Future manuscripts will address such major issues as extrusion rates, motility and patient satisfaction.

Methods

The COMS protocol has been previously described[1]. The Manual of Procedures[2] and sample data collection forms[3] are available. Prior to enrollment, patients undergo detailed ophthalmic, photographic, echographic, and general medical evaluations. All patients gave written informed consent prior to randomization. Exclusion criteria are outlined in Table 1.

Table 1. Exclusion criteria for COMS randomized trials

Patient:	age <21
	any social, mental or physical condition that impairs ability to give consent or to return for follow-up
Tumor:	bilateral choroidal melanoma
	extrascleral extension greater than 2 mm
	diffuse, multifocal or "ring" melanoma
	involvement of one half or more of tumor with the ciliary body
	apical height <2.5 mm
Prior treatment:	use of immunosuppressive therapy
	previous treatment for ocular melanoma
	previous intervention for ocular conditions secondary to the tumor
	previous fine needle biopsy
Medical:	other known malignancy (other than carcinoma *in situ* of the uterine cervix or superficial non-melanotic skin cancers)
	co-existing disease likely to compromise survival
	contraindications to surgery, radiation therapy or general anesthesia

A standard, gentle enucleation procedure using general anesthesia is performed utilizing the following steps:

- 360 degree limbal peritomy
- inspection of quadrants for extraocular extension
- disinsertions of rectus muscles and sectioning of oblique muscles either before or after sectioning of optic nerve
- optic nerve sectioning, generally from a nasal approach, while proptosing globe anteriorly by traction or medial rectus stump
- non-metallic implant (hydroxyapatite implants permitted).

All COMS personnel, including the diagnosing ophthalmologist, echographer, and enucleating surgeon, are certified as knowledgeable and skilled in study procedures prior to examination and treatment of study patients. Data concerning complications noted at the time of surgery and during the immediate 24 hour postoperative period are recorded on a standard form and are entered in the central COMS database maintained at the COMS Coordinating Center in Baltimore, Maryland. Summaries of complication rates are reviewed periodically by the COMS Quality Assurance Committee, the participating ophthalmologists, and the Data and Safety Monitoring Committee.

Results

COMS investigators had reported data for 981 enucleations as of June 30, 1992, the cutoff date for data included in this report. Three hundred and fourteen enucleations were for medium sized tumors (height greater than 3 mm, less than 8 mm*, maximal basal dimension no larger than 16 mm) and 667 procedures for large tumors. Of the 981 enucleations, 777 (79.0%) were performed within two weeks of enrollment; the majority of those enucleations that took place more than two weeks after enrollment were in patients with large tumors who were assigned to preoperative radiation. As shown in Table 2, slightly more than half of all cases enucleated were male; almost all were non-Hispanic whites. Mean age at surgery was 60 years. Intraoperative complications are summarized in Table 3 by tumor size. Rates within the two size categories are similar. Patients with large tumors who had preoperative radiation were not at increased risk of complications.

Table 2. Demographic characteristics of patients

Characteristic	*Medium tumors*		*Large tumors*	
	No.	*(%)*	*No.*	*(%)*
Gender				
Male	156	(49.7)	389	(58.3)
Female	158	(50.3)	278	(41.7)
Race/Ethnicity				
White, not Hispanic	305	(97.1)	646	(96.8)
Hispanic	5	(1.6)	13	(2.2)
Black, not Hispanic	2	(0.6)	5	(0.7)
Asian or Pacific Islander	2	(0.6)	1	(0.1)
American Indian	0	(0.0)	2	(0.3)
Age, years				
<30	9	(2.9)	18	(2.7)
30-39	13	(4.1)	49	(7.3)
40-49	39	(12.4)	78	(11.7)
50-59	69	(22.0)	147	(22.0)
60-69	95	(30.3)	199	(29.8)
70-79	72	(22.9)	141	(21.1)
≥80	17	(5.4)	35	(5.2)
Total number of patients	314		667	

The most important complications associated with enucleation related to anesthesia and cardiopulmonary problems (Table 3). These complications were: transient postoperative pulmonary edema in one patient with pre-existing cardiac disease who had been approved for surgery by both cardiology and anesthesiology consultants; one patient with exacerbation of chronic obstructive pulmonary disease; four patients with transient hypertension, myocardial ischemia or arrhythmias requiring intraoperative medications; one patient each with blood aspiration during a difficult intubation who was kept in the hospital longer than the norm; acute postoperative urinary retention; and prolonged post-

*In 1991 the maximum allowed height for enrollment in the medium tumor protocol was increased from 8.0 mm to 10.0 mm and the minimum height was decreased to 2.5 mm.

Table 3. Frequency of complications

Type of complication	*Medium tumors* No.	(%)	*Large tumors* No.	(%)	*Total* No.	(%)	[95% CI]*
Anesthesia or cardiopulmonary	4	(1.3)	5	(0.7)	9	(0.9)	[0.4-1.7]
Surgical site							
Unanticipated extrascleral extension of more than 2 mm	2	(0.6)	13	(1.9)	15	(1.5)	[0.8-2.5]
Extrusion of implant	1	(0.3)	0	(0.0)	1	(0.1)	[0.0-0.6]
Marked conjunctival chemosis	1	(0.3)	0	(0.0)	1	(0.1)	[0.0-0.6]
Central dehiscence	1	(0.3)	0	(0.0)	1	(0.1)	[0.0-0.6]
Any surgical site complication	5	(1.6)	13	(1.9)	18	(1.8)	[1.1-2.9]
Any of above	9	(2.9)	18	(2.7)	27	(2.8)	[1.8-4.0]

*Approximate 95% confidence interval (CI) on percentage of enucleations with specified complication derived from Poisson distribution[12]

operative apnea which resolved spontaneously without sequelae.

An unusual amount of intraoperative orbital hemorrhage was reported for 15 cases (7 medium and 8 large). However, because minimum standards or definitions for reporting these observations have not been adopted by the COMS investigators, such observations are difficult to classify. Similarly, prolonged postoperative nausea or vomiting was noted in five cases (1 medium and 4 large), probably attributable to use of general anesthesia.

Discussion

The COMS group has chosen this time to report our observations concerning complications of enucleation surgery seen in a prospective series of nearly 1,000 patients because a very large number of procedures have been performed and the complication rates reported should be representative of the overall rates when recruitment is completed. As shown in Table 3, the 95% confidence intervals on the rates of complications are quite narrow as a result of the large number of cases. Data concerning the frequency of complications of enucleation surgery are of obvious value to ophthalmologists, their patients and to third parties such as insurance organizations, quality assurance and peer review organizations. As outlined in the methods section of this report, a straightforward enucleation procedure was selected by the COMS surgeons. Incorporation of uniform certification procedures assured that experienced surgeons performed the procedures. Using the COMS protocol, complications have been observed in less than three percent of enucleations.

The most important intraoperative events that might occur include death and major medical problems such as myocardial infarction or cerebrovascular accident. Fortunately, these events are rare; none occurred among the 981 cases enucleated to date in the COMS. It is unlikely that altering the surgical technique will alter perioperative death rates or major anesthetic or cardiovascular complication rates. Undoubtedly, exclusion of patients with medical problems who are unlikely to survive (exclusive of their melanoma) for at least five years, as prescribed by the COMS protocol, favorably influenced the major systemic complication rate.

The most important intraoperative local complications of enucleation surgery relate to the unanticipated discovery of extraocular tumor extension or rupture of the globe exposing the orbit to the tumor. Careful examination, including detailed echographic study, can identify those patients with gross extraocular extension preoperatively. Using the COMS protocol, which incorporates standardized A scan and contact B scan echography by certified examiners to complement expert ophthalmic examinations, less than 1% of medium tumor patients and 2% of large tumor patients thus far have had unanticipated gross extrascleral extension (Table 3). Among the 15 cases in which this complication occurred, the Echography Center graders had correctly designated one case of extrascleral extension based on the photoechograms submitted, had indicated possible extrascleral extension for seven cases, and had observed no evidence of extrascleral extension for six cases. One set of echograms had not yet been reviewed at the Echography Center. It is possible that these last six cases could have been diagnosed echographically during the dynamic examination but no extraocular tumor was visible on the polaroid photographs submitted to the Echography Center for review. Extraocular tumor may have been overlooked by the examiner and not photographed.

The rates of extraocular extension compare favorably with large pathology series where rates of extrascleral extension of 8-14% were seen[4]. In a report from the Mayo Clinic[5] extraocular extension was found in 50 (8.2%) of 610 patients, of whom 16 had only microscopic extraocular extension. The COMS protocol was designed to exclude patients with extrascleral extension greater than 2 mm, because, if gross extraocular tumor were noted preoperatively, a different treatment such as exenteration or enucleation and therapeutic postoperative radiation (not prophylactic preoperative radiation) might have been recommended. Rupture of the globe (including inadvertent cutting off of the back of the globe at the time of sectioning of the optic nerve) may relate to the surgical technique. This serious complication did not occur in our series.

There was only one report of early implant extrusion among 981 enucleations. Early extrusion of the ocular implant most commonly results from poor wound apposition[6] or wound tension from the use of an oversized implant[7]. A conformer that is too large may put excessive pressure on the fornices and pull the wound apart. Conjunctival epithelial ingrowth may result in orbital cyst formation[8] or epithelialization of the implant cavity and ultimate extrusion. Cyst formation may also be seen with infection, hemorrhage, and suture granuloma formation[9,10]. Excessive trauma to Tenon's capsule during closure can cause necrosis and wound dehiscence. Rates of implant extrusion and such important cosmetic issues as ptosis, superior sulcus deformity and prosthetic mobility will be subjects of reports dealing with long-term findings following enucleation surgery. This report has been restricted to intraoperative and perioperative complications.

Erie *et al.*[11] have reported that 17% of enucleations among the population of a defined community were attributed to intraocular tumor. The COMS experience has revealed that standard enucleation, using minimal manipulation among patients without major medical problems, has few immediate complications. Long-term postoperative complications and survival rates among COMS patients will be the subjects of future reports. The COMS Data and Safety Monitoring Committee reviews both data accumulated within the COMS and data externally generated at least twice each year to determine whether continued enrollment and randomization of patients is justified both scientifically and ethically. To date, this committee has not made a recommendation to stop patient accrual or randomization.

References

1. Schachat AP: Collaborative ocular melanoma study. In: Ryan SJ (ed) Retina 1, pp 733-736. St Louis: CV Mosby Co 1989
2. Collaborative Ocular Melanoma Study Group: COMS Manual of Procedures. Springfield, Virginia, National Technical Information Service, August 1, 1989, Accession # PB90-115536
3. Collaborative Ocular Melanoma Study Group: COMS Study Forms Book. Springfield, Virginia, National Technical Information Service, August 1, 1989, Accession # PB91-217315
4. Seddon IM, Egan KM, Gragoudas ES: Choroidal melanoma: prognosis. In: Ryan SJ (ed) Retina 1, pp 663-673. St Louis: CV Mosby Co 1989

5. Pach JM, Robertson DR, Taney BS, Martin JA, Campbell RI, O'Brien PC: Prognostic factors in choroidal and ciliary body melanomas with extrascleral extension. Am J Ophthalmol 101:325-331, 1986
6. Dryden R, Leibsohn J: Postenucleation orbital implant extrusion. Arch Ophthalmol 96:2064-2065, 1978
7. McGehee FO, Constance G: Complications of enucleation. In: Guibor P, Guibor M (eds) Complications of Enucleation, pp 215-217. New York: Stratton 1976
8. Hanig CJ, Hornblass A: Treatment of postenucleation orbital implant extrusion. Ann Ophthalmol 15:191-193, 1986
9. Siliquini JJ: Migration and extrusion of the implant. Int Ophthalmol Clin 10:843-849, 1970
10. Iliff CE: The extruded implant. Arch Ophthalmol 78:742-744, 1967
11. Erie JC, Nevitt MP, Hodge D, Ballard DJ: Incidence of enucleation in a defined population. Am J Ophthalmol 113:138-144, 1992
12. Beyer WH (ed): Standard Probability and Statistics Tables and Formulae. Boca Raton: CRC Press 1991
13. Collaborative Ocular Melanoma Study Group: Accuracy of diagnosis of choroidal melanoma in the Collaborative Ocular Melanoma Study. Arch Ophthalmol 108:1268-1273, 1990

COLLABORATIVE OCULAR MELANOMA STUDY GROUP

June 30, 1992

Participating Clinical Centers, Principal Investigators, Ophthalmic Surgeons, Clinic Coordinators, and Echographers are listed below. A complete listing of the Collaborative Ocular Melanoma Study Group has been published[13].

Kellogg Eye Center, Ann Arbor, MI – Andrew K. Vine, MD; Scott R. Sneed, MD; Susan G. Elner, MD; Bartley R. Frueh, MD; Mark W. Johnson, MD; Julie M. Willis, LPN, COMA; Kathleen A. Meyer, RDMS.

Emory Eye Center, Atlanta, GA – Paul Sternberg, MD; Thomas M. Aaberg, MD; Antonio Capone, MD; Ted H. Wojno, MD; Jayne M. Brown; Rhonda G. Waldron, COMT.

Piedmont Hospital, Atlanta, GA – William H. Jarrett, II, MD; William S. Hagler, MD; Jayne M. Brown; Rhonda G. Waldron, COMT.

Wilmer Institute, Baltimore, MD – Andrew P. Schachat, MD; Morton F. Goldberg, MD; Lenard H. Hammer, MD; Nicholas T. Iliff, M.D.; Marguerite Alexander, RN; Ellen F. Greenberg, COT; Cathy DiBernardo, RN.

Retina Associates of Cleveland, Beachwood, OH – Thomas A. Rice, MD; Michael A. Novak, MD; Lawrence J. Singerman, MD; Daniel Weidenthal, MD; Z. Nicholas Zakov, MD; Hernando Zegarra, MD; Mike Hartnett, COT; Susan E. Lichterman, RN; Pamela Rowe, CRA; Kelly Smith, COT.

Retina Associates, Inc., Boston, MA – Clement Trempe, MD; John Weiter, MD; Jay S. Duker, MD; Zena F. Nies; Fernando Acosta, MD; Alex Jalkh, MD.

University of Virginia, Charlottesville, VA – Brian P. Conway, MD; Marianne Cowley, MD; Mary J. Henofer, RN.

Northwestern University, Chicago, IL – Lee M. Jampol, MD; Robert Schroeder, MD; Mark Daily, MD; Richard G. Gieser, MD; David V. Weinberg, MD; Gail Daubert, RN; William Myers, MD.

University of Illinois, Chicago, IL – Norman P. Blair, MD; Kenneth I. Resnick, MD; Dorris Brown-Hutchins; Leonard Kut, MD.

Cleveland Clinic Foundation, Cleveland, OH – Froncie A. Gutman, MD; Umberto Albanese, MD; John V. Linberg, MD; Vivian Tanner, COT; LuAnne Sculley.

Ohio State University, Columbus, OH – Frederick H. Davidorf, MD; Robert B. Chambers, DO; Joseph J. Fammartino, MD; Susan E. Cornetet; Cynthia Taylor.

Texas Retina Associates, Dallas, TX – Dwain Fuller, MD; Gary Edd Fish, MD; William Snyder, MD; Theresa Anderson, Beth A. Pieczynski, COA; Randal Straach.

Porter Memorial Hospital, Denver, CO – Kenneth R. Hovland, MD; Douglas L. Holmes, MD; Stephen T. Petty, MD; John D. Zilis, MD; Richard O. Hammond, MD; Suzette Compton, RN; David Beers; Sandra R. Sall, AAS.

Duke Eye Center, Durham, NC – Jonathan J. Dutton, MD, PhD; Barbara A. Schuh, COT.

Hermann Eye Center, Houston, TX – Richard S. Ruiz, MD; Graham P. Avery, MD; William L. Decker, MD; Paul C. Salmonsen, MD; Robert Johnson, RDO, COA; Thomas C. Prager, PhD.

Midwest Eye Institute, Indianapolis, IN – John T. Minturn, MD; Ronald T. Martin, MD; William R. Nunery, MD; Donna Agugliaro, RN; Margaret Kirby, RN.

University of Iowa, Iowa City, IA – Thomas A. Weingeist, MD, PhD; Christopher F. Blodi, MD; Keith D. Carter, MD; Jeffrey A. Nerad, MD; Connie Fountain; Marcia Griffin; Tom Fisher; Karl C. Ossoinig, MD; Laura Warner.

Estelle Doheny Eye Foundation, Los Angeles, CA – A. Linn Murphree, MD; Donald Frambach, MD; A. Frances Walonker, CO, COMT; Ronald L. Green, MD.

Jules Stein Eye Institute, Los Angeles, CA – Bradley R. Straatsma, MD; Hector Sulit, MD; Robert Caldwell, PA; Barry Kerman, MD; Nancy London, COA; Joel N. Moral, COT; Ron Smith, COT.

University of Wisconsin, Madison, WI – Suresh R. Chandra, MD; Frank Myers, MD; Richard Dortzbach, MD; Bradley Lemke, MD; Betty Lewis; Margo Blatz; Thomas Stevens, MD.

North Shore University Hospital, Manhasset, NY – Samuel Packer, MD; Paul T. Finger, MD; Cynthia Pearlberg.

Bascom Palmer Eye Institute, Miami, FL – Timothy G. Murray, MD; Donald H. Nicholson, MD; Mary Lou Lewis, MD; Patrick E. Rubsamen, MD; Leonard Berg, MD; Harold J. Berger, MD; William R. Burks, MD; Howard A. Doyle, Jr., MD; Alfred H. Rivera, MD; David R. Simon, MD; David A. Snyder, MD; Barry S. Taney, MD; Marianela Castellanos; Ana M. Soler; Sandra Frazier Byrne; Fiona Ehlies; E. Kym Gendron; J. Randall Hughes.

Medical College of Wisconsin, Milwaukee, WI – William F. Mieler, MD; Gerald J. Harris, MD; Sharon A. Rekow, COMA; Gary W. Abrams, MD; Michael Lewandowski, RDMS.

Royal Victoria Hospital and Hôpital Notre-Dame, Montreal, Canada – Christine Corriveau, MD; Jean Deschenes, MD; Mikael A. Sebag, MD; Marie Carole Boucher, MD; Francois Codere, MD; Darlene O'Connor; Liette Bousquet, COA; Diane Chialant, RN.

Touro Infirmary, New Orleans, LA – Kurt A. Gitter, MD; Gerald Cohen, MD; Susy A. Steib; Sandra W. Palao.

Tulane Medical Center, New Orleans, LA – Barrett Haik, MD; Zeynel A. Karcioglu, MD; Elaine M. Eckols, COA; Mary E. Smith, RDMS.

Cornell University, New York, NY – David H. Abramson, MD; Camille A. Servodidio, RN, MPH, CRNO.

McGee Eye Institute, Oklahoma City, OK – Reagan H. Bradford, Jr., MD; Janie M. Shofner, COA; Jaime Rodriguez.

Southern California Permanente Group, Panorama City, CA – Man M. Singh Hayreh, MD; Robert Caldwell, PA; Barry Kerman, MD; Nancy London, COA; Joel N. Moral, COT; Ron Smith, COT.

Retina Vitreous Consultants, Pittsburgh, PA – Jeffrey S. Rinkoff, MD; Karl R. Olsen, MD; Randall L.Beatty, MD; Scott R. Hobson, MD; Gary Weinstein, MD; Barbara J. Bahr, LPN; Donna Green, RN.

Devers Eye Clinic, Portland, OR – Richard G. Chenoweth, MD; Richard F. Dreyer, MD; Mark Evans; Patrick B. Rice, CRA.

Oregon Health Sciences University, Portland, OR – David J. Wilson, MD; Frederick Fraunfelder, MD; Michael Klein, MD; Joseph Robertson, MD; Robert C. Watzke, MD, FACS; Roger A. Dailey, MD; John L. Wobig, MD, FACS; Shirley Ira, COT; Mark Evans.

Mayo Foundation, Rochester, MN – Dennis M. Robertson, MD; Helmut Buettner, MD; John Pach, MD; Margaret J. Ruszczyk; Mary Schumann, COMT.

Associated Retinal Consultants, P.C., Royal Oak, MI – Raymond R. Margherio, MD; Patrick L. Murphy, MD; Kristi Cumming, RN; Patricia Manatrey, RN; Beth Mitchell, RN; William Park, OD.

Washington University, Saint Louis, MO – Morton E. Smith, MD; Philip L. Custer, MD; Henry J. Kaplan, MD; Mary V. Gaines; William Hart, MD.

University of Texas, San Antonio, TX – Wichard van Heuven, MD; Lina M. Marouf MD; James W. Speights, MD; Brian B. Berger, MD; Lt. Colonel Donald A. Hollsten, MD; Kenneth L. Piest, MD; Christopher Westfall, MD; Debbie Schifanella; Jacalyn McAdam, ARDMS.

Northern California COMS Group, San Francisco, CA – Howard Schatz, MD; Robert N. Johnson, MD; Karen Laughlin, LPN; Anne Miller; Margaret M. Stolarczuk, OD.

Ophthalmic Consultants Northwest, Seattle, WA – Edward B. McLean, MD; J. Timothy Heffernan, MD; R. Toby Sutcliffe, MD; Marilyn M. Teeter, MA; Craig G. Wells, MD.
University of Washington, Seattle, WA – Craig G. Wells, MD; Robert E. Kalina, MD; James L. Kinyoun, MD; Betty Lawrence, COA.
Northern Florida COMS Group, Tampa, FL – William S. Grizzard, MD; Mark E. Hammer, MD; Peter R. Pavan, MD; Aaron P. Appiah, MD; Mark Greenwald; Janet Traynom, COT.
Scott and White Memorial Hospital, Temple, TX – J. Paul Dieckert, MD; Glen O. Brindley, MD; Juanice R. Hamm, RN; Suzann M. Whatley.
Ontario Cancer Institute, Toronto, Canada – E. Rand Simpson, MD; Martin Kazdan, MD; Hugh McGowan, MD; Herbert Tanzer, MD; Andrea Mackie, COA; Barbara Japp; Charles J. Pavlin, MD.
Retina Associates Southwest, Tucson, AZ – Leonard Joffe, MD; Denis M. Carroll, MD; Reid F. Schindler, MD, FRCS; Christine Hanson, RN; Larry M. Wilson.

Participating Resource Centers

Coordinating Center, The Wilmer Ophthalmological Institute, Baltimore, MD – Barbara S. Hawkins, PhD (*Principal Investigator*); Marie Diener-West, PhD (*Study Statistician*); George T. Allen; Craig E. Belongie; Renée Y. Church; Townes C. Coates; Paul B. Connor; Joyce L. Fritsch; Irene L. Goldsborough; Patricia A. James; Jonathan S. Kerman; Kelly S. Manos, MAS; Jan A. Markowitz, PhD; B. Michele Melia, ScM; Claudia S. Moy, PhD; M. Marvin Newhouse; Katasha R. Smart-Davis.
Echography Center, Bascom Palmer Eye Institute, Miami, FL – Sandra Frazier Byrne (*Principal Investigator*); Fiona Ehlies; E. Kym Gendron; J. Randall Hughes; Maria Rivera; Pat Superfine Rivera; Jeanette L. Moreno.
National Eye Institute, Bethesda, MD – Carl Kupfer, MD (*Director*); Jeanne King; Gaye Lynch; Jack A. McLaughlin, PhD; Richard L. Mowery, PhD.
Pathology Center, Massachusetts Eye and Ear Infirmary, Boston, MA – Daniel M. Albert, MD (*Principal Investigator*); Emily Hajar; Bartholomew Johnson; Nancy L. Robinson.
Photograph Reading Center, The University of Iowa Hospitals and Clinics, Iowa City, IA – Thomas A. Weingeist, MD, PhD (*Principal Investigator*); Paul R. Montague; Jose S. Pulido, MD; Diane Anderson; Christine Taylor; Carolyn Vogel.
Radiological Physics Center, M.D. Anderson Hospital, Houston, TX – William F. Hanson, PhD (*Principal Investigator*); Paula Kennedy; Ramesh C. Tailor, PhD.
Study Chairman's Office, Scheie Eye Institute, Philadelphia, PA – Stuart L. Fine, MD (*Principal Investigator*); Lee McCaffrey, MA; Virginia Nido; Debbie Russo.
Steering Committee – Stuart L. Fine, MD (*Chairman*); John D. Earle, MD; Barbara S. Hawkins, PhD; Richard L. Mowery, PhD; Bradley R. Straatsma, MD.
Executive Committee – *Permanent Members:* Stuart L. Fine, MD (*Chairman*); Daniel M. Albert, MD; Sandra Frazier Byrne; Marie Diener-West, PhD; John D. Earle, MD; Peter Fitzpatrick, MB, BS; William F. Hanson, PhD; Barbara S. Hawkins, PhD; John N. Kirkwood, MD; Lee McCaffrey, MA; Richard L. Mowery, PhD; Claudia S. Moy, PhD; Dennis M. Robertson, MD; Marvin Rotman, MD; Andrew P. Schachat, MD; James Schwade, MD; Bradley R. Straatsma, MD; Thomas A. Weingeist, MD, PhD; *Rotating Members (1992):* Gail Daubert, RN; Ellen F. Greenberg, COT; Robert N. Johnson, MD; Paul Sternberg, MD.

Data and Safety Monitoring Committee – *Voting Members:* Matthew D. Davis, MD (*Chairman*); Thomas E. Davis, MD*, Frederick L. Ferris, MD; J. Donald M. Gass, MD; Laël C. Gatewood, PhD; Gerald E. Hanks, MD; Robert J. Levine, MD; Robert W. Makuch, PhD; *Non-Voting Members:* Marie Diener-West, PhD; Stuart L. Fine, MD; Barbara S. Hawkins, PhD; Richard L. Mowery, PhD.

Quality Assurance Committee – Claudia S. Moy, PhD (*Chairman*); Daniel M. Albert, MD; Sandra Frazier Byrne; Renée Y. Church; Marie Diener-West, PhD; John D. Earle, MD; Stuart L. Fine, MD (*ex officio*); William F. Hanson, PhD; Barbara S. Hawkins, PhD; Kelly S. Manos, MAS; B. Michele Melia, ScM; William F. Mieler, MD; Paul R. Montague; Andrea Mackie, COT (*1992-1993*); Dennis M. Robertson, MD.

* Now deceased

CHOROIDAL MELANOMA: A PRACTICAL APPROACH FOR THE 1990's

Stuart L. Fine

Department of Ophthalmology, Scheie Eye Institute, Philadelphia, Pennsylvania, USA

Although choroidal melanoma accounts for less than 1% of all ocular cancers, it is of profound interest to ophthalmologists for three reasons. First, it is the commonest primary intraocular malignancy in adults. Second, it is one of the few conditions seen in ophthalmic practice which is life threatening as well as sight threatening. Third, it is a condition about which there has been considerable controversy regarding both diagnosis and preferred management.

Until the 1970's, up to 20% of eyes enucleated for suspected melanoma were found to harbor a simulating, usually non-malignant lesion. The widespread application of both indirect ophthalmoscopy and ultrasonography has substantially improved the diagnostic ability of practicing ophthalmologists such that the diagnostic accuracy is now between 95% and greater in large centers. In fact, among the 44 clinical centers participating in the Collaborative Ocular Melanoma Study (COMS) the diagnostic accuracy is greater than 99%. Additionally, it has become standard practice among ophthalmologists not to recommend or perform enucleation, or other therapy, for melanoma without seeking consultation concerning diagnosis. Moreover, in unusual cases, fine needle tumor biopsy has become an accepted mode of practice to aid with diagnosis. Thus, while diagnosis is no longer the problem that it was in the 197O's, controversy about management continues to this day. In the late 1970's Dr. Lorenz Zimmerman proposed that enucleation surgery might promote metastasis of viable malignant cells and thus increase mortality. While this hypothesis was not widely accepted, it suggested the desirability for gentle manipulation during enucleation surgery performed by an expert rather than by a beginning ophthalmic surgeon. However, the decision as to when a patient requires treatment is still an unresolved issue. Unfortunately, there are no good long-term natural history data concerning survival of untreated patients with choroidal melanoma. For over a century, patients with ocular melanoma have been treated and for most of those 100 years, the standard method of treatment has been enucleation. Thus, it is survival after enucleation which provides the largest data base on mortality.

In the 1970's, alternative therapies utilizing various forms of radiation began to be performed so that there now exists mortality information for up to eight years on substantial numbers of patients. It appears that for the first five years after treatment, survival is comparable with either enucleation or plaque radiation. However, since the patients treated with enucleation and with radiation were not randomized, it is far from certain that the groups treated by either of those methods are truly comparable. In fact, the possibility exists of a substantial survival advantage for one therapy or the other. To address this issue, vital for both patients and for ophthalmologists, the National Eye Institute de-

Address for correspondence: Stuart L. Fine, M.D., Department of Ophthalmology, University of Pennsylvania, Scheie Eye Institute, Myrin Circle, 51 North 39th Street, Philadelphia, PA 19104, USA

Retina and Vitreous, pp. 191-192
Proceedings of the Symposium on Retina and Vitreous,
organized by the New Orleans Academy of Ophthalmology
New Orleans, LA, USA, March 12-15, 1992
edited by Rudolph M. Franklin

cided to undertake support of the Collaborative Ocular Melanoma Study in 1986. Since 1988, more than 40 clinical centers participating in the COMS have been enrolling patients with both medium tumors and large tumors. Medium tumors are defined as those between 2.5 mm and 10 mm in height with a basal diameter not greater than 16 mm. Patients with tumors meeting these size criteria who are otherwise eligible are assigned at random either to standard enucleation or to treatment with external plaque irradiation using ^{125}I as the radiation source. To date approximately 750 patients have been enrolled in this randomized trial. These patients will be followed up annually for 10 years or until the time of death.

For patients with tumors larger than those eligible for the medium tumor category, enrollment into the study is followed by randomization to either standard enucleation or to enucleation preceded by external beam radiation, specifically 20 gy in 5 divided doses. To date, approximately 800 patients have been enrolled in this trial, and these patients will be followed for 10 years or until death.

A Data and Safety Monitoring Committee including epidemiologists, biostatisticians, bioethicists and ophthalmologists meets regularly to review the accumulating data with regard to survival and complications from both forms of treatment. If and when clinically important data are developed, this information will be made available to the patients, the study investigators, and to the ophthalmic community. Until that time, ophthalmologists are encouraged to refer potentially eligible patients to study centers so that those patients can be considered for enrollment in the trial.

The epidemiologic studies, the retrospective case control studies, and experimental studies have provided no useful information concerning how to reduce the risk of death from melanoma, how to identify individuals likely to develop ocular melanoma, or patients likely to develop metastases early in the course with or without treatment. Consequently, the randomized controlled clinical trial now in progress, with the support of the National Eye Institute, not only will provide useful information concerning preferred management but also will develop information concerning risk factors, rates of progression, and optimal timing for intervention. With the continued support of the ophthalmic community these answers will be forthcoming.

V

PROLIFERATIVE VITREORETINOPATHY

PERIRETINAL PROLIFERATION

W. Richard Green

Eye Pathology Laboratory, The Johns Hopkins Hospital, Baltimore, MD, USA

There is a wide spectrum of periretinal proliferation that can be classified into simple epiretinal membranes without contraction features, intermediate epiretinal membranes with contraction features, and complex membranes with contraction and retinal detachment.

There are two principal cells which are involved in this proliferation[1]. One is the retinal glial cell (fibrous astrocyte) and the other is retinal pigment epithelium. Fibrous astrocytes gain access to the inner surface of the retina where Müller cells and internal limiting membrane are absent. The cell body of Müller cells is located in the inner nuclear layer

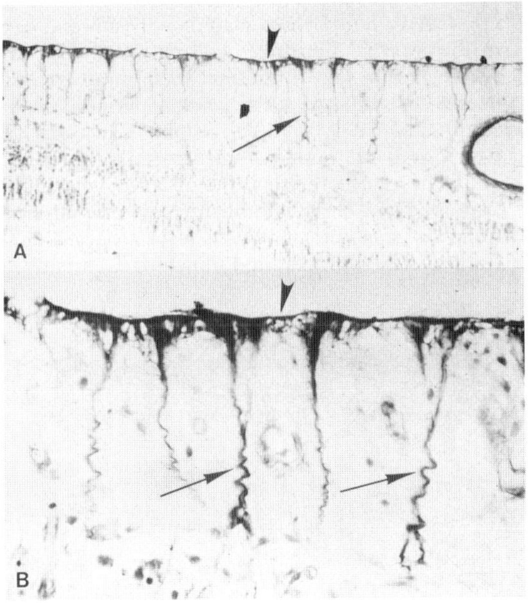

Fig. 1. Low (A) and higher (B) power view of Müller cells (arrows) and internal limiting membrane (arrowheads) (periodic acid-Schiff: A, ×137; B, ×328).

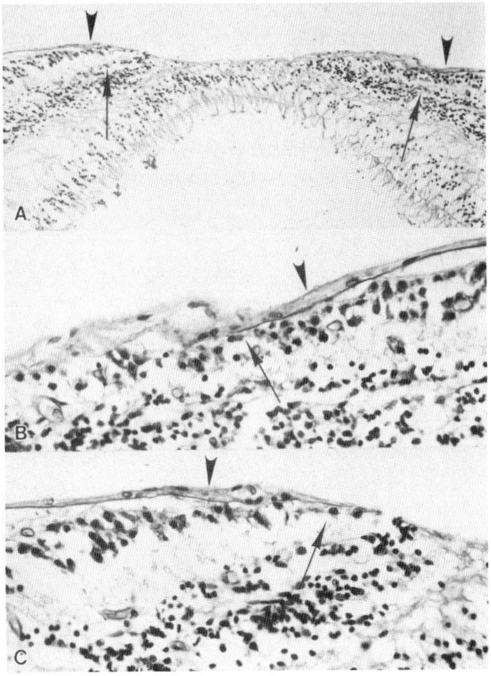

Fig. 2. Foveal area where the internal limiting membrane (arrows) becomes discontinuous nasal (B) and temporal (C). At these points glial cells (arrowheads) extend onto the inner surface of the retina (periodic acid-Schiff: A, ×100; B and C, ×300).

Address for correspondence: W. Richard Green, MD, Eye Pathology Laboratory, The Johns Hopkins Hospital, 600 N. Wolfe Street, Baltimore, MD 21287-9248, USA

Retina and Vitreous, pp. 195-222
Proceedings of the Symposium on Retina and Vitreous,
organized by the New Orleans Academy of Ophthalmology
New Orleans, LA, USA, March 12-15, 1992
edited by Rudolph M. Franklin

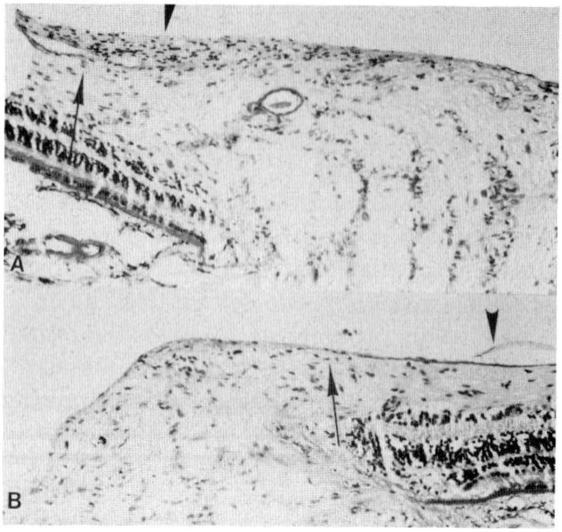

Fig. 3. Optic nerve head where the internal limiting membrane is discontinuous (arrows) and a fibroglial membrane (arrowheads) extends onto the inner surface of the retina (periodic acid-Schiff: A and B, ×137).

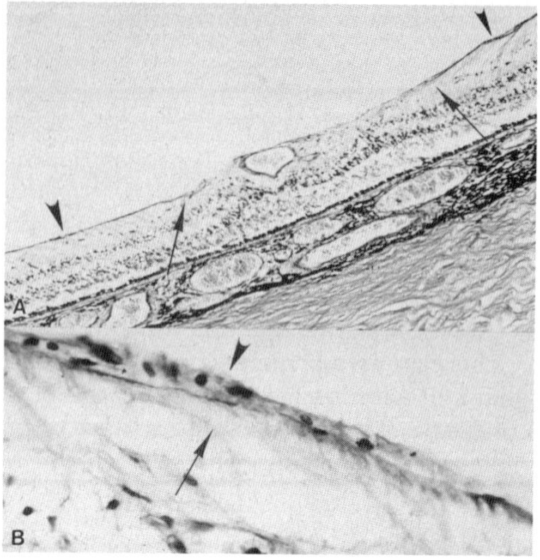

Fig. 4. Area temporal to macula with a broad gap in the internal limiting membrane (between arrows). A thin glial preretinal membrane (arrowheads) extends to either side (periodic acid-Schiff: A, ×137; B, ×528). (From: Clarkson JG, Green WR, Massof D: A histopathologic review of 168 cases of preretinal membrane. Am J Ophthalmol 84:1-17, 1977. Published with permission from *The American Journal of Ophthalmology*. Copyright by The Ophthalmic Publishing Company.)

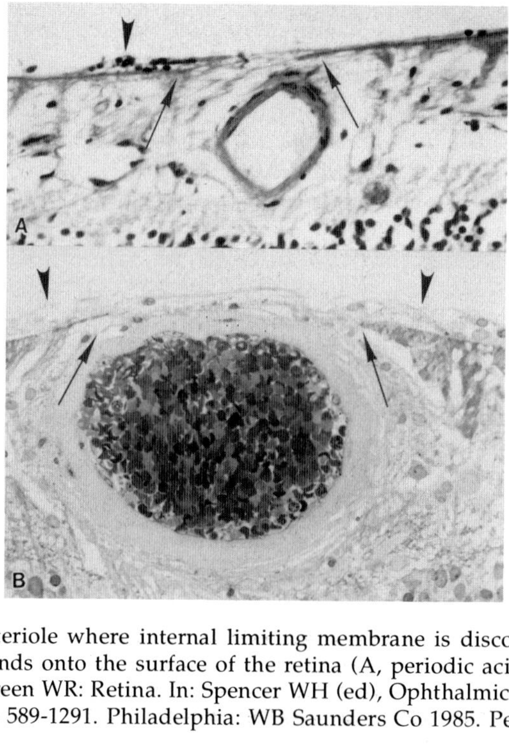

Fig. 5. Area of retinal arteriole where internal limiting membrane is discontinuous (arrows) and a fibroglial membrane extends onto the surface of the retina (A, periodic acid-Schiff ×70; B, toluidine blue, ×390). (B is from: Green WR: Retina. In: Spencer WH (ed), Ophthalmic Pathology: An Atlas and Textbook, Vol 2, Ch 8, pp 589-1291. Philadelphia: WB Saunders Co 1985. Permission courtesy of WB Saunders Co.)

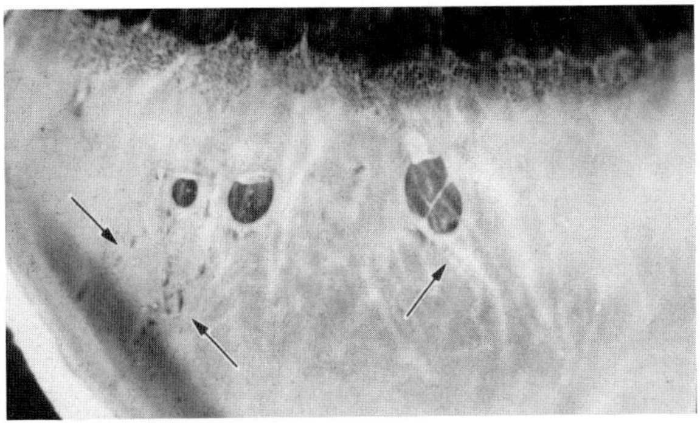

Fig. 6. Gross appearance of retinal pits (arrows) and retinal tears.

and it has processes that span nearly the full thickness of the retina (Fig. 1). Internally, Müller cells have a basement membrane which forms much of the internal limiting membrane of the retina (Fig. 1). Müller cells are reduced in number and the internal limiting membrane is thin or absent in several areas. Areas where this occurs naturally include the foveola, optic nerve head, over major retinal blood vessels, and at retinal tufts. The internal limiting membrane is absent in the foveola (Fig. 2). This is the site where fibrous astrocytes may extend into the surface of the retina for a variable distance (Fig. 2). Foos

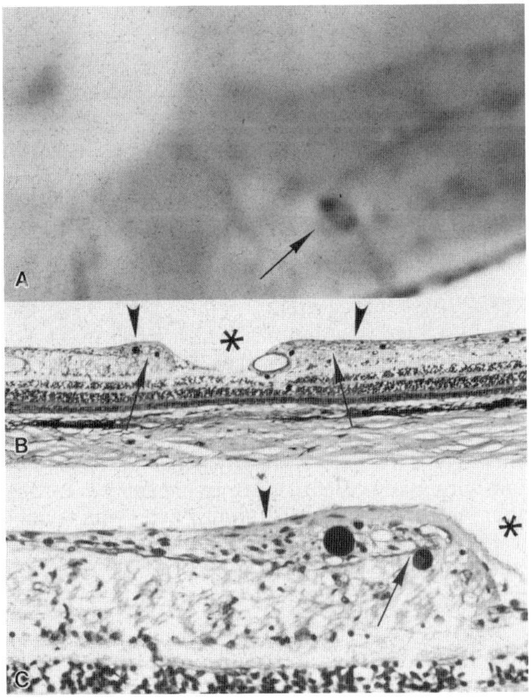

Fig. 7. A: Gross appearance of a retinal pit near the optic nerve head. B: Retinal pit (asterisk) with glial cells extending from the retina through the defect in the internal limiting membrane (arrows) to form a preretinal membrane (arrowheads) (PAS, ×75). C: Higher power of posterior margin of retinal pit (asterisk) showing direct continuity of the glial preretinal membrane (arrowhead) with the retina through a break in the internal limiting membrane. Arrow indicates the end of the internal limiting membrane. The spherical globules are corpora amylacea (periodic acid-Schiff, ×185). (From: Clarkson JG, Green WR, Massof D: A histopathologic review of 168 cases of preretinal membrane. Am J Ophthalmol 84:1-17, 1977. Published with permission from *The American Journal of Ophthalmology*. Copyright by The Ophthalmic Publishing Company.)

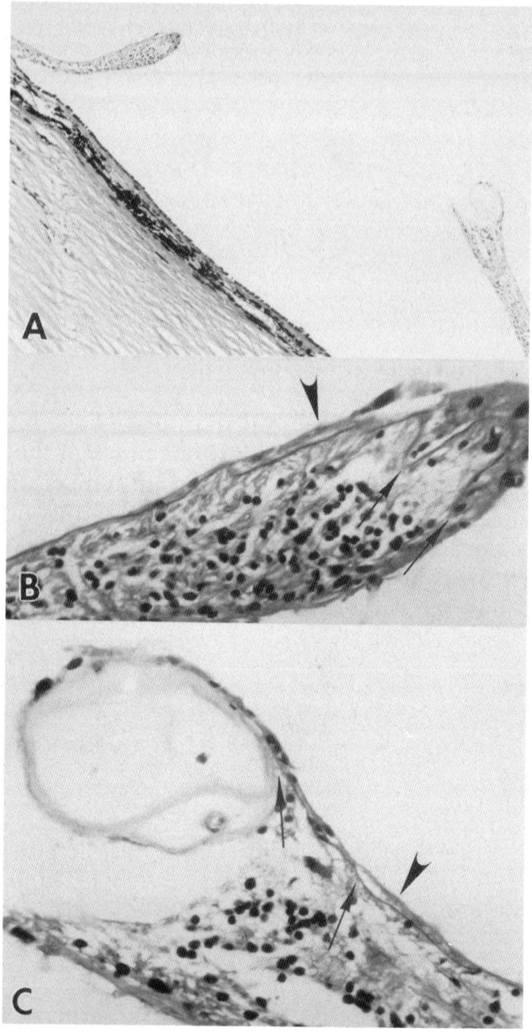

Fig. 8. A: Low-power view of a peripheral retinal tear with glial preretinal membrane extending on the inner surface of the retina anteriorly and posteriorly (PAS, ×65). Higher power of anterior (B) and posterior (C) margins of hole with glial preretinal membrane (arrowheads) extending along the inner surface of the internal membrane (arrowheads) (B and C, PAS, ×390). (From: Clarkson JG, Green WR, Massof D: A histopathologic review of 168 cases of preretinal membrane. Am J Ophthalmol 84:1-17, 1977. Published with permission from *The American Journal of Ophthalmology*. Copyright by The Ophthalmic Publishing Company.)

and co-workers[2] have noted that this occurs without contraction features in up to 20% of persons over the age of 70 years.

Another site where glial cells readily grow onto the inner surface of the retina is at the optic nerve head (Fig. 3). The internal limiting membrane stops at the margin of the optic nerve head where Müller cells are absent. At that point fibroglial tissue may extend onto the inner surface of the retina. A basement membrane, formed by fibrous astrocytes, incompletely covers the optic nerve head[3]. Another site where there are defects in the internal limiting membrane is along major retinal blood vessels. Here Müller cells are pushed off to the side and the internal limiting membrane may be discontinuous (Figs. 4 and 5). This is a site where fibrous astrocytes may extend onto the inner surface of the

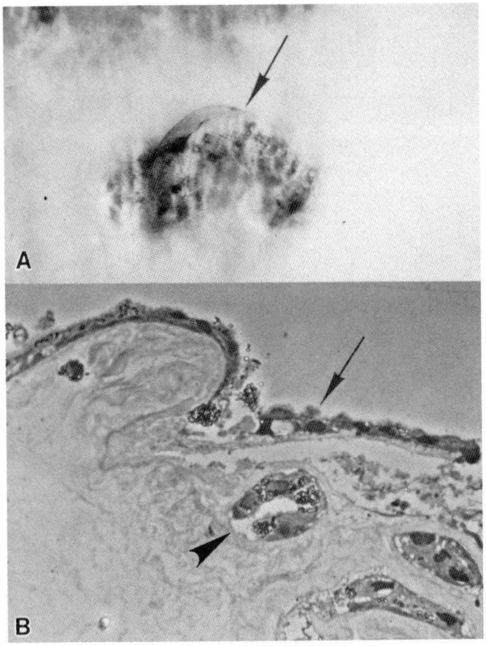

Fig. 9. A: Gross appearance of lattice degeneration with a portion of the pocket of vitreous lined by a pigmented membrane. (From: Green WR: Retina. In: Spencer WH (ed), Ophthalmic Pathology: An Atlas and Textbook, Vol 2, Ch 8, pp 589-1291. Philadelphia: WB Saunders Co 1985. Published courtesy of WB Saunders Co.) B: Area of lattice degeneration with retinal pigment epithelium in a monolayer (arrow) and an acinar pattern (arrowhead) lining the inner aspect of the vitreous pocket associated with lattice degeneration (paraphenylenediamine ×525).

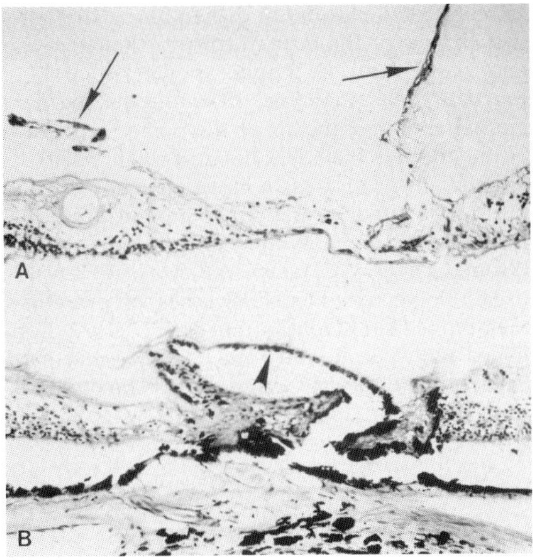

Fig. 10. A: Area of lattice degeneration with fibrous astrocytes (arrows) partially lining the pocket of fluid vitreous (hematoxylin and eosin ×737). B: Small area of lattice degeneration with retinal pigment epithelium (arrowhead) lining the entire pocket of fluid vitreous (hematoxylin and eosin ×137). (From: Green WR: Retina. In: Spencer WH (ed), Ophthalmic Pathology: An Atlas and Textbook, Vol 2, Ch 8, pp 589-1291. Philadelphia: WB Saunders Co 1985. Published courtesy of WB Saunders Co.)

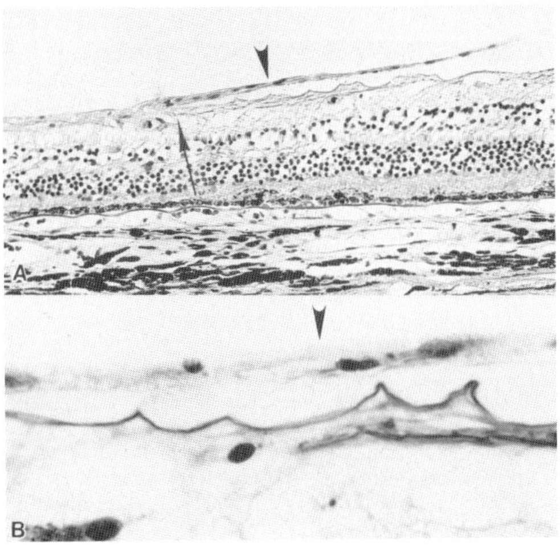

Fig. 11. A: Margin of area of lattice degeneration with discontinuity of the internal limiting membrane (arrow) and fibrous astrocytes (arrowheads) line the inner aspect of the formed vitreous (periodic acid-Schiff: A, ×185; B, ×800). (From: Green WR: Retina. In: Spencer WH (ed), Ophthalmic Pathology: An Atlas and Textbook, Vol 2, Ch 8, pp 589-1291. Philadelphia: WB Saunders Co 1985. Published courtesy of WB Saunders Co.)

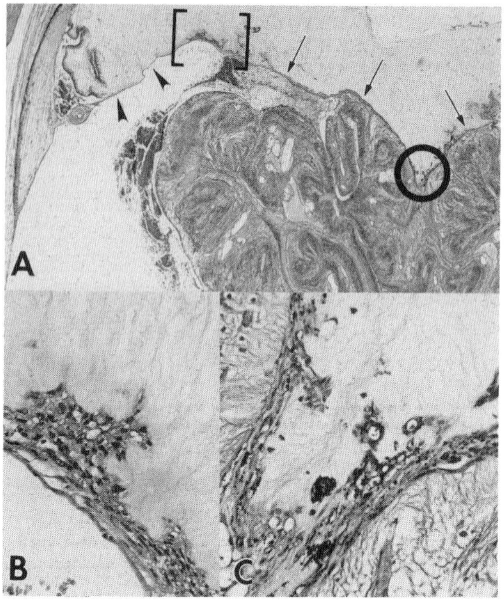

Fig. 12. A: Retinal dialysis at ora serrata with retinal pigment epithelium extending through the dialysis, along the posterior surface of the vitreous (arrowheads) and then along the anterior surface of the retina (arrows) (hematoxylin and eosin, ×20). B: Higher power of area in brackets (A) showing the retinal pigment epithelial membrane along the posterior surface of the vitreous (hematoxylin and eosin, ×200). C: Higher power of area in circle (A) showing the multi-laminated preretinal pigment epithelial membrane (hematoxylin and eosin, ×180). (From: Clarkson JG, Green WR, Massof D: A histopathologic review of 168 cases of preretinal membrane. Am J Ophthalmol 84:1-17, 1977. Published with permission from *The American Journal of Ophthalmology*. Copyright by The Ophthalmic Publishing Company.)

retina. Retinal tufts are an additional natural occurring area where fibrous astrocytes can gain access to the inner surface of the retina.

Acquired areas where fibrous astrocytes can gain access to the inner surface retina include: retinal pits, retinal tears and holes, avulsed retinal vessels, areas of regenerative remodeling, lattice degeneration and random sites of vitreous traction. A retinal pit occurs as a result of posterior vitreous detachment and vitreous traction with avulsion of inner retinal layers (Figs. 6 and 7). With the defect in the inner retina, fibrous astrocytes may extend onto the inner surface of the retina (Fig. 7). A similar process may occur at retina tears (Fig. 8).

Lattice degeneration, a vitreoretinal degenerative process, is characterized by the absence of Müller cells and internal limiting membrane and the presence of an overlying pocket of fluid vitreous. Vitreoretinal adhesion at the margin of the lattice may be fortified by hyperplasia of fibrous astrocytes and retinal pigment epithelium (Figs. 9-11).

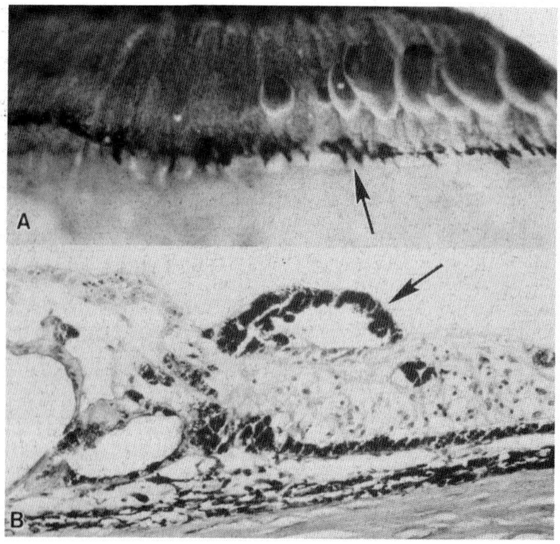

Fig. 13. Hyperplasia of pigment epithelium at ora serrata. A: Hyperplastic epithelium has a spiculate appearance and is located at ora serrata (arrow). B: Appearance of hyperplastic pigment epithelium (arrow) as it extends into the vitreous cavity at the ora serrata. PAS, ×220.

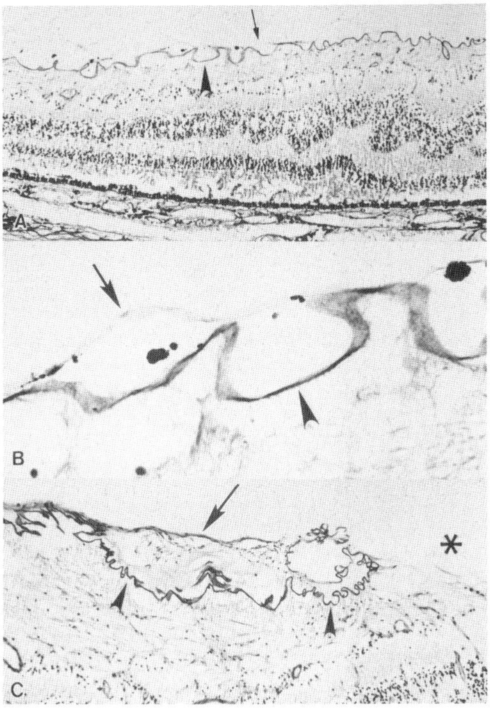

Fig. 14. Post-retinal detachment macular pucker. A and B: Thin, hypocellular preretinal membrane (arrow) with wrinkling of internal limiting membrane (arrowhead) (periodic acid-Schiff: A, ×70, B, ×328). C: Contraction of preretinal membrane (arrow) with marked wrinkling of internal limiting membrane (arrowheads). A large area of retina has been stripped of internal limiting membrane (asterisk) by contraction of the preretinal membrane (periodic acid-Schiff; ×90). (From: Clarkson JG, Green WR, Massof D: A histopathologic review of 168 cases of preretinal membrane. Am J Ophthalmol 84:1-17, 1977. Published with permission from *The American Journal of Ophthalmology*. Copyright by The Ophthalmic Publishing Company.)

Retinal pigment epithelium gains access to the vitreous cavity and inner surface of the retina at retinal tears, holes, dialysis (Fig. 12), at the ora serrata (Fig. 13), within the vitreous base, and at areas of lattice degeneration (Figs. 9 and 10).

Three clinical conditions with periretinal proliferation following retinal detachment surgery include macular pucker, proliferative vitreoretinopathy and retroretinal membranes. An example of macular pucker after a successful retinal detachment procedure is illustrated in Fig. 14. A thin hypocellular epiretinal membrane that has apparently contracted leading to wrinkling of the internal limiting membrane. The contraction was so marked that it has stripped and gathered a large portion of the internal limiting membrane. The predominate cell in macular pucker is the fibrous astrocyte, but about half the cases following retinal detachment surgery also have retinal pigment epithelium.

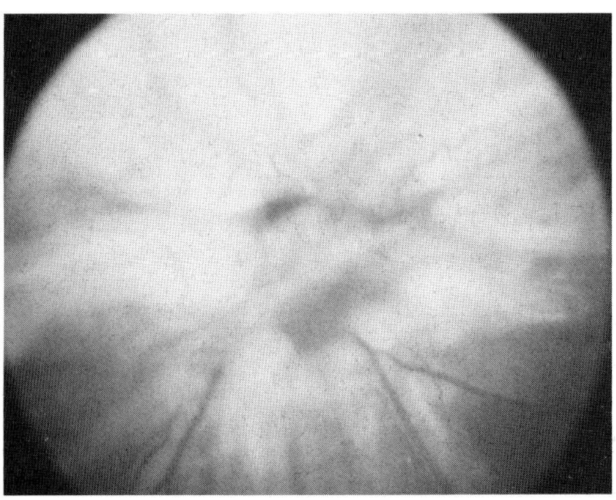

Fig. 15. Closed funnel retinal detachment from proliferative vitreoretinopathy.

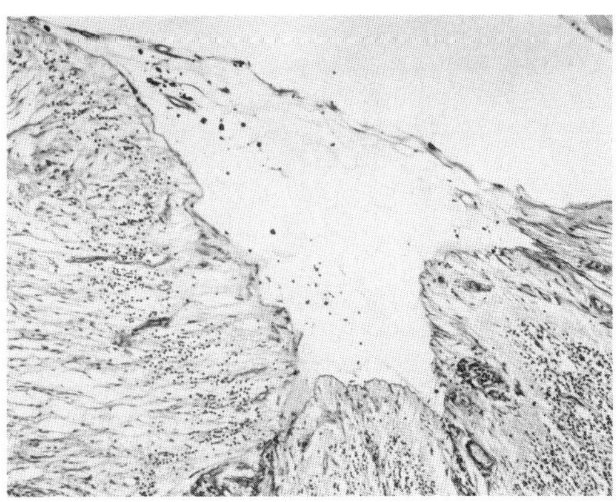

Fig. 16. Fixed retinal fold from proliferative vitreoretinopathy (periodic acid-Schiff, ×137).

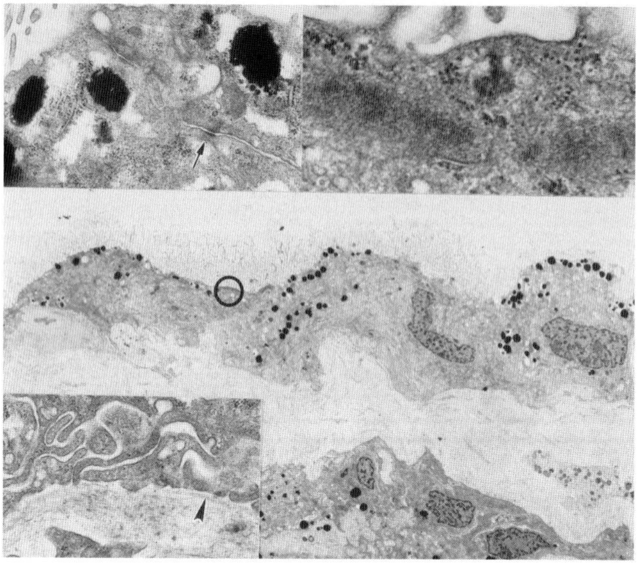

Fig. 17. Epiretinal membrane after prior retinal detachment, composed of new collagen and retinal pigment epithelial cells. Some cells are arranged in monolayer and have spotty basement membrane (arrowhead) and basal plasma membrane infoldings (bottom inset). Numerous apical villous processes are present on vitreal side, and melanin pigment granules are concentrated in apical portion of cells. Junctional complexes are present near apices of cells (arrow). Apical subplasmalemmal microfilaments measuring 4 to 5 nm and with fusiform densities are present in some cells (circle and top right inset) (main figure, ×2700; top left inset, ×20,000; top right inset, ×45,000; bottom inset, ×20,000). (From: Michels RG: A clinical and histopathologic study of epiretinal membrane affecting the macula and removed by vitreous surgery. Trans Am Ophthalmol Soc 80:580-656, 1982. Permission courtesy of the American Ophthalmological Society.)

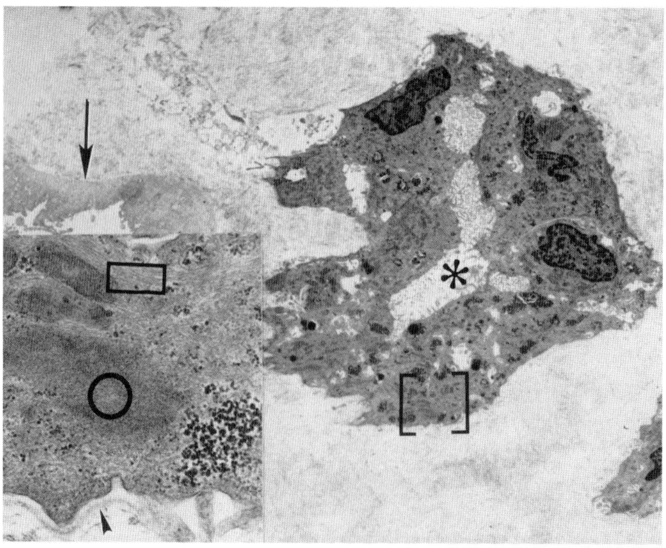

Fig. 18. Epiretinal membrane, after retinal detachment, containing new collagen, fragments of internal limiting membrane (arrow), and retinal pigment epithelium arranged in tubulo-acinar pattern. Apical portion of pigment epithelium lines lumen (asterisk). Pigment epithelial cells show myoblastic differentiation with peripheral dense aggregates of microfilaments measuring 4 to 5 nm (circle). Occasional cytoplasmic filaments measuring 10 nm are also present (rectangle). Inset is high-power magnification of bracketed area in main figure (arrowhead, basement membrane) (main figure, ×3300; inset, ×30,000). (From: Michels RG: A clinical and histopathologic study of epiretinal membrane affecting the macula and removed by vitreous surgery. Trans Am Ophthalmol Soc 80:580-656, 1982. Permission courtesy of the American Ophthalmological Society.)

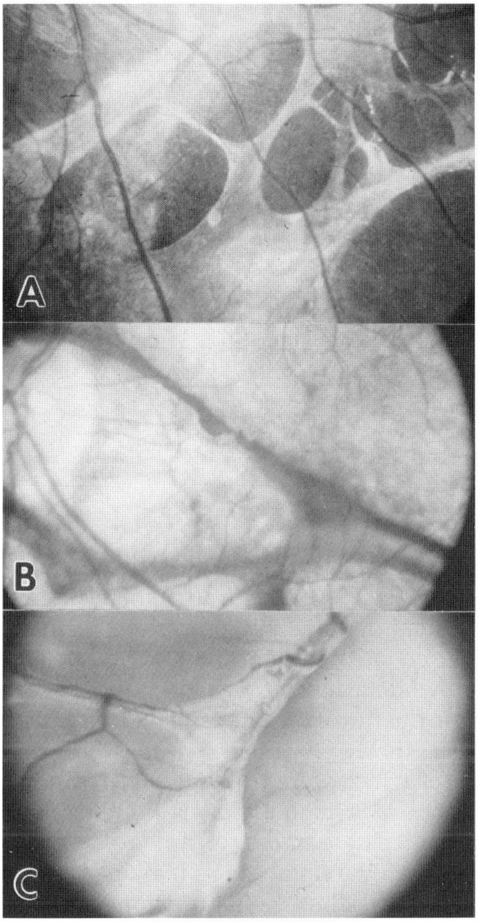

Fig. 19. A: Ophthalmoscopic appearance of retroretinal membrane that appears like a sheet with oval dehiscences. (From: Wallyn RH, Hilton GF: Subretinal fibrosis in retinal detachment. Arch Ophthalmol 97:2128-2129, 1979. Copyright 1979, American Medical Association.) Strands of retroretinal membranes with the retina flat (B) and held up in a tented and detached configuration (C). (From: Green WR: Retina. In: Spencer WH (ed), Ophthalmic Pathology: An Atlas and Textbook, Vol 2, Ch 8, pp 589-1291. Philadelphia: WB Saunders Co 1985. Permission courtesy of WB Saunders Co.)

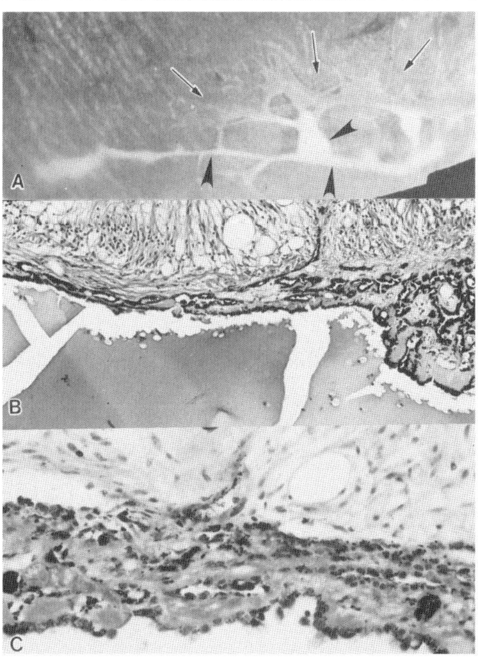

Fig. 20. A. View of choroid with retina removed, showing hyperplastic retinal pigment epithelium (RPE) in a sheet (arrows) which is continuous with *in situ* RPE anteriorly and strands of RPE with fibrous tissue (arrowheads) posteriorly. (From: Green WR: Retina. In: Spencer WH (ed), Ophthalmic Pathology: An Atlas and Textbook, Vol 2, Ch 8, pp 589-1291. Philadelphia: WB Saunders Co 1985. Permission courtesy of WB Saunders Co.) B and C: Multi-laminated retroretinal membrane composed of hyperplastic retinal pigment epithelium (Masson trichrome: B ×110; C, ×310).

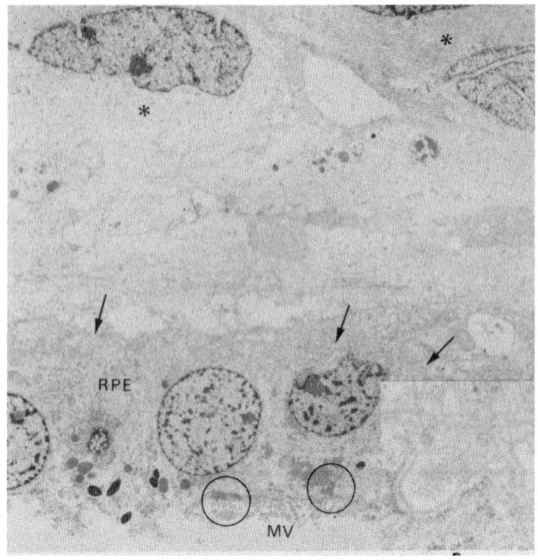

Fig. 21. Retroretinal membrane composed of glial cells internally and a single layer of retinal pigment epithelium externally. The glial cells have large aggregates of cytoplasmic filaments (asterisks) which measure 8-10 nm at a higher power. The retinal pigment epithelial cells are arranged in a single polarized layer. The base of the cell is located internally and has marked plasma membrane infoldings and well-developed basement membrane (arrows and inset). The apex of the cells is located externally and has apically located junction complexes (circles) and microvilli (MV) (×4200; inset, ×29,000). (From: Wilkes SR, Mansour AM, Green WR: Proliferative vitreoretinopathy. Histology of retroretinal membranes. Retina 7:94-101, 1987. Published courtesy of *Retina*.)

Another syndrome or condition of cellular proliferation occurring after retinal detachment surgery is proliferative vitreoretinopathy (PVR) (Fig. 15). This was first considered to be due to contraction of the vitreous and was called massive vitreous retraction. This complication could occur in a relatively short period of time after a successful scleral buckling procedure. In a study of experimental retinal detachment Machemer and Laqua[4] found that this was not due to innate retraction of the vitreous, but rather to a cellular proliferation that contracts and detaches the retina. In Fig. 16, there is a fold of retina bridged by proliferative tissue. In most of these cases which were studied by electron microscopy[5,6], hyperplastic retinal pigment epithelium in a monolayer (Fig. 17) or in a tubulo-acinar pattern (Fig. 18) was the most common cell observed.

Another clinical category of periretinal proliferation in the setting in retinal detachment is retroretinal membranes (Figs. 19 and 20)[7,8]. This starts first as a continuous sheet of proliferation of retinal pigment epithelium and then dehiscences occur (Fig. 19A) and eventually only a strand(s) (Fig. 19B) may persist in a contracted state and cause retinal detachment (Fig. 19C). In the electron microscopic study of a surgically enucleated eye, an upside-down retinal pigment epithelium on the under surface of the retina can be seen (Fig. 21). In some of these retroretinal membranes, glial cells predominate (Figs. 22 and 23). In one consecutive series of retinal detachment, Wallyn and Hilton[9] observed retroretinal membranes in about 3% of retinal detachments.

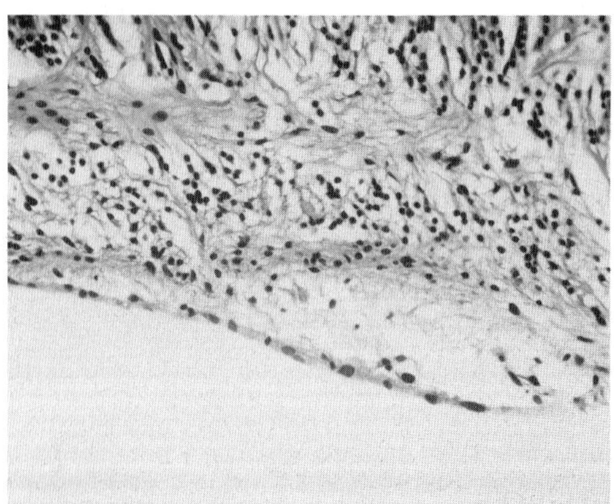

Fig. 22. One layer of glial cells is situated under a gliotic retina, showing loss of the photoreceptor cell layer in an eye with chronic uveitis of 24 years' duration and chronic retinal detachment (hematoxylin and eosin, ×270). (From: Wilkes SR, Mansour AM, Green WR: Proliferative vitreoretinopathy. Histology of retroretinal membranes. Retina 7:94-101, 1987. Published courtesy of *Retina*.)

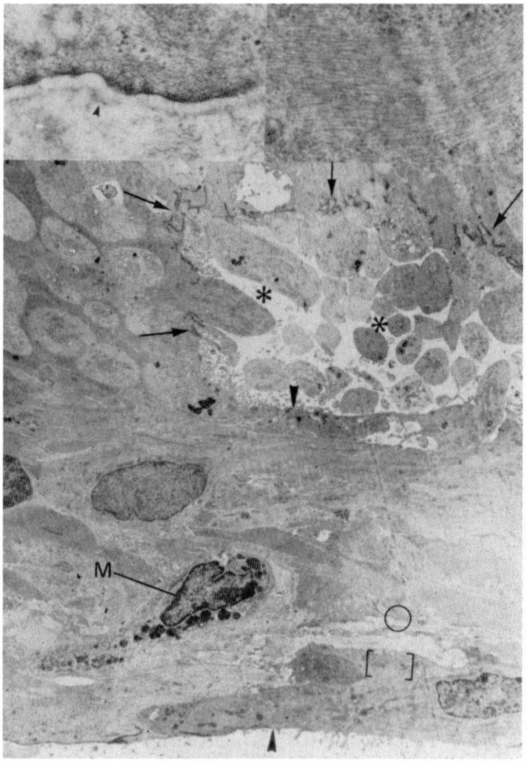

Fig. 23. Transmission electron microscopy of a glial retroretinal membrane in an eye with retinal dialysis and chronic retinal detachment. A multilayered membrane (between arrowheads) is composed of cells with aggregates of 8-10 nm cytoplasmic filaments (bracket and upper right inset) and well-developed basement membrane (circle and upper left inset, arrowhead). A macrophage (M) is entrapped in the membrane. The retina has been puckered externally, forming a cavity (asterisks) containing remaining photoreceptor inner segments. The cavity is bound by the retroretinal membrane externally and by the inner segments and junctional complexes of the external limiting membrane (arrows) to the sides and internally. The glial cells in the inner aspect of the membrane are randomly oriented, whereas those on the external surface are polarized, with the base located internally, and the apex with the villous processes located externally (×2000; both insets, ×51,000). (From: Wilkes SR, Mansour AM, Green WR: Proliferative vitreoretinopathy. Histology of retroretinal membranes. Retina 7:94-101, 1987. Published courtesy of *Retina*.)

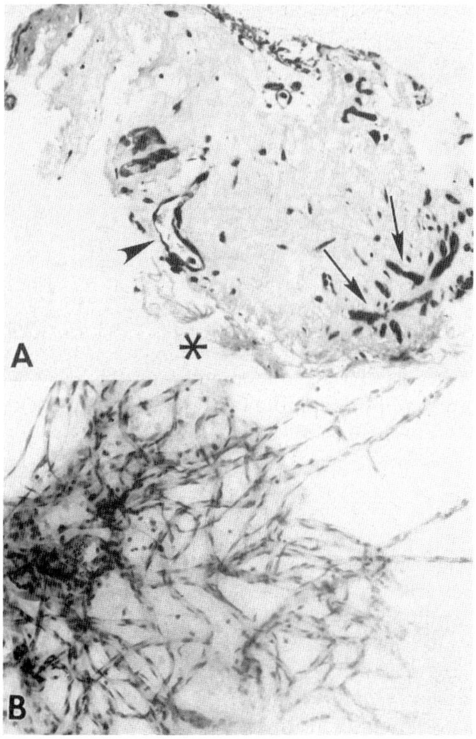

Fig. 24. Proliferative vitreoretinopathy. A: A 44-year-old man developed proliferative vitreoretinopathy after a repair of a retinal detachment. A pars plana vitrectomy and peeling of an epiretinal membrane were performed. The ocular fluid specimen contained a dense fibrovascular membrane with a coiled fragment of internal limiting membrane at one edge (asterisk). Cells in a tubuloacinar pattern (arrows) were suggestive of hyperplastic RPE. Erythrocytes were found in the blood vessels (arrowhead) (celloidin bag, Van de Grift, ×240). (From: Engel HM, Green WR, Michels RG, Rice TA, Erozan YS: Diagnostic vitrectomy. Retina 1:121-149, 1981. Published courtesy of *Retina*.) B: A 53-year-old male with proliferative diabetic retinopathy and tractional retinal detachment underwent vitrectomy. A fibrovascular membrane is present (celloidin bag preparation, hematoxylin and eosin, ×160). (From: Engel KM, De la Cruz Z, Jimenez-Abalahin LD, Green WR, Michels RG: Cytopreparatory techniques for eye fluid specimens obtained by vitrectomy. Acta Cytol 26:551-560, 1982. Published courtesy of *Acta Cytologica*.)

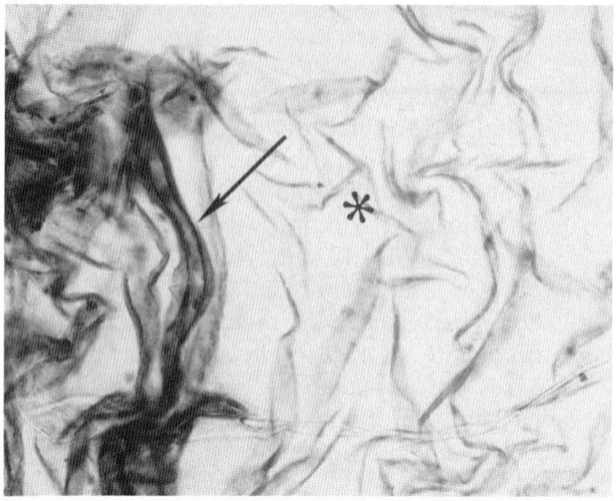

Fig. 25. Glial preretinal membrane (by electron microscopy) with blood vessels (arrow) and attached wrinkled internal limiting membrane (asterisk). Millipore filter; modified Papanicolaou stain; ×265. (From: Green WR, Kenyon KR, Michels RG, Gilbert HD, De la Cruz Z: Ultrastructure of epiretinal membranes causing macular pucker after retinal detachment surgery. Trans Ophthalmol Soc UK 99:63-77, 1979. Published courtesy of *Eye*.)

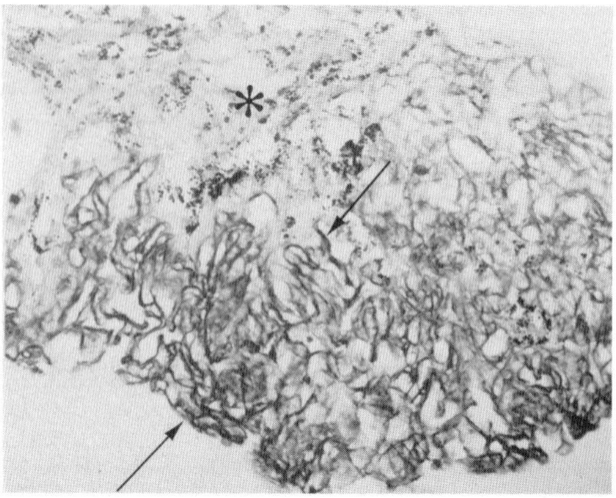

Fig. 26. Glial preretinal membrane (asterisk) (verified by electron microscopy in same case) with entrapped melanin pigment and a large fragment of greatly gathered internal limiting membrane (between arrows). Celloidin bag concentrate; periodic acid-Schiff; ×410). (From: Green WR, Kenyon KR, Michels RG, Gilbert HD, De la Cruz Z: Ultrastructure of epiretinal membranes causing macular pucker after retinal detachment surgery. Trans Ophthalmol Soc UK 99:63-77, 1979. Published courtesy of *Eye*.)

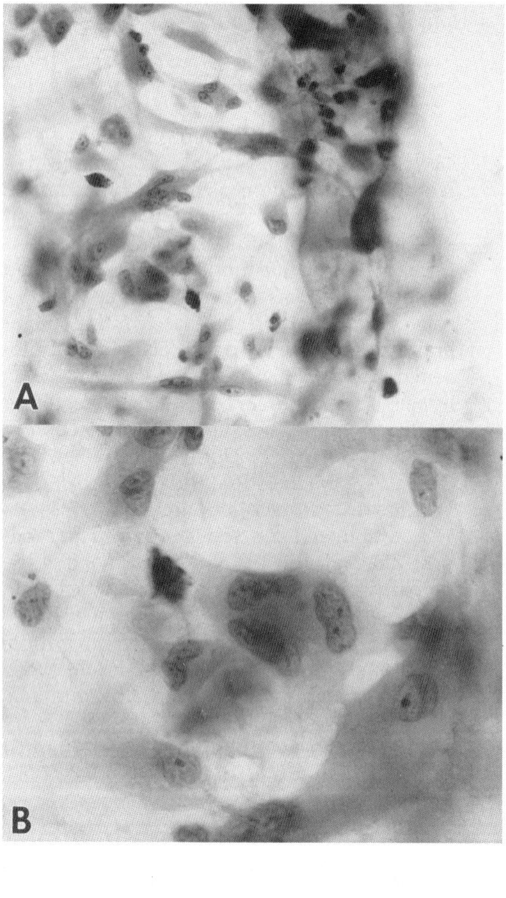

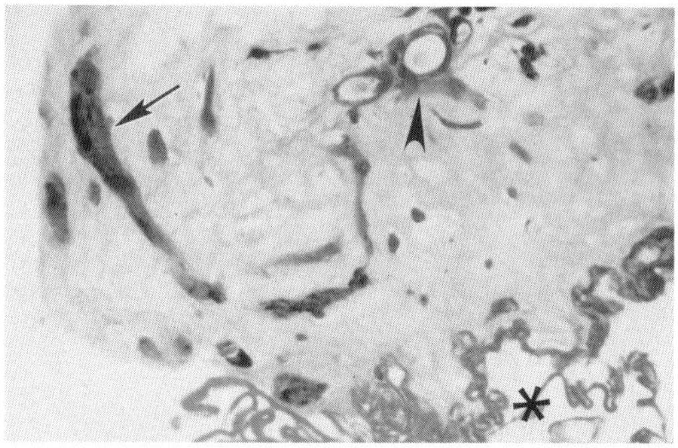

Fig. 27. (left) Cellular membrane fragment with large plump spindle and stellate-shaped cells with multinucleation (modified Papanicolaou: A, ×300; B, ×900).

Fig. 28. (right) Dense fibrocellular membrane fragment with some cells arranged in an acinar pattern (arrow) blood vessels (arrowhead) and a large segment of gathered internal limiting membrane (asterisk) (Celloidin bag technique, periodic acid-Schiff ×400). (From: Green WR: Diagnostic cytopathology of ocular fluid specimens. Ophthalmology 91:726-748, 1984. Published courtesy of *Ophthalmology*.)

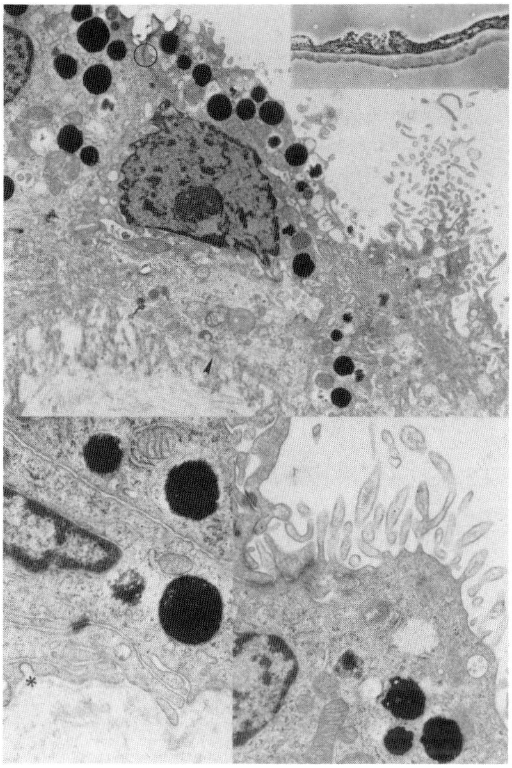

Fig. 29. Retinal pigment epithelial cells of epiretinal membrane occurring after retinal reattachment surgery. Inset: continuous monolayer of pigmented cells overlying collagenous component of membrane (paraphenylenediamine, ×400). Main figure: polarization of pigment-containing cells with respect to junctional complexes (circled) and numerous fine processes of free-surface apical cell membrane and to nearly continuous basement membrane (arrowhead) closely apposed to basal cell surface (×7500). Bottom left: intracytoplasmic melanin granules and extracellular basement membrane (asterisk) (×25,000). Bottom right: numerous junction complexes and apical surface processes (×20,000). (From: Kampik A, Kenyon KR, Michels RG, De la Cruz Z: Epiretinal and vitreous membranes: comparative study of 56 cases. Arch Ophthalmol 99:1445-1454, 1981. Copyright 1981, American Medical Association.)

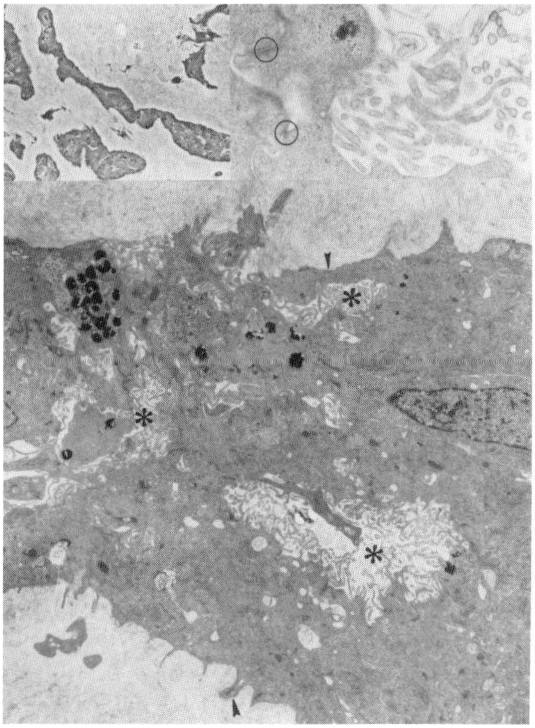

Fig. 30. Top left: phase-contrast photomicrograph demonstrates tendency of epithelial-like cells to assume a tubulo-acinar configuration surrounded by collagenous material. Paraphenylenediamine; ×600. Main figure: electron micrograph of corresponding area shows polarized configuration of cells within an acinar-like structure with apical surfaces facing a central "lumen" (asterisks) while their basal surfaces are invested by well-defined basement membranes (arrowheads) adjacent to the extracellular collagen fibrils. ×5500. Top right: detail of apical area resolves several junctional complexes (circled) and multiple surface projections, ×22,000. (From: Green WR, Kenyon KR, Michels RG, Gilbert HD, De la Cruz Z: Ultrastructure of epiretinal membranes causing macular pucker after retinal detachment surgery. Trans Ophthalmol Soc UK 99:63-77, 1979. Published courtesy of *Eye*.)

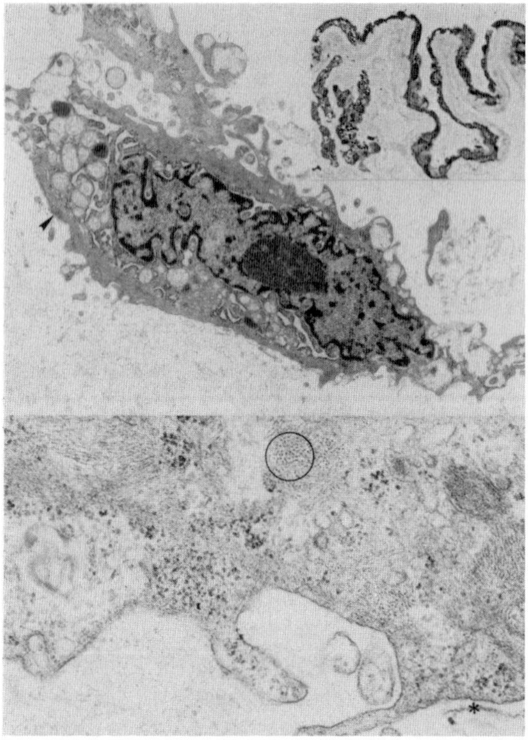

Fig. 31. Inset, top right: phase-contrast photomicrograph shows typical configuration of glia. There is proliferation of a continuous layer of glial cells along the inner surface of a collagenous epiretinal membrane. Paraphenylenediamine; ×500. Top: electron micrograph of corresponding area includes fusiform glial cell with numerous cytoplasmic processes and extracellular basement membrane (arrowhead). ×14,000. Bottom: detail of fibrous astrocyte discloses distinguishing cytoplasmic feature of numerous bundles of intermediate filaments, about 10 nm in diameter (circled) and basement membrane (asterisk). Adjacent collagen fibrils are approximately 25 nm in diameter (significantly larger than vitreous collagen fibrils) and therefore represent newly synthesized collagen. ×54,000. (From: Green WR, Kenyon KR, Michels RG, Gilbert HD, De la Cruz Z: Ultrastructure of epiretinal membranes causing macular pucker after retinal detachment surgery. Trans Ophthalmol Soc UK 99:63-77, 1979. Published courtesy of *Eye*.)

With the development of vitreous surgery, we have over the past 15 years or more obtained specimens from a variety of clinical settings of periretinal proliferation. These are situations where the surgeon, principally Dr. R.G. Michels, isolated and placed various portions of the periretinal proliferative tissue in fixative for electron microscopy. This included: proliferative vitreoretinopathy[5,6]; some specimens with anterior PVR[10]; secondary epiretinal membranes including macular pucker following retinal detachment[6,11]; after other surgery or trauma[12]; associated with ocular inflammatory disease[13-16]; pigmented epiretinal membranes[17]; recurrent epiretinal membranes[18]; retroretinal membranes[7,8]; vitreomacular traction syndrome[19,20]; idiopathic progressive unilateral vitreous fibrosis and secondary traction retinal detachment[21]; and impending macular hole[20,22]. Another category is idiopathic epimacular membranes in adults with no other features in the eye, including lattice degeneration[20,23-25]. Idiopathic epiretinal membranes may occur in children[26]. These may occasionally be congenital and in rare instances there may be retinal prolapse[26].

With membranes which are examined by light microscopy their constituents can often be determined. A fibrovascular membrane is usually clearly evident (Fig. 24). The crinkled appearance of internal limiting membrane of the retina is characteristic (Fig. 25). We see some internal limiting membrane (ILM) fragments (Fig. 26) in up to 70% of specimens of macular epiretinal membranes[6]. The absence of ILM does not seem to effect function and there is little tendency for regeneration[27]. It is not possible to determine whether cells such as those in Fig. 27 are retinal pigment epithelium or fibrous astrocytes. When cells have a tubulo-acinar pattern, it strongly suggests that they are retinal pigment epithelium as in the dense fibrocellular membrane with a large gathered segment of the internal limiting membrane in Fig. 28.

The various cell types can be identified by ultrastructural features[1,5,6]. Both retinal pigment epithelium and fibrous astrocyte maintain polarity with a basement membrane and

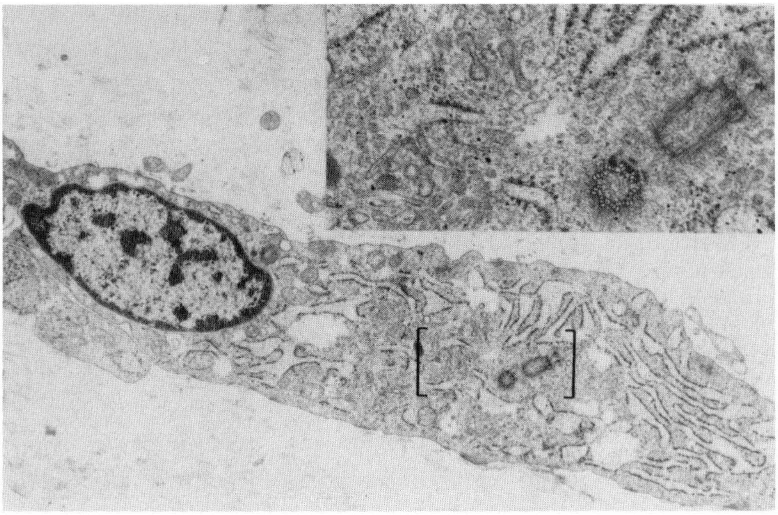

Fig. 32. Fibrocytes in epiretinal membrane associated with retinal detachment. Identifying characteristics include fusiform configuration of cell containing numerous profiles of rough-surfaced endoplasmic reticulum and absence of polarity (×11,500). Inset: higher magnification of bracketed area in top figure resolves round and smooth reticulum cisternae, plus prominent centriole (×45,000). (From: Kampik A, Kenyon KR, Michels RG, De la Cruz Z: Epiretinal and vitreous membranes: comparative study of 56 cases. Arch Ophthalmol 99:1445-1454, 1981. Copyright 1981, American Medical Association.)

apical villous processes. Fig. 29 illustrates retinal pigment epithelium in a monolayer with basement membrane, apical villous processes and junctional complexes. Retinal pigment epithelium may also proliferate in a tubulo-acinar pattern (Fig. 30).

Fibrous astrocytes also have polarity with basement membrane but the distinguishing feature of this cell is the presence of bundles of intermediate cytoplasmic filaments (Fig. 31). We also see fibrocytes which are usually spindle-shaped, have no basement membrane and have abundant endoplasmic reticulum (Fig. 32). Similar cells to fibrocytes are myofibrocytes which additionally have contraction features such as a corkscrew nucleus and subplasmalemmal aggregates of microfilaments with fusiform densities (Fig. 33).

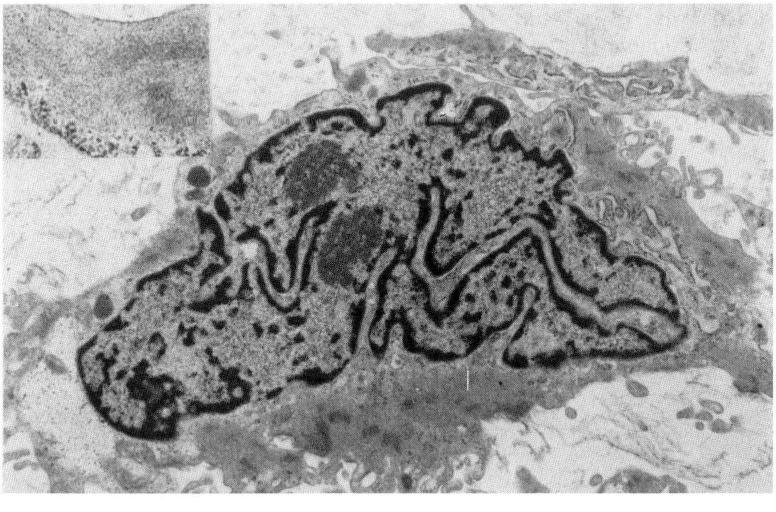

Fig. 33. Myofibrocyte with cork screw nucleus and marked subplasmalemmal aggregates of microfilaments with fusiform densities (×15,000; inset ×52,000).

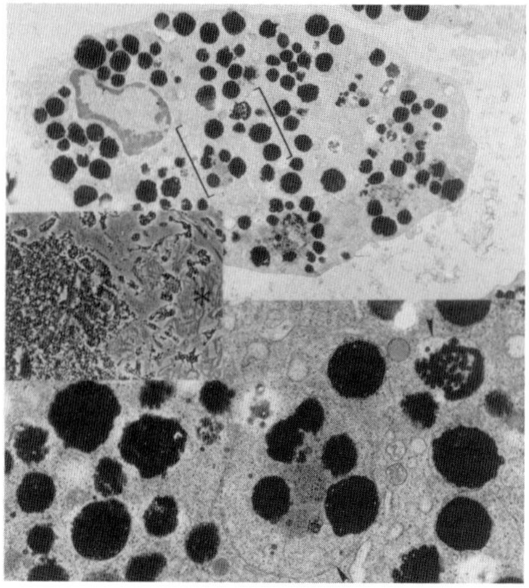

Fig. 34. Macrophage of epiretinal membrane associated with retinal reattachment surgery. Inset: mass of densely pigmented cells at left and extensive segment of inner limiting membrane (asterisk) (paraphenylenediamine, ×400). Top: large epithelioid cell containing pigment among other pleomorphic inclusions (×8000). Bottom: higher magnification of bracketed area in top figure resolves melanin granules, in various stages of degradation, contained within membrane-limited secondary lysosomes (arrowheads) or residual bodies (×25,000). (From: Kampik A, Kenyon KR, Michels RG, De la Cruz Z: Epiretinal and vitreous membranes: comparative study of 56 cases. Arch Ophthalmol 99:1445-1454, 1981. Copyright 1981, American Medical Association.)

Both retinal pigment epithelium and fibrous astrocytes may have aggregates of microfilaments with fusiform densities (myoblastic differentiation). This feature is associated with the ability of cells to migrate and contract.

Another cell type seen in surgical specimens is the macrophage which is large, round and has polymorphic membrane-bound phagosomes (Fig. 34).

Now consider the histopathologic features of some of the clinical categories of periretinal proliferation. Lindsey and co-workers[28] provided clinicopathologic correlation of a starfold of the retina (Fig. 35) following a retinal detachment procedure. This is an example of early proliferative vitreoretinopathy. We observed retinal pigment epithelium

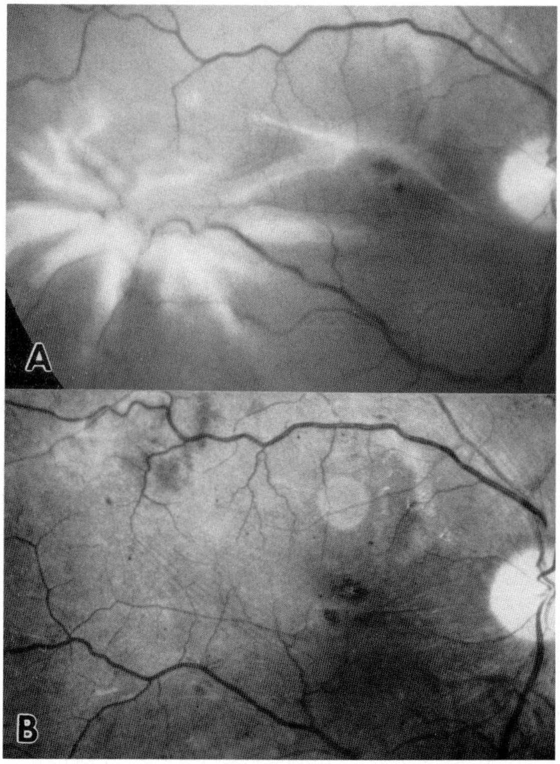

Fig. 35. A: Rhegmatogenous retinal detachment of the right eye with prominent, fixed starfold inferotemporal to the macula. B: appearance of the right eye after successful retinal reattachment surgery and subsequent epiretinal membrane removal by pars plana vitrectomy. (From: Lindsey PS, Michels RG, Luckenbach M, Green WR: Ultrastructure of epiretinal membrane causing retinal starfold. Ophthalmology 90:578-583, 1983. Published courtesy of *Ophthalmology*.)

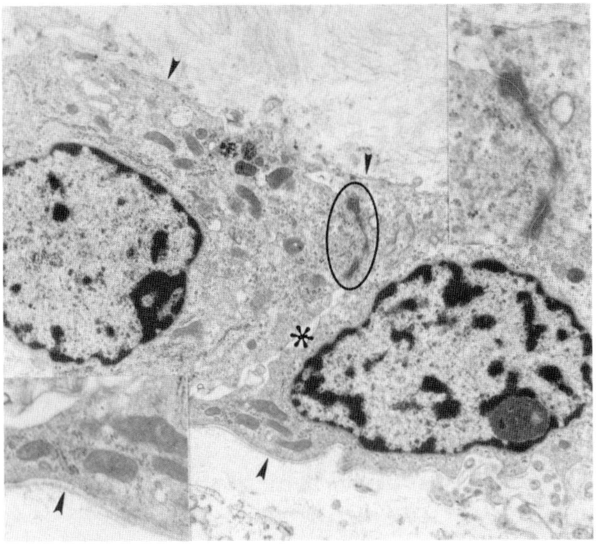

Fig. 36. Retinal pigment epithelium forming a luminal structure (asterisk). Well-developed basement membrane (arrowheads and left lower inset) is present at the base of the cells on either side opposite the lumen. The cells are joined by junctional complexes (oval and upper right inset; main figure ×11,300; lower left inset, ×23,300; upper right inset, ×22,600). (From: Lindsey PS, Michels RG, Luckenbach M, Green WR: Ultrastructure of epiretinal membrane causing retinal starfold. Ophthalmology 90:578-583, 1983. Published courtesy of *Ophthalmology*.)

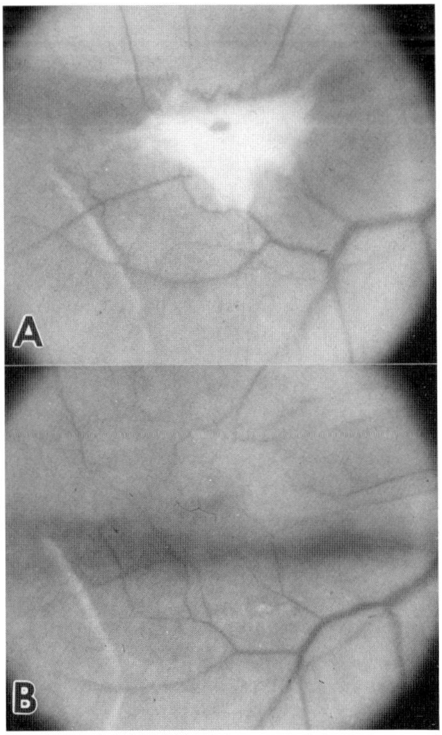

Fig. 37. Pre- (A) and (B) postoperative appearance of a thick, fibrous epiretinal membrane that developed after anterior segment surgery and ocular inflammation.

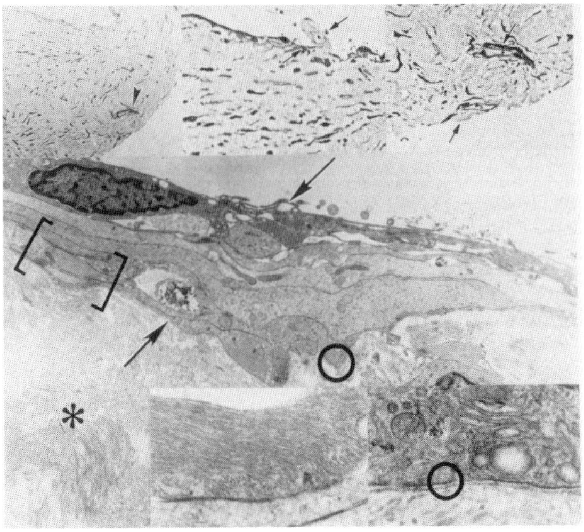

Fig. 38. Membrane from case illustrated in Fig. 37 is thick and composed of fibrous astrocytes, fibrocytes and new collagen. Multiple layers of fibrous astrocytes line inner (vitreal) surface (between arrows). These cells show polarity with basement membrane (circles and bottom right inset), and cells contain numerous cytoplasmic filaments measuring 8 to 10 nm (bracket and bottom left inset). Blood vessels (arrowheads) are also present in membrane (top left and top right insets) (main figure, ×66,600; top insets, paraphenylenediamine, top left inset, ×160; top middle and top right insets, ×250. Bottom left inset, ×50,000; bottom right inset, ×41,000). (From: Michels RG: A clinical and histopathologic study of epiretinal membrane affecting the macula and removed by vitreous surgery. Trans Am Ophthalmol Soc 80:580-656, 1982. Published courtesy of The American Ophthalmological Society.)

with new collagen in this case (Fig. 36).

Anterior proliferative vitreoretinopathy is the condition in which the vitreous is collapsed and condensed along its base and has contribution by fibrous astrocytes with the production of new collagen, blood vessels coming from the peripheral retina and minor contributions of ciliary epithelium. This tissue contracts and leads to traction on the peripheral retina which is drawn forward. This is an identical picture to that described previously as the snow bank in pars planitis[29,30].

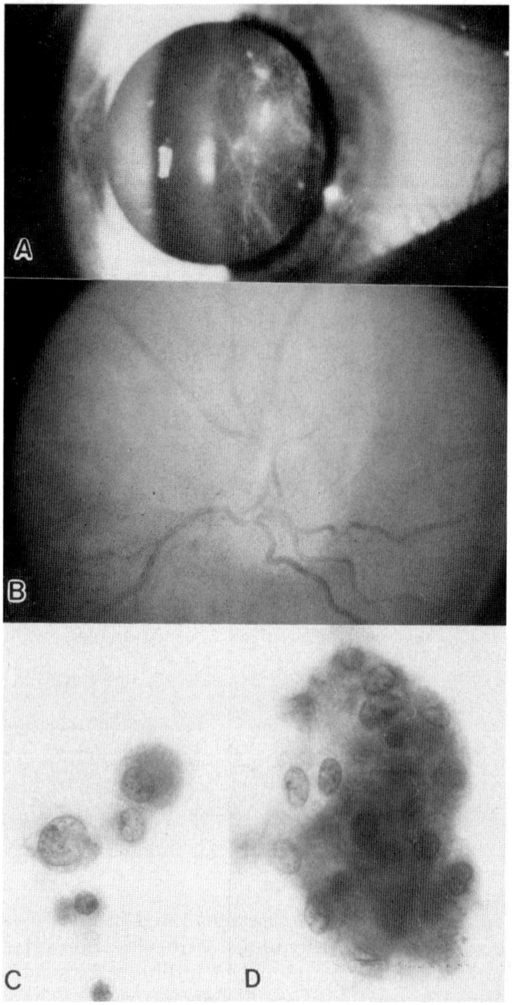

Fig. 39. Pars planitis. Vitrectomy and removal of preretinal membrane in a nine-year-old girl with pars planitis. A: Vitreous contains much debris. B: Epiretinal membrane extends from optic nerve head along superotemporal arcade and distorts macula. Vitreous specimen concentrated by millipore-filter technique showed fragments of fibrocellular membranes and granulomatous inflammation with epithelioid cells, giant cells and lymphocytes. (C,D, ×1000). (From: Green WR: Diagnostic cytopathology of ocular fluid specimens. Ophthalmology 91:726-748, 1984. Published courtesy of *Ophthalmology*.)

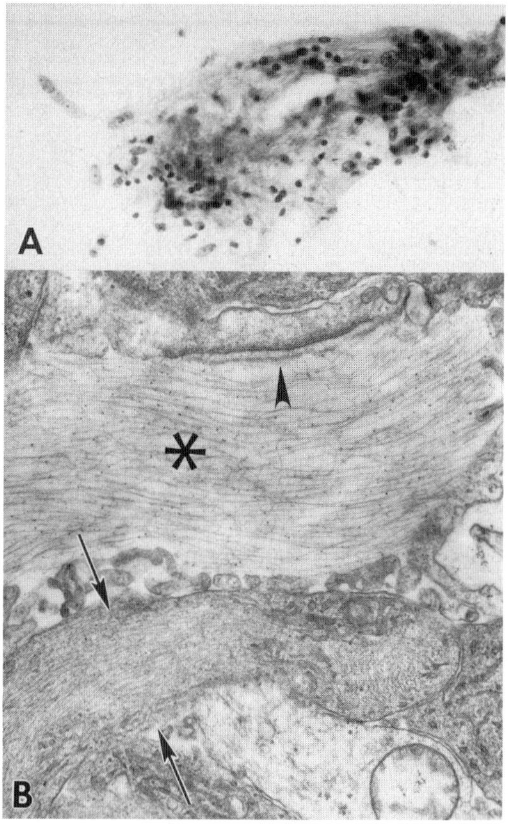

Fig. 40. Same case as in preceding figure. A: Fibrocellular membrane fragment (membrane filter, modified Papanicolaou stain, ×328). B: Ultrastructural appearance of membrane with native collagen (asterisk) fibrous astrocytes with bundles of intermediate filaments (between arrows) and basement membrane (arrowhead) (×33,000).

Macular epiretinal membranes may be idiopathic[5,20,23-25] and can occur after retinal detachment surgery[6,11,32], after accidental and other surgical trauma[12,31,32], and can be associated with impending macular holes[22] and macular holes[33,34], and ocular inflammatory disease[13-16,29,35]. This particularly thick epiretinal membrane had a fibrous appearance (Fig. 37) and followed intracapsular cataract extraction and penetrating kerato-

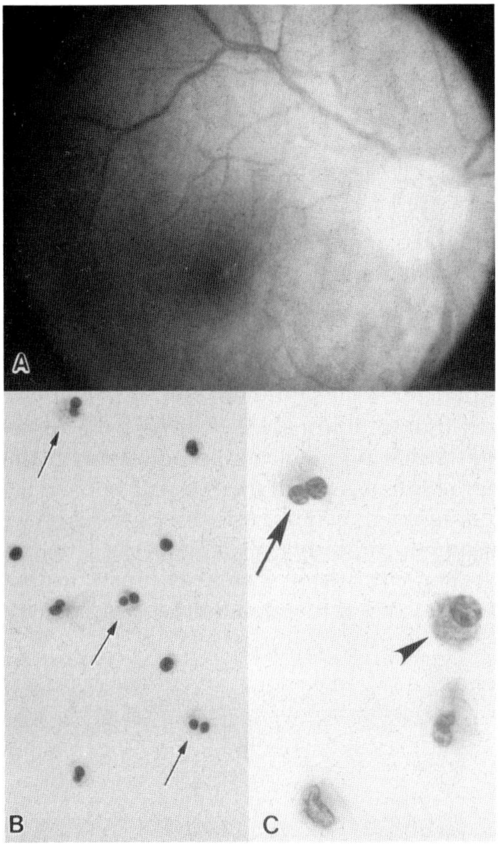

Fig. 41. Nematode endophthalmitis. A seven-year-old girl with presumed *Toxocara canis* had unilateral uveitis, inferior peripheral mass, superior epiretinal membrane (A). Enzyme-linked immunosorbent assay (ELISA) titer was positive at 1:64. Vitrectomy and epiretinal membrane dissection were performed. Examination using the millipore-filter technique disclosed eosinophils (arrows) with typical bilobed nuclei, plasma cells (arrowhead), and lymphocytes (membrane filter, modified Papanicolaou stain, B, ×525; C, ×1200). (From: Green WR: Diagnostic cytopathology of ocular fluid specimens. Ophthalmology 91:726-748, 1984. Published courtesy of *Ophthalmology*.)

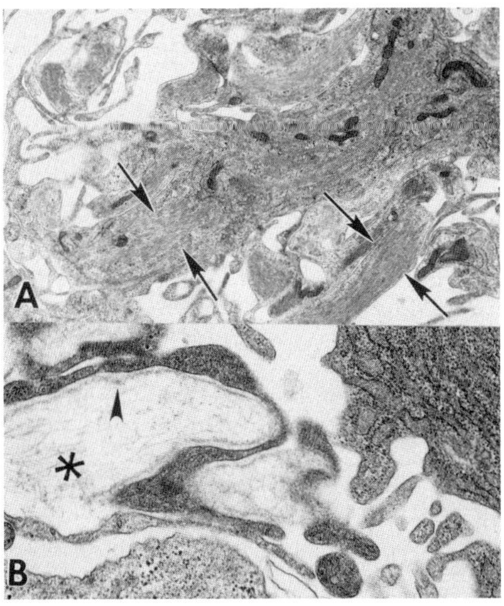

Fig. 42. Preretinal membrane is composed of fibrous astrocytes with bundles of 10 nm filaments (between arrows) and basement membrane (arrowhead) and native collagen (asterisk) (A, ×11,200; B, ×30,000).

plasty. The membrane was removed (Fig. 37B) and examination disclosed a thick fibrocellular tissue (Fig. 38). The principal cell type was the fibrous astrocyte with bundles of intermediate cytoplasmic filaments and basement membrane.

An 11-year-old girl with pars planitis with vitreous opacities (Fig. 39A) developed an epipapillary and preretinal membrane with contraction features (Fig. 39B). Pars plana vitrectomy with removal of vitreous and the membrane disclosed granulomatous inflammation (Fig. 39C,D), and fibrocellular membrane fragments (Fig. 40A) which were composed mostly of fibrous astrocytes (Fig. 40B).

Another example of secondary epiretinal membrane is a child with a peripheral lesion that was considered to be a Toxocara infestation. The patient had an epiretinal membrane with traction features distorting the macula with reduction of vision (Fig. 41A). Examination of the vitreous specimen concentrated with the millipore filter disclosed typical bilobed eosinophiles and some plasma cells (Fig. 41B,C). A portion of the epiretinal membrane, studied by electron microscopy, disclosed eosinophiles and plasma cells and fibrous astrocyte with the typical bundles of intermediate filaments and the basement membrane (Fig. 42).

Idiopathic epiretinal membranes are uniformly associated with posterior vitreous detachment (Fig. 43)[25]. In an electron microscopic study of 101 idiopathic epiretinal membranes, Smiddy and co-workers[25] observed retinal pigment epithelium in 67% of these membranes and retinal pigment epithelium was the predominate cell in half the cases. This observation raises the question of how the retinal pigment epithelium gets on the inner surface of the retina without a hole or other features, as seen in eyes with secondary membranes. It could be postulated that the retinal pigment can migrate through the intact retina or that it could be ectopic and represent some form of dysembryogenesis. Another possibility is that proliferating cells may change characteristics[36-38]. Fig. 44 illustrates the pre- and postoperative appearance of an idiopathic epiretinal membrane. Fig. 45 il-

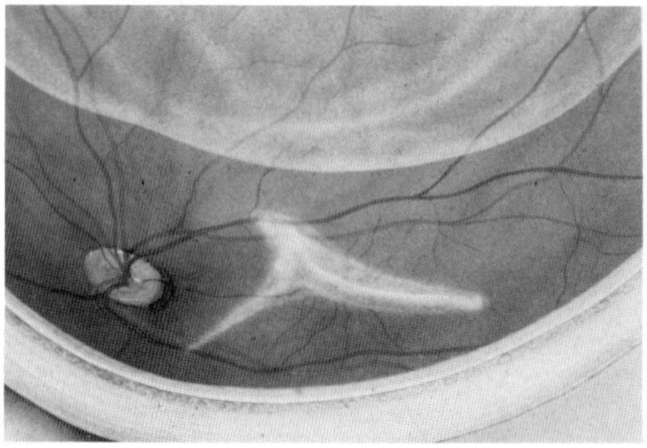

Fig. 43. (left) Features of idiopathic epiretinal membrane. There is a pre-existing posterior vitreous detachment, with an epiretinal membrane covering the macular area and obscuring the distortion of the retinal vasculature. (From: Smiddy WE, Michels RG, Green WR: Morphology, pathology, and surgery of idiopathic vitreoretinal macular disorders. A review. Retina 10:288-296, 1990. Published courtesy of *Retina*.)

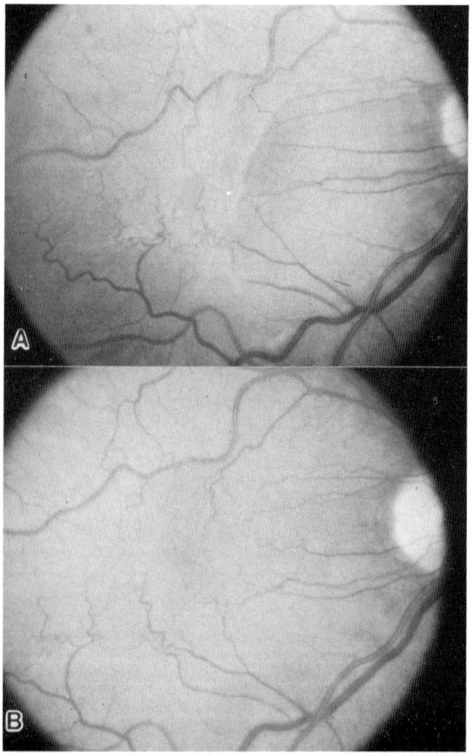

Fig. 44. (right) Pre- (A) and postoperative (B) appearance of a patient with an idiopathic preretinal membrane.

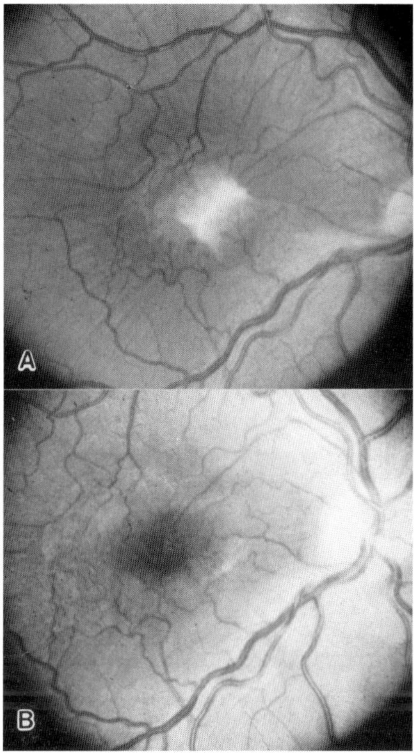

Fig. 45. Pre- (A) and postoperative (B) appearance of a patient with an idiopathic preretinal membrane.

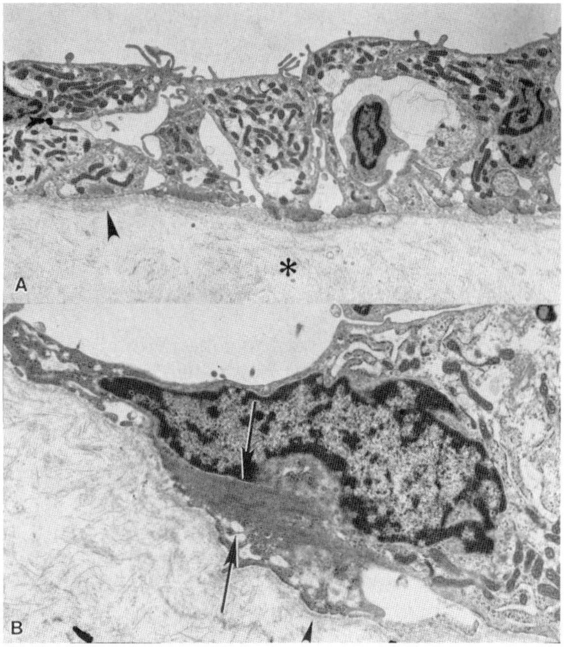

Fig. 46. Retinal pigment epithelial cells with multilayered basement membrane (arrowhead) on a collagen base (asterisk) (×6000). B: Higher power of monolayer of retinal pigment epithelial cells with basement membrane (arrowhead) and aggregates of marginal 5- to 7-nm microfilaments with fusiform densities (between arrows) (×11,000). (From: Smiddy WE, Michels RG, Green WR: Morphology, pathology, and surgery of idiopathic vitreoretinal macular disorders. A review. Retina 10:288-296, 1990. Published courtesy of *Retina*.)

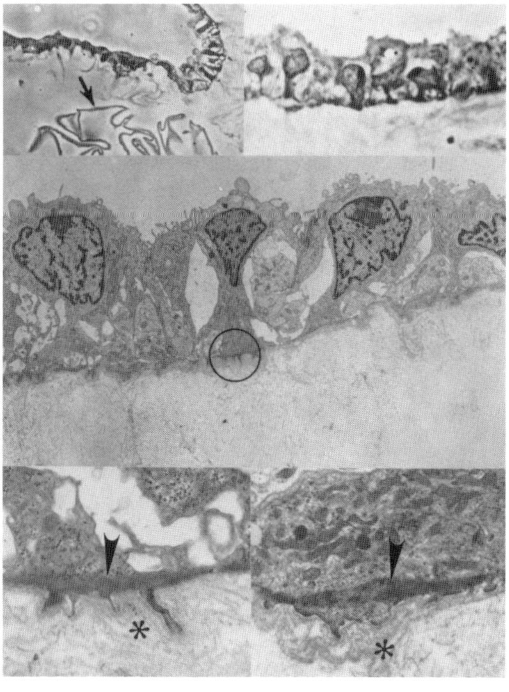

Fig. 47. Idiopathic epiretinal membrane in a 56-year-old woman. Membrane contains new collagen and retinal pigment epithelial cells arranged in monolayer. Cell bases are located externally and have multiple layers of basement membrane (circle and asterisks). Basal aggregates of subplasmalemmal microfilaments measuring 4 to 5 nm and containing linear densities are present (arrowheads). Plasma membrane and associated basement membrane in area of these microfilaments are redundant in villous or finger-like configuration (circle and lower insets). Large fragment of gathered internal limiting membrane is present (arrow, top inset) (main figure, ×4500; bottom left inset, ×12,000; bottom right inset, ×13,500, paraphenylenediamine, top left inset ×160; top right inset, ×1000). (From: Michels RG: A clinical and histopathologic study of epiretinal membrane affecting the macula and removed by vitreous surgery. Trans Am Ophthalmol Soc 80:580-656, 1982. Published courtesy of The American Ophthalmological Society.)

lustrates a more dense idiopathic epiretinal membrane. Fig. 46 is an example of an idiopathic epiretinal membrane with retinal pigment epithelium. There is tissue culture-like monolayer of retinal pigment epithelium with a multilayered basement membrane (Fig. 47). The retinal pigment epithelium in this case has subplasmalemmal aggregates of microfilaments with fusiform densities. Idiopathic epiretinal membranes in children and young adults[26] are more likely to have cells with contractile features (Fig. 48). Rare idiopathic epiretinal membranes in children may have holes in the epiretinal membrane with prolapse of retinal tissue[26]. It was considered that contraction of the cellular ele-

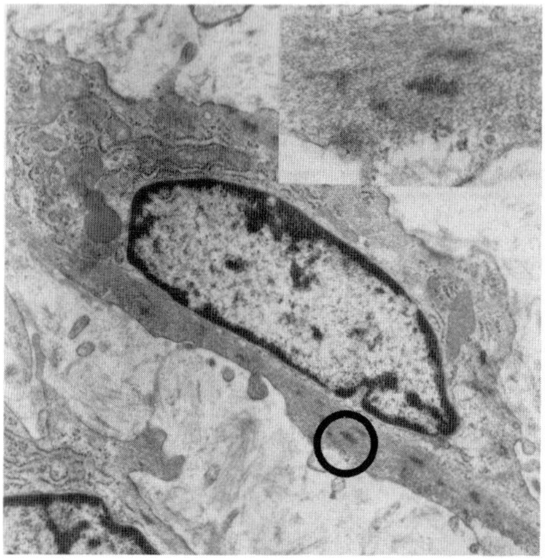

Fig. 48. Idiopathic preretinal membrane in a young person contains myofibrocytes with characteristic spindle shape and containing large aggregates of subplasmalemmal microfilaments measuring 4 to 5 nm and containing small fusiform densities (circle and inset) (main figure, ×14,000; inset, ×44,000). (From: Michels RG: A clinical and histopathologic study of epiretinal membrane affecting the macula and removed by vitreous surgery. Trans Am Ophthalmol Soc 80:580-656, 1982. Published courtesy of The American Ophthalmological Society.)

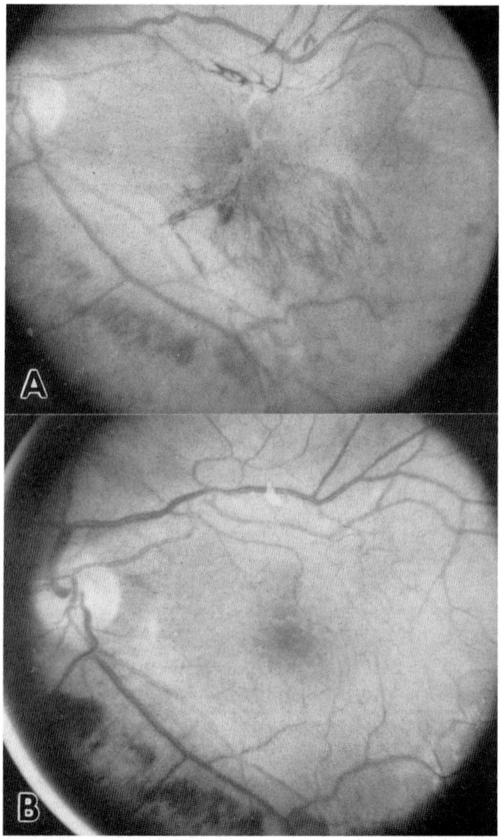

Fig. 49. Pre- (A) and postoperative (B) appearance of a secondary pigmented preretinal membrane. (From: Cherfan GM, Smiddy WE, Michels RG, De la Cruz Z, Wilkenson CP, Green WR: Clinicopathologic correlation of pigmented epiretinal membranes. Am J Ophthalmol 106:536-545, 1988. Published with permission from *The American Journal of Ophthalmology*. Copyright by The Ophthalmic Publishing Company.)

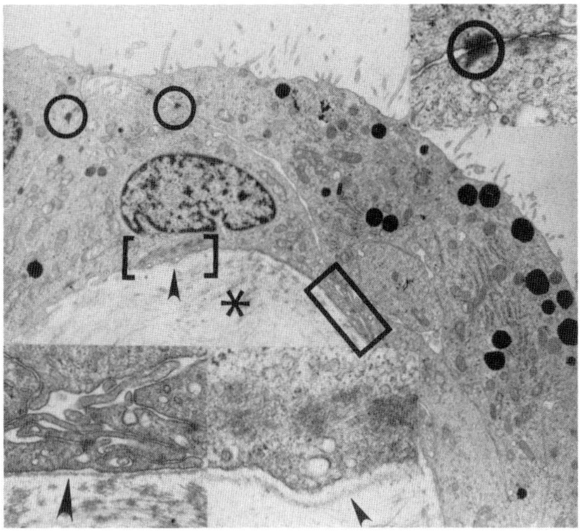

Fig. 50. Retinal pigment epithelial cells in pigmented epiretinal membrane after prior retinal detachment. Cells are arranged in monolayer with cell bases and adjacent basement membrane (arrowheads) located on retinal side. The cellular layer rests on a base of new collagen (asterisk). Cell apices have villous processes, and junctional complexes (circles), are present near apex. Melanin pigment granules are located mainly in apical portions of cells. Occasional subplasmalemmal microfilaments measuring 4 to 5 nm and containing fusiform densities are present (brackets and lower right inset). Basal plasma membrane infoldings are also present (rectangle and lower left inset) (main figure, ×8000; top right inset, ×27,000; bottom left inset, ×20,000; bottom right inset, ×40,000).

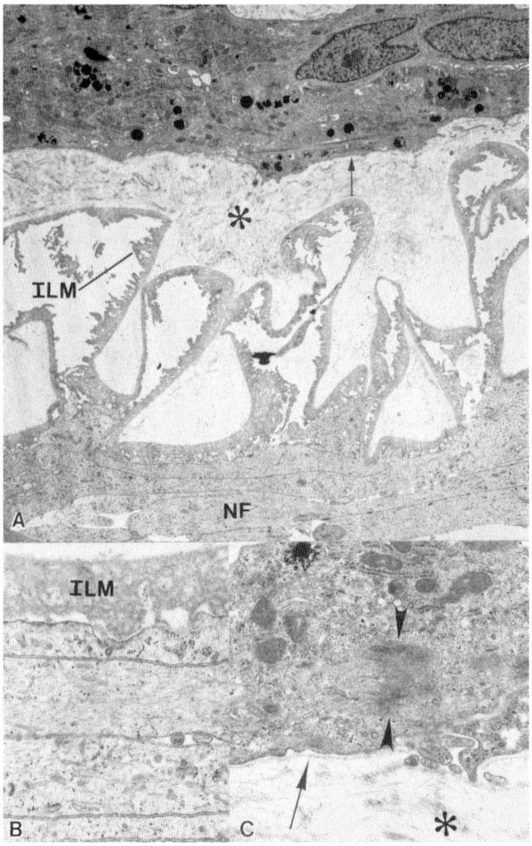

Fig. 51. Thick specimen composed of multiple layers including retinal pigment epithelium with basement membrane (arrow and bottom right inset) and aggregates of 5- to 7-nm filaments with fusiform densities (arrowheads, bottom right); a layer of native collagen (asterisks); gathered internal limiting membrane (ILM); and retinal nerve fibers (NF and bottom left) (×14,000). (From: Cherfan GM, Smiddy WE, Michels RG, De la Cruz Z, Wilkenson CP, Green WR: Clinicopathologic correlation of pigmented epiretinal membranes. Am J Ophthalmol 106:536-545, 1988. Published with permission from *The American Journal of Ophthalmology*. Copyright by The Ophthalmic Publishing Company.)

ments produced tangential traction on the retina which led to prolapse of a nubbin or retina through a defect in the epiretinal membrane.

Another clinical category is pigmented epiretinal membranes (Fig. 49), as reported by Cherfan *et al*[17]. All ten cases in the series were considered secondary as eight had had previous retinal detachment surgery and two were associated with retinal tears. Retinal pigment epithelium was the predominate cell type in all ten cases and in nine the retina

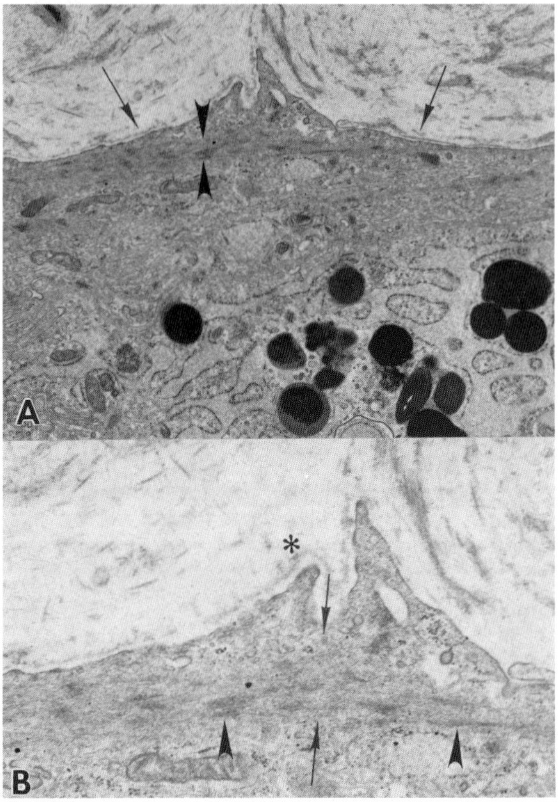

Fig. 52. Upside-down retinal pigment epithelium along the undersurface of a collagenous retroretinal membrane has basement membrane (arrows) and aggregates of microfilaments (between arrowheads) with fusiform densities. B: Higher power of retinal pigment epithelial cell with myoblastic features has basement membrane (asterisk) and subplasmalemmal aggregates of 5 nm filaments (between arrows), with fusiform densities (arrowheads). (A, ×12,000; B, ×26,500). (From: Schwartz D, De la Cruz Z, Green WR, Michels RG: Proliferative vitreoretinopathy: ultrastructural study of 20 retroretinal membranes removed by vitreous surgery. Retina 8:275-281, 1988. Published courtesy of *Retina.*)

pigment epithelium had myoblastic features (Fig. 50). Fibrous astrocytes were present in only two cases and new collagen in only one case. Macrophages with pigment were present in four cases and, in part, accounted for some of the pigmentation. We observed segments of internal limiting membrane in seven cases and nerve fiber layer in four of the ten cases. Fig. 51 illustrates one of the cellular membranes with native collagen, gathered internal limiting membrane, and a segment of nerve fibers.

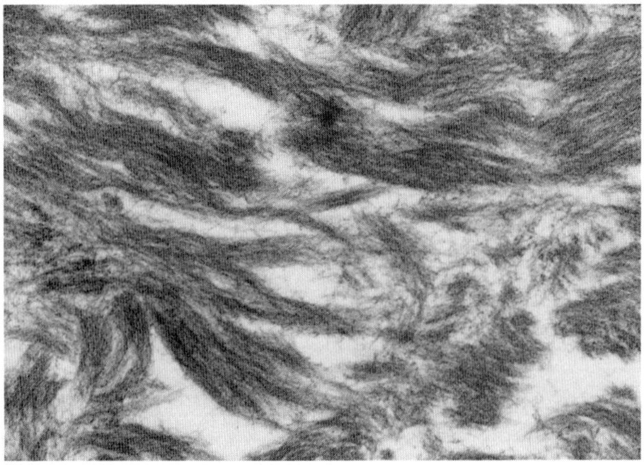

Fig. 53. Abundant fibrin deposition in a retroretinal membrane from a 67-year-old woman with retinal detachment present for three months (×60,000). (From: Schwartz D, De la Cruz Z, Green WR, Michels RG: Proliferative vitreoretinopathy: ultrastructural study of 20 retroretinal membranes removed by vitreous surgery. Retina 8:275-281, 1988. Published courtesy of *Retina.*)

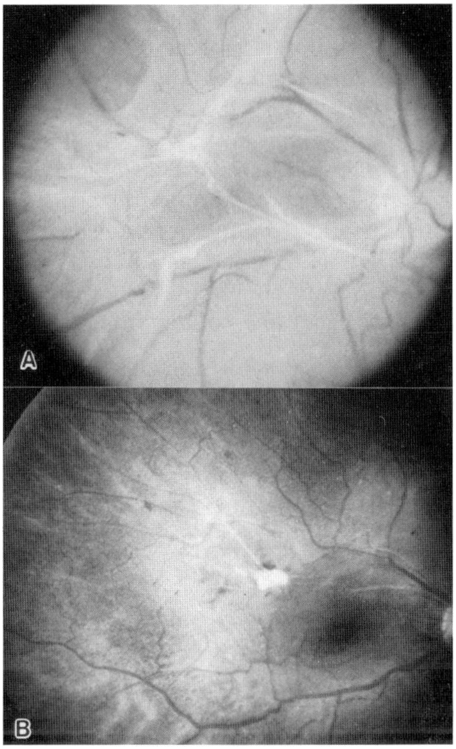

Fig. 54. Pre- (A) and postoperative (B) appearance of vitreous condensation in the vitreomacular traction syndrome.

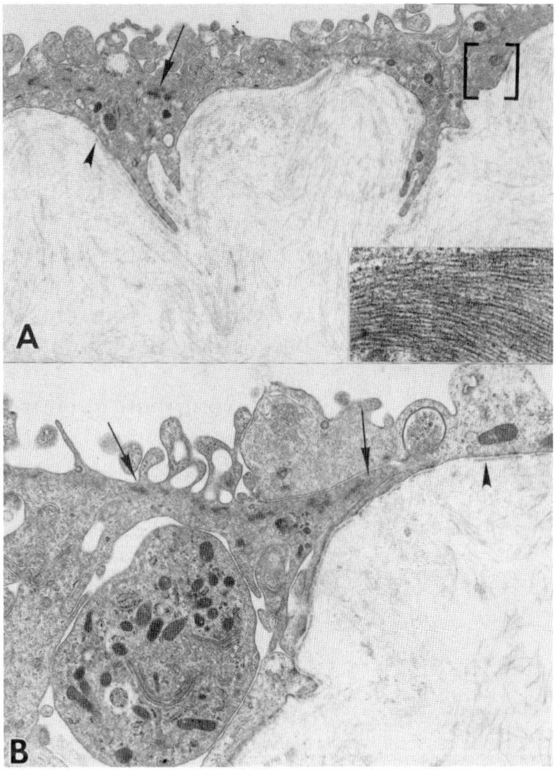

Fig. 55. Tissue removed from patient with the vitreomacular traction syndrome. A: Monolayer of fibrous astrocytes with basement membrane (arrowhead), aggregates of 5- to 7-nm microfilaments (arrow), and large bundles of 10-nm filaments (bracket and inset). Apparent contraction of cellular layer had a gathering effect on the collagen base (×10,000; inset, ×54,000). B: Another fibrous astrocyte showing basement membrane (arrowhead) and an apparent tension line of marginal aggregates of 5- to 7- nm microfilaments with fusiform densities (arrows) (×12,000).

Schwartz and co workers[8] reported the histopathologic features of 20 cases of surgically removed retroretinal membranes. Retinal pigment epithelium was the principal cell type. Fibrous astrocytes were present in 13 cases. In 11 of the cases, cells with myoblastic features were present – either myofibroblast (six) or RPE with myoblastic differentiation (five). Fig. 52 is an example of a retroretinal membrane with retinal pigment epithelium. We found a conspicuous component of fibrin in four of the specimens (Fig. 53). The fibrin is considered to act as a scaffold on to which retinal pigment epithelium can grow and produce a retroretinal membrane.

The vitreomacular syndrome is the condition in which there is partial posterior detachment with remaining attachment in the macular and optic nerve areas (Fig. 54)[19,20]. In cases where membranes were isolated for electron microscopy, Smiddy and co-workers[19] observed fibrous astrocytes as the principal cell in all cases (Fig. 55). Fibrocytes were present in two specimens, myofibrocytes in three, macrophages in four and segments of internal limiting membrane were removed along with the epiretinal membrane and vitreous membranes in six. All seven specimens had native collagen and one additionally had new collagen.

The idiopathic unilateral vitreous fibrosis with traction detachment syndrome is characterized by partial posterior vitreous detachment with remaining attachment at the optic nerve head and macula, secondary fibrosis, traction and distortion of the posterior pole (Fig. 56). Myofibrocytes (Fig. 57), fibrocytes and possible fibrous astrocytes were identified by electron microscopy.

Smiddy and co-workers[22] have studied specimens from 29 cases of impending macular holes. We observed vitreous strands in all 29 cases, fibrocellular membrane fragments in three and segments of internal limiting membrane in four. Electron microscopic study of seven of the cases disclosed native collagen in six, new collagen in one, and in one there was some fibrocellular tissue and a segment of internal limiting membrane. The collagen is considered native because the fiber diameter is 8 to 10 nm. New collagen has a fiber diameter of 16 to 20 nm[39].

The principal cells which contribute to periretinal proliferation are retinal fibrous astrocytes and retinal pigment epithelium. The retinal glial cells gain access to the inner surface of the retina and vitreous in natural occurring areas where the internal limiting membrane of the retina is absent – at the foveola, optic nerve head, along major retinal blood vessels, and in the vitreous base of the area of retinal tufts. Acquired lesions where

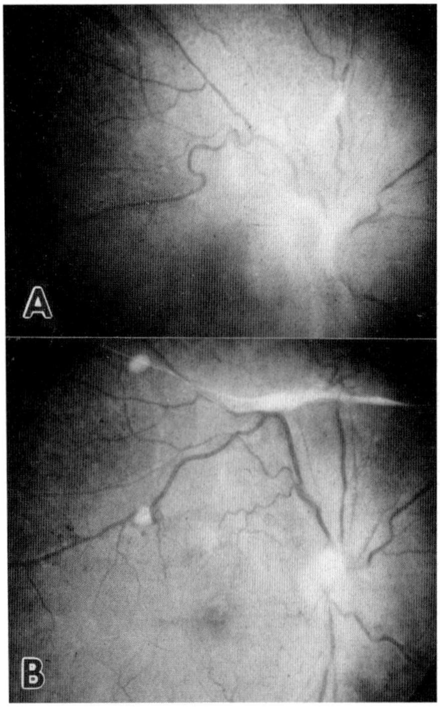

Fig. 56. A: Fibrocellular proliferation has progressed and covers proximal portion of superior temporal arcade and maculopupillary bundle area. The macula is detached and pulled toward the disc. B: Cut edge of cellular tissue above the optic nerve head where vitreous was firmly adherent to retina. (From: Thomas EL, Michels RG, Green WR, Malouf G: Idiopathic progressive unilateral fibrous fibrosis and secondary traction retinal detachment. Retina 2:134-144, 1982. Published courtesy of *Retina*.)

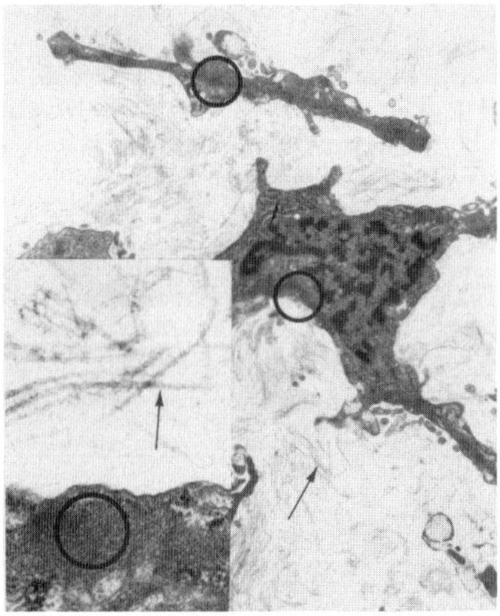

Fig. 57. Ultrastructural appearance of spindle- and stellate-shaped cells with an irregularly shaped nucleus, moderate amount of rough endoplasmic reticulum and marginally located aggregates of microfilaments (circles and inset) measuring 4 nm in diameter. New collagen with fibrils measuring 20 to 25 nm (arrows, main figure and inset) is located between the cells (×11,000; inset, ×60,000). (From: Thomas EL, Michels RG, Green WR, Malouf G: Idiopathic progressive unilateral fibrous fibrosis and secondary traction retinal detachment. Retina 2:134-144, 1982. Published courtesy of *Retina*.)

fibrous astrocytes gain excess to the inner surface of the retina and vitreous include retinal tags, pits, holes and tears, sites of avulsed retinal vessels, areas of degenerative remodelling, lattice degeneration, and random sites of vitreous traction. Retinal pigment epithelium gains access to the inner surface of the retina and vitreous at retinal tears, holes, dialysis, areas of lattice degeneration, the ora serrata, and perhaps by migration through the retina.

Some generalizations concerning the principal cell types in the various clinical setting of periretinal proliferation can be made. The retinal pigment epithelium is the predominate cell in proliferative vitreoretinopathy, idiopathic and pigmented preretinal membrane and retroretinal membranes. It is also present in up to 50% of post-retinal detachment macular puckers. Fibrous astrocytes are the predominate cells in proliferative diabetic retinopathy, secondary epiretinal membranes after surgery, trauma, ocular inflammatory disease and in the vitreomacular traction syndrome. Myofibrocytes have slight predominance in the idiopathic progressive unilateral vitreous fibrosis with secondary traction detachment and in idiopathic membranes in children.

Periretinal proliferation is a dynamic cell-mediated process that goes through the evolution of cellular proliferation, contraction, and collagen production. The contracted site is perpetuated by collagen.

Some of the molecular biological features of periretinal proliferation are being unravelled and the roles of the breakdown of the blood-ocular barrier, fibronectin, platelet derived growth factor and transforming growth factor-beta are being investigated.

References

1. Green WR: Vitreomacular juncture. In: Ryan SJ (ed) Retina, Vol 3, Ch 117, pp 13-69. St Louis: CV Mosby 1989
2. Foos RY: Vitreoretinal juncture: simple epiretinal membranes. Albrecht von Graefe's Arch Klin Exp Ophthalmol 189:231-250, 1974
3. Haeguard S, Jensen OA, Prause JO: Structure of the vitreal face of the monkey disc (Macacca mulatta) SEM on frozen-crushed optic nerve heads supplemented by TEM and immunohistochemistry. Graefe's Arch Clin Exp Ophthalmol 226:377-383, 1988
4. Machemer R, Laqua K: pigment epithelium proliferation in retinal detachment (massive periretinal proliferation). Am J Ophthalmol 80:1-23, 1975
5. Kampik A, Kenyon KR, Michels RG, De la Cruz Z: Epiretinal and vitreous membranes: comparative study of 56 cases. Arch Ophthalmol 99:1445-1454, 1981
6. Michels RG: A clinical and histopathologic study of epiretinal membrane affecting the macula and removed by vitreous surgery. Trans Am Ophthalmol Soc 80:580-656, 1982
7. Wilkes SR, Mansour AM, Green WR: Proliferative vitreoretinopathy. Histology of retroretinal membranes. Retina 7:94-101, 1987
8. Schwartz D, De la Cruz Z, Green WR, Michels RG: Proliferative vitreoretinopathy: ultrastructural study of 20 retroretinal membranes removed by vitreous surgery. Retina 8:275-281, 1988
9. Wallyn RH, Hilton GF: Subretinal fibrosis in retinal detachment. Arch Ophthalmol 97:2128-2129, 1979
10. Zarbin MA, Michels RG, Green WR: Dissection of epiciliary tissue to treat hypotomy after surgery for retinal detachment with proliferative vitreoretinopathy. Retina 11:208-213, 1991
11. Green WR, Kenyon KR, Michels RG, Gilbert HD, De la Cruz Z: Ultrastructure of epiretinal membranes causing macular pucker after retinal detachment surgery. Trans Ophthalmol Soc UK 99:63-77, 1979
12. Kampik A, Green WR, Michels RG, Rice TA: Epiretinale Membrane nach Photokoagulation (postkoagulative Maculopathie). Ber Dtsch Ophthalmol Des 78:593-598, 1981
13. Engel HM, Green WR, Michels RG, Rice TA, Erozan YS: Diagnostic vitrectomy. Retina 1:121-149, 1981
14. Engel HM, De la Cruz Z, Jimenez-Abalahin LD, Green WR, Michels RG: Cytopreparatory techniques for eye fluid specimens obtained by vitrectomy. Acta Cytol 26:551-560, 1982
15. Green WR: Diagnostic cytopathology of ocular fluid specimens. Ophthalmology 91:726-748, 1984

16. Michels RG, Green WR, Engel HM, Rice TA, Erozan YS: Diagnostic vitrectomy. In: Jakobiec FA, Sigelman J (eds) Advanced Techniques in Ocular Surgery, pp 224-281. Philadelphia: WB Saunders 1984
17. Cherfan GM, Smiddy WE, Michels RG, De la Cruz Z, Wilkenson CP, Green WR: Clinicopathologic correlation of pigmented epiretinal membranes. Am J Ophthalmol 106:536-545, 1988
18. Maguire AM, Smiddy WE, Nanda SK, Michels RE, De la Cruz Z, Green WR: Clinicopathologic correlation of recurrent epiretinal membranes after previous surgical removal. Retina 10:213-222, 1990
19. Smiddy WE, Green WR, Michels RG, De la Cruz Z: Ultrastructural studies of vitreomacular traction syndrome. Am J Ophthalmol 107:177-185, 1989
20. Smiddy WE, Michels RG, Green WR: Morphology, pathology, and surgery of idiopathic vitreoretinal macular disorders. A review. Retina 10:288-296, 1990
21. Thomas EL, Michels RG, Green WR, Malouf G: Idiopathic progressive unilateral fibrous fibrosis and secondary traction retinal detachment. Retina 2:134-144, 1982
22. Smiddy WE, Michels RG, De Bustros S, De la Cruz Z, Green WR: Histopathology of tissue removed during vitrectomy for impending macular hole. Am J Ophthalmol 108:360-364, 1989
23. Kampik A, Green WR, Michels RG: Ultrastructural features of progressive idiopathic epiretinal membrane removed by vitreous surgery. Am J Ophthalmol 90:797-809, 1980
24. Smiddy WE, Michels RG, Gilbert HD, Green WR: Clinicopathologic study of idiopathic macular pucker in children and young adults. Retina 12:232-236, 1992
25. Smiddy WE, Maguire AM, Green WR, Michels RG, De la Cruz Z, Enger C, Jaeger M, Rice TA: Idiopathic epiretinal membrane: ultrastructural characteristics and clinicopathologic correlation. Ophthalmology 96:811-821, 1989
26. Zarbin MA, Michels RG, Green WR: Epiretinal membrane contractive associated with macular prolapse. Am J Ophthalmol 110:610-618, 1990
27. Mittelman D, Green WR, Michels RG, De la Cruz Z: Clinicopathologic correlation of an eye after surgical removal of an epiretinal membrane. Retina 9:143-147, 1989
28. Lindsey PS, Michels RG, Luckenbach M, Green WR: Ultrastructure of epiretinal membrane causing retinal starfold. Ophthalmology 90:578-583, 1983
29. Pederson JE, Kenyon KR, Green WR, Maumenee AE: Pathology of pars planitis. Am J Ophthalmol 86:762-774, 1978
30. Green WR, Kincaid MC, Michels RG, Pederson JE, Kenyon KR, Maumenee AE: Pars planitis. Trans Ophthalmol Soc UK 101:361-367, 1981
31. Lang GK, Green WR, Maumenee AE: Clinicopathologic studies of keratoplasty eyes obtained postmortem. Am J Ophthalmol 101:28-40, 1986
32. Wilson DJ, Green WR: Histopathologic study of the effect of retinal detachment surgery on 49 eyes obtained postmortem. Am J Ophthalmol 103:167-179, 1987
33. Fragieh GT, Green WR, Engel HM: A histopathologic study of macular holes and cysts. Retina 1:311-336, 1981
34. Guyer DR, Green WR, De Bustros S, Fine SL: Histopathologic features of idiopathic macular holes and cysts. Ophthalmology 97:1045-1051, 1990
35. Green WR: Retina. In: Spencer WH (ed), Ophthalmic Pathology: An Atlas and Textbook, Vol 2, Ch 8, pp 589-1291. Philadelphia: WB Saunders Co 1985
36. Müller-Jensen K, Machemer R, Azarnia R: Autotransplantation of retinal pigment epithelium in intravitreal diffusion chamber. Am J Ophthalmol 80:530-537, 1975
37. Vinores SA, Campochiaro PA, Conway BP: Ultrastructural and electron-immunocytochemical characterization of cells in epiretinal membranes. Invest Ophthalmol Vis Sci 31:14-28, 1990
38. Vinores SA, Campochiaro PA, McGehee R, Orman W, Hackett SF, Hjelmeland LM: Ultrastructural and immunocytochemical changes in retinal pigment epithelium, retinal glia, and fibroblasts in vitreous culture. Invest Ophthalmol Vis Sci 31:2529-2545, 1990
39. Hogan MJ, Alvarado JA, Wedell JE: Histology of the Human Eye: An Atlas and Textbook, pp 632-636. Philadelphia: WB Saunders Co 1971

INTRAVITREAL USE OF PERFLUORO-N-OCTANE IN THE MANAGEMENT OF RETINAL DETACHMENT WITH PROLIFERATIVE VITREORETINOPATHY

Antonio Capone, Jr., H. Michael Lambert, Thomas M. Aaberg, Sr., Paul Sternberg, Jr., Pedro F. Lopez and Barry A. Mandell

Retina Service, Department of Ophthalmology, Emory University, Atlanta, Georgia, USA

Abstract

The perfluorocarbon liquids are an important new intraoperative adjunct which complement currently available surgical tools and techniques for managing retinal detachment complicated by proliferative vitreoretinopathy (PVR). Their utility derives from their physical properties and chemical inertness. The vitreoretinal surgeon anticipating the use of perfluoro-N-octane (PFO) should familiarize himself with techniques for instilling and maintaining control of the liquid perfluorocarbon, the management of subretinal fluid (SRF), and techniques for PFO removal.

Prior to the advent of PFO in vitreous surgery, the surgical approach to PVR consisted first of release of pre-equatorial traction, followed by release of that posterior to the equator. When PFO is employed, this order is reversed. Instillation of PFO reposits the detached retina posteriorly, and retinal mobility is minimized. The resultant anteroposterior traction renders the anterior component more accessible and facilitates meticulous dissection. Subretinal fluid is displaced through anterior breaks, obviating the need for iatrogenic posterior retinotomies.

Complications associated with the use of these substances consist of intraoperative subretinal PFO or inadvertent intraocular retention at the conclusion of surgery. The incidence of these complications diminishes as the surgeon gains experience with these agents.

Introduction

Improvement of the surgical treatment of PVR is in the process of evolution. The newest addition to the surgeon's armamentarium for the management of this disease is the family of perfluorocarbon liquids. These substances have modified the contemporary surgical approach to PVR, as well as a number of other retinal conditions[1-8].

Of the various perfluorocarbon liquids, perfluoro-N-octane (PFO), perfluorodecalin, perfluorotributylamine and perfluorophenanthrene have been used clinically. PFO is the most widely used. Its low viscosity renders it the easiest member of this group to handle, and its high vapor pressure enhances evaporation of residual liquid perfluorocarbon during fluid-air exchange. Herein we discuss the techniques for intraoperative use of PFO and its role in contemporary vitreoretinal surgery, with emphasis on the management of PVR.

Supported in part by a departmental grant from Research to Prevent Blindness, Inc.

Address for correspondence: Antonio Capone, Jr., MD, Retina Service, Department of Ophthalmology, Emory University, 1327 Clifton Road, NE, 4th Floor, Atlanta, GA 30322, USA

Retina and Vitreous, pp. 223-236
Proceedings of the Symposium on Retina and Vitreous,
organized by the New Orleans Academy of Ophthalmology
New Orleans, LA, USA, March 12-15, 1992
edited by Rudolph M. Franklin

Perfluorocarbon liquids

Physicochemical properties (Table 1)

Table 1. Physical and chemical properties of commonly used perfluorocarbon liquids

	Perfluoro-octane	*Perfluoro-decalin*	*Perfluoro-tributylamine*
Formula	C_8F_{18}	$C_{10}F_8$	$C_{12}F_{27}N$
Appearance	clear/ colorless	clear/ colorless	clear/ colorless
Purity	99.9%	100%	94%
Molecular weight	438	462	671
Density	1.76	1.942	1.89
Index of refraction	1.27	1.31	1.29
Viscosity*	0.8	2.7	2.8
Surface tension**	14	16	16
Vaporization pressure***	57	13.5	1.14
Boiling point	100°C	142.9°C	177°C

*centistokes at 25°C; **dyne/cm at 25°C; ***mm mercury at 37°C

Perfluorocarbon liquids are comprised of highly stable carbon-fluorine bonds which render them virtually inert·[9]. Foremost among the physical properties which render them useful in vitreoretinal surgery is their density. With a specific gravity of approximately 1.8, PFO is heavier than water or saline. The force exerted by 5 ml of perfluorotributylamine against the retina is 4.3 g, more than 14 times that exerted by the same volume of silicone oil[2]. Its greater relative weight is used to advantage to displace subretinal fluid (SRF) and reposit the retina posteriorly. By virtue of their lower relative specific gravities, loose subretinal blood, nuclear or cortical lens fragments, intraocular lenses, vitreous, retinal pigment epithelial cells or the retina itself may all be anteriorly displaced by PFO as well.

PFO is optically clear and has an index of refraction close to that of saline. Visibility is thus clear and virtually free of optical aberration. The aqueous interface is clearly visible. Its low viscosity facilitates intraocular insertion and removal. The surface tension of PFO is lower than that of water at body temperature. The resultant high interfacial tension renders it immiscible. The boiling point of PFO is high enough that photocoagulation may be performed with little risk of vaporization.

Toxicology

It is axiomatic that a suitable vitreous substitute should neither be toxic to ocular tissues nor augment cellular proliferation[10]. The importance of perfluorocarbon liquid purity has been duly emphasized[10,11]. *In vitro* studies suggest that the perfluorocarbon liquids are indeed biologically inert, as various cell lines have been grown without abnormality on the fluorochemical interface[12-14].

In vivo animal studies have similarly shown little evidence of clinical, electroretinographic or light/electron microscopic adverse effects of the perfluorocarbon liquids after up to 48 hours of intravitreal placement, depending on the agent. No adverse histologic changes have been noted in eyes harboring small residual amounts of PFO for up to six months[10].

Following intravitreal placement of two days or more, histologic changes are generally seen in the inferior retina. These include photoreceptor outer segment distortion, thinning of the outer plexiform layer and preretinal macrophage collection[15]. Similar, albeit milder, changes are seen in the superior retina of eyes wherein silicone oil is used for long-term tamponade[16]. These changes are reversible in the case of perflurotributyline if removed after two days[17].

Exposure of six to 60 days produces morphologic alterations of Müller cells, with bump-like protrusions extending into the inter-photoreceptor space resulting in photoreceptor disarray, infolding of the external limiting lamina and the adjacent outer nuclear layer, loss of photoreceptor segments and nuclei, RPE hypertrophy and drusen formation. Macrophages with remnants of photoreceptor outer segments are seen inferiorly as well. All these findings are restricted to the inferior retina[11]. Only perfluorophenanthrene has been reported to be free of clinical, electroretinographic, or light/electron microscopic evidence of retinal toxicity in rabbit eyes when left in place for six weeks[14].

Instrumentation and general techniques

Instrumentation

A syringe containing PFO is attached to a short span of connector tubing (accompanying the vitreoretinal viscodissector, VISTEC Company, #5092), in turn attached to a blunt-tipped 20-gauge needle. The interval of connector tubing frees the surgeon to control the intraocular needle throughout the course of instillation. Injection is performed by the assistant upon the surgeons cue.

Instillation

Prior to using PFO, all breaks expected to come into contact therewith should be freed of traction, as the high interfacial tension which renders PFO immiscible in saline limits, but does not absolutely restrict, its passage through retinal breaks. If a break cannot be flatly apposed to the subjacent RPE by PFO, and thereby functionally closed, there is considerable risk of subretinal passage of PFO.

Instillation should proceed at a site remote from any retinal break(s) until the spherical collection of intraocular perfluorocarbon well exceeds them in size. Slow, controlled injection with the tip positioned just over the optic nerve head minimizes dispersion into smaller satellite droplets. Maintaining PFO as a single globule preserves clear visualization of the posterior pole. The advantage of PFO's high interfacial tension is lost if collections of PFO smaller than extant breaks gain access thereto. This is rarely a concern for pre-equatorial breaks due to the size of the sphere of PFO by the time it approaches the equator. The anterior edge of PFO should be kept below the level of the infusion port to avoid turbulence and the resultant dispersion which occur as infusate jets through the perfluorocarbon.

Management of subretinal fluid

The most important consideration with regard to management of SRF in cases utilizing PFO is the location of retinal breaks. In procedures performed without PFO, SRF drainage is usually the last step prior to photocoagulation. Following fluid-air exchange, removal of residual SRF is performed either with a Flynn cannula[18] or via a posterior drainage retinotomy. The use of PFO obviates the necessity of posterior retinotomies for the SRF evacuation.

In the setting of anterior retinal breaks, whether isolated or in combination with posterior breaks, instillation of PFO will result in apposition of the traction-free postequatorial retina to the subjacent RPE with displacement of SRF anteriorly. However, when the level of PFO is brought above the most anterior retinal break, displaced SRF is afforded no route of egress. This may result in detachment of the anterior retina and pars plana.

There are three options available at this juncture. The first is simply to remove PFO until the most anterior break is again open. This option improves but often does not remedy the situation, and may be impractical in the setting of isolated posterior pole breaks.

A second option is to perform an air-fluid exchange. Complete removal of PFO may be necessary temporarily for successful execution of this maneuver, and traction anterior to the break should be minimal or have been addressed previously. The globe is rotated away from the most anterior break. PFO is then reintroduced into the eye slowly under direct visualization while the eye is rotated to its normal position. This "steamroller" maneuver serves to displace any residual SRF from the subretinal space into the central vitreous cavity via the anterior retinal defect. PFO is then brought anterior to the break, thereby functionally closing it. Surgery may then proceed either under air or fluid (following reinstillation of fluid in the latter instance), as preferred by the surgeon.

A third option is to perform an anterior endodrainage retinotomy through an area of retina supported by the scleral buckle. SRF may then be removed either by raising the level of PFO or by fluid-air exchange. Given the known complications of endodrainage retinotomies[19], this third option is the least preferred.

Photocoagulation

Following evacuation of SRF, posterior pole breaks are endophotocoagulated. Apposition of the postequatorial retina to the subjacent RPE under PFO is superior to that under air insufflation alone. Photocoagulation of the postequatorial retina is thereby facilitated, with lower overall energy requirements. Furthermore, visualization necessary for photocoagulation is superior in the PFO/balanced saline solution-filled eye compared to the air-filled eye. With air in the aphakic eye there may be folds in Descemet's membrane which must be managed prior to photocoagulation. In the pseudophakic eye, water vapor precipitation on the anterior or posterior lens must be managed as well. Visualization problems associated with the use of air are avoided by the use of PFO tamponade.

When photocoagulation of the pre-equatorial retina is necessary PFO remains in the eye, as the posterior placement of the retina enhances anterior retinal apposition. If there is residual SRF anterior to the collection of PFO it is first addressed as described above.

Removal

PFO is easily removed from the central vitreous cavity employing conventional instrumentation for active or passive fluid extrusion. When removal is performed under saline the collection of PFO retains its spherical shape by virtue of interfacial tension. Complete removal with an extrusion needle under direct visualization is straightforward.

The air:PFO interfacial relationship differs from that between saline and PFO. Forces which work to maintain the collection of PFO as a discrete sphere in saline are not operative for small volumes of PFO in air. As a result, PFO will tend to layer on the posterior retina in a shallow meniscus as does water. Unaware of this, the surgeon may incompletely remove PFO under the mistaken assumption that only a small amount of saline had been left behind. This eventuality may be prevented by infusing a small volume (0.5-1.0 ml) of irrigating solution into the air-filled eye. Once immersed in saline, PFO will again coalesce into droplets. Care is exercised first to remove the PFO, and then the remaining irrigating solution. This procedure may be repeated to confirm complete PFO removal.

Removal of PFO which has passed into the subretinal space intraoperatively is somewhat more problematic. When this occurs in a fluid-filled eye, spheroid subretinal droplets may be apparent in the posterior pole. Complete removal of intravitreal PFO is often necessary, as the retina generally must be artifactually redetached in order for an extrusion tip to access the subretinal accumulation of PFO. Subretinal PFO in an air-filled eye may be more difficult to detect due to subretinal layering. Complete removal in this setting requires at least partial air-fluid exchange with saline neurosensory redetachment.

Proliferative vitreoretinopathy

General considerations

Several authors have reported their experience with the use of perfluorocarbon liquids in the surgical management of PVR[2-6,20]. Most cases of PVR seen at our institution are in advanced stages (CP-6, type 1,2 plus CA-6, type 4,5, or worse)[21]. A scleral buckle is placed first if not already present (Fig. 1). A previously placed buckle is revised, if necessary, to ensure both circumferential support of the vitreous base as well as adequate support of new or inadequately supported preexisting breaks. A broad scleral buckle of moderate height is desired. The resultant central vitreous base displacement improves visualization of and access to pre-equatorial pathology.

Vitreous surgery is performed via the standard 20-gauge, three port pars plana approach. The crystalline lens is spared, when possible, yet is generally sacrificed to provide access to anterior pathology. A core vitrectomy is performed in primary vitreous procedures. Prior to the advent of perfluorocarbon liquids in vitreous surgery, the surgical approach to PVR consisted first of release of pre-equatorial traction, followed by release

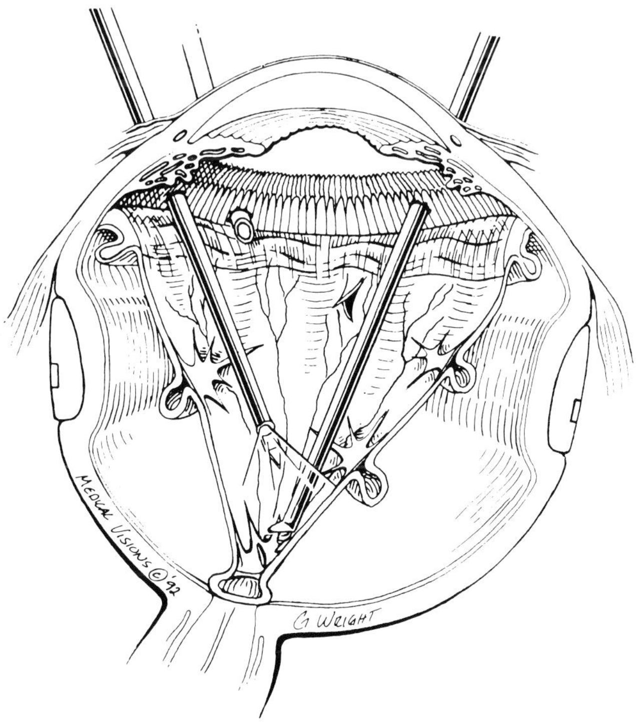

Fig. 1. Cross-section of the globe following placement of #276 scleral buckle on a #240 encircling band, lensectomy and vitrectomy. Posterior pole delamination is performed first. Prepapillary proliferation is grasped with the intraocular microforceps. With the aid of an illuminated pick, the dissection plane is established and delamination extended bimanually in all four quadrants to the equator. Any preexisting or iatrogenic retinal breaks must be freed of traction. Pre-equatorial and equatorial traction have yet to be addressed.

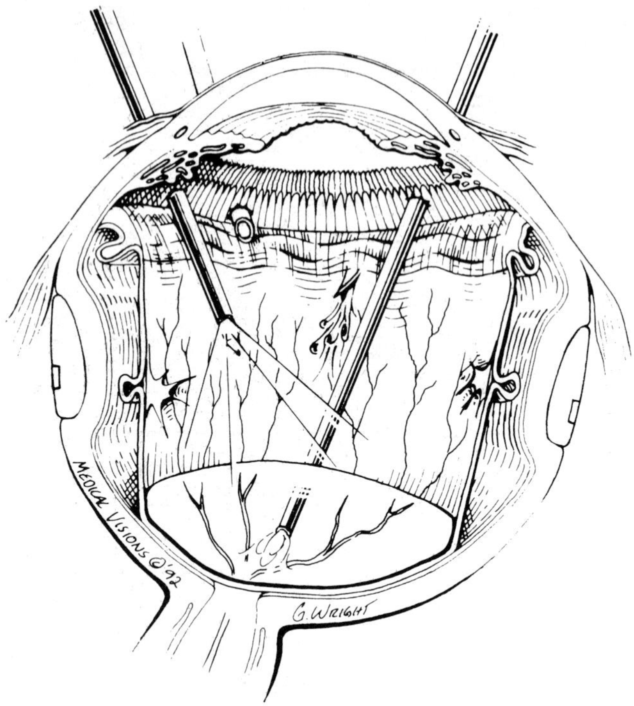

Fig. 2. The blunt infusion needle is positioned over the optic nerve head. Controlled injection is performed, maintaining the tip of the needle in the growing globule of PFO to minimize dispersion into satellite bubbles. SRF exits the subretinal space via a preexisting anterior break.

of that posterior to the equator. When a perfluorocarbon liquid is employed, this order is reversed.

If a peripapillary posterior vitreous detachment is not present, as is typically the case unless PVR develops following trauma or iatrogenically following posterior segment surgery, the posterior hyaloid is separated from the optic disc employing a bimanual maneuver utilizing an illuminated pick and active suction[22,23]. In a previously vitrectomized eye, the dissection is begun by incising confluent pre- and peripapillary proliferation, when present. The posterior pole is delaminated bimanually, employing an illuminated pick and microforceps, and the dissection extended to the equator in all four quadrants (Fig. 1). Considerable mobility of the detached retina may ensue following separation of the posterior hyaloid or delamination of the posterior pole. It is at this juncture that PFO is typically first introduced into the eye.

Postequatorial traction

As stated above, membrane delamination in an eye with PVR begins posteriorly, at or near the disc, and is extended toward the equator in all four quadrants prior to the instillation of PFO (Fig. 2). The adequacy of the postequatorial delamination is then reassessed. Persistent retinal folds under PFO indicate areas of traction which have not been adequately released (Fig. 3). An illuminated pick or analogous instrument may be used to "run" the retinal fold in an attempt to engage residual preretinal proliferative tissue. Once structurally significant traction is eliminated, the normal anatomic relationship of the retina to the subjacent RPE is restored.

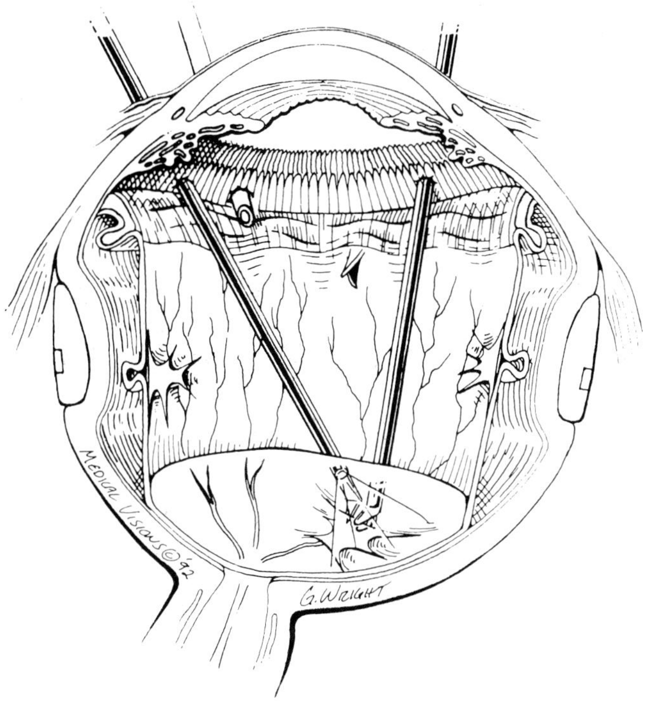

Fig. 3. Flat retinal apposition to the subjacent RPE indicates adequate relief of structurally significant preretinal and subretinal PVR. Such residual, structurally significant PVR is typically apparent under PFO. Preretinal proliferation is removed. Relief of subretinal traction requires removal of PFO and a retinotomy for subretinal access.

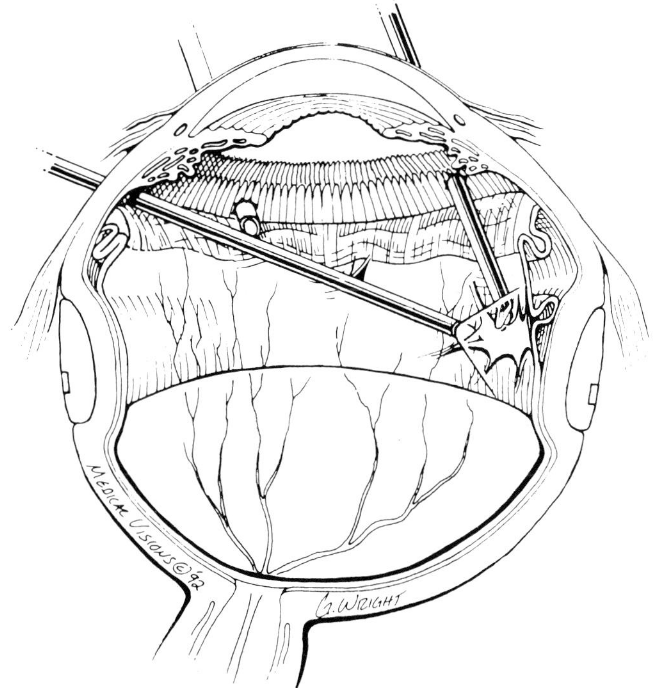

Fig. 4. Equatorial proliferation is addressed next.

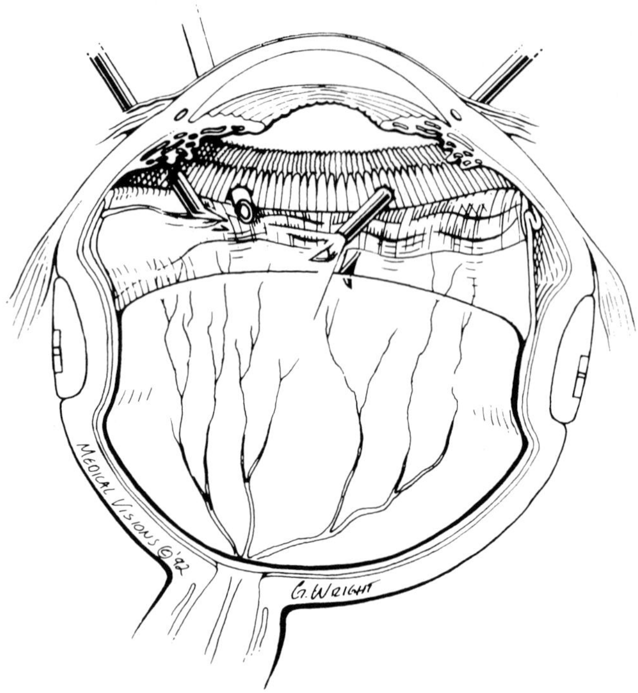

Fig. 5. Anterior proliferation is addressed last.

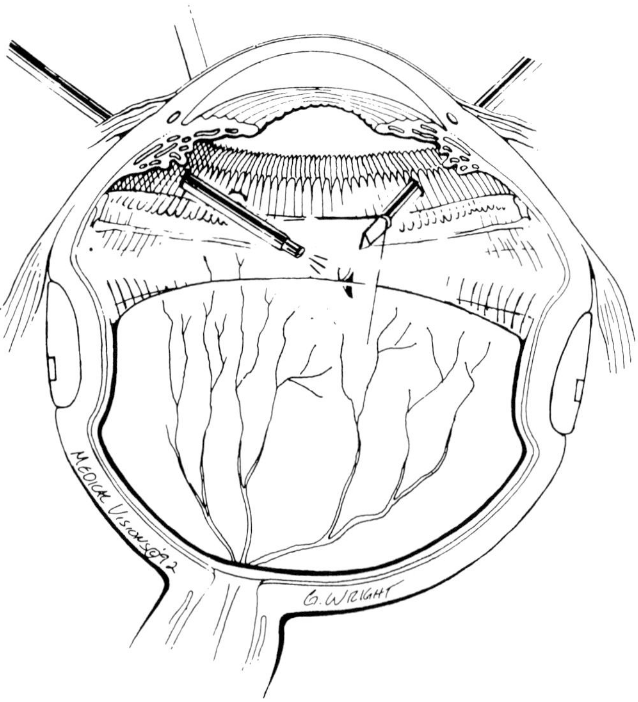

Fig. 6. Air-fluid exchange is performed. Removal of the aqueous layer anterior to the perfluorocarbon results in re-attachment of anterior retina and pars plana.

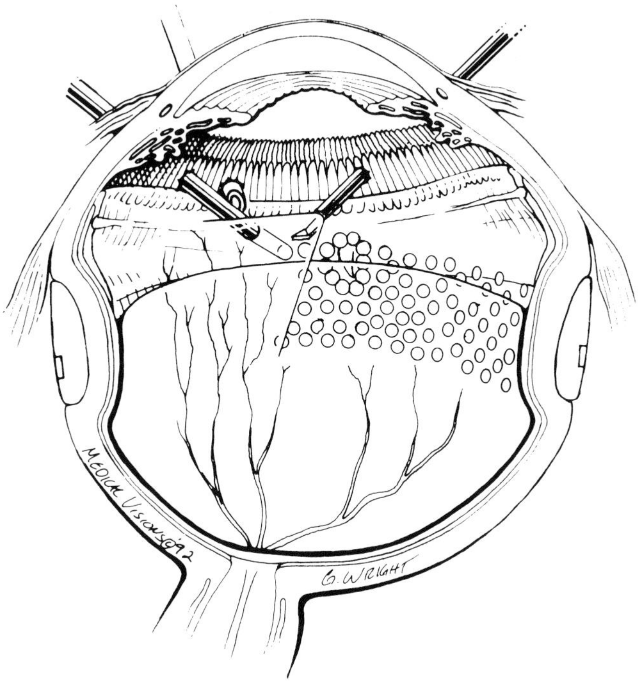

Fig. 7. Circumferential photocoagulation is applied to pre-equatorial retina.

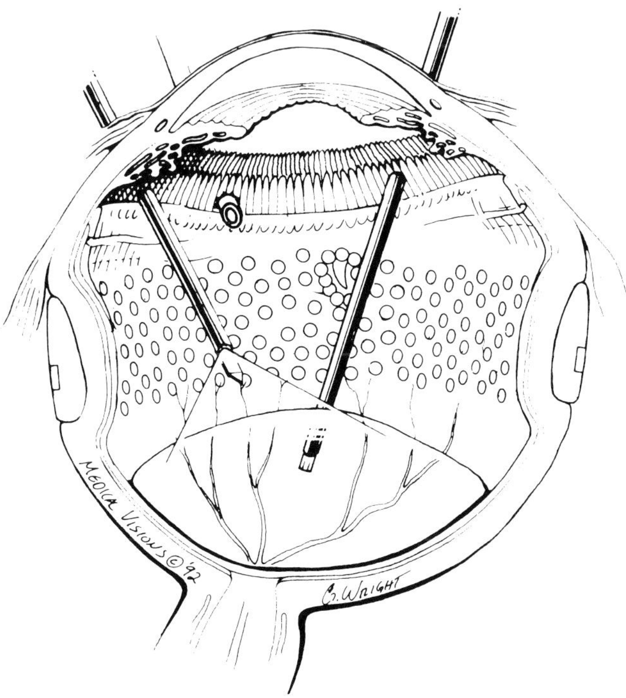

Fig. 8. PFO is then removed passively from the vitreous cavity under air, with the extrusion tip positioned over the disc.

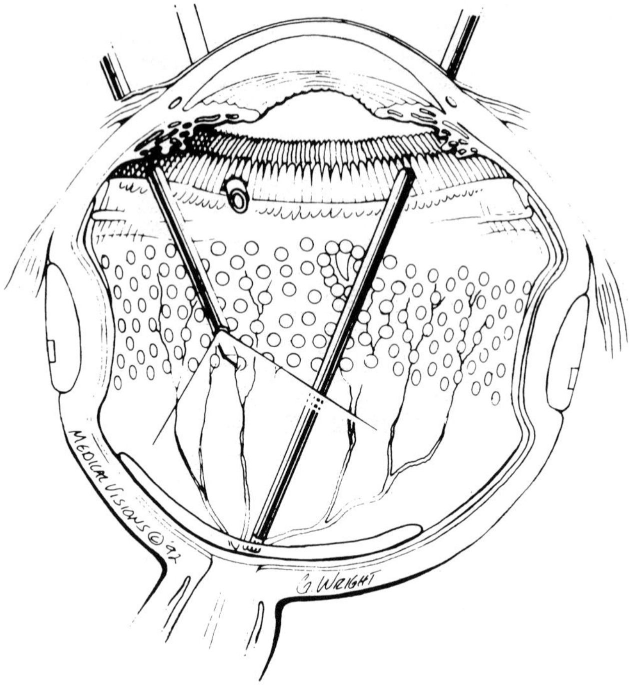

Fig. 9. Small amounts of PFO lay flatly on the retina under air.

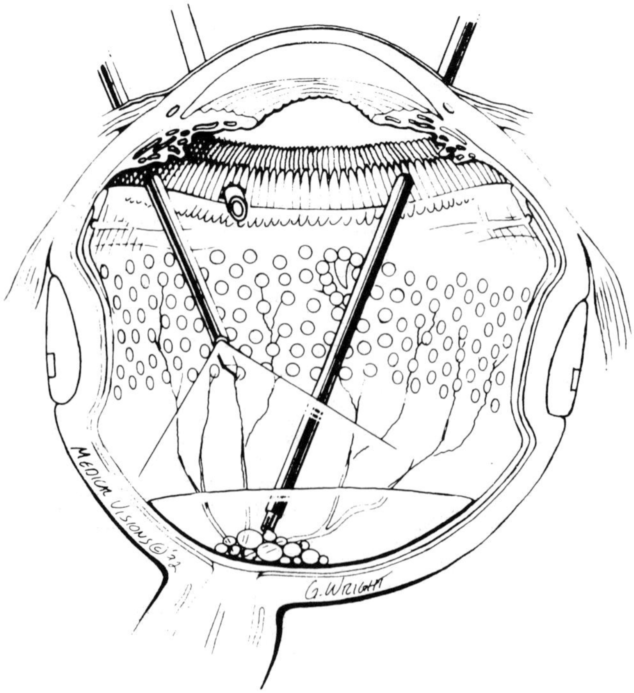

Fig. 10. Saline irrigation causes residual PFO to coalesce into small droplets. The PFO droplets are removed first, then the saline.

PFO may render subretinal PVR dramatically apparent, as in the case of previously unrecognized linear or "napkin-ring" strands, both derived from contracted sheets of proliferative tissue[24,25]. Conversely, subretinal PVR may be only subtly apparent, particularly in the setting of long-standing, highly viscous subretinal fluid which is not readily displaced from the subretinal space by PFO. On occasion a retinal fold under PFO will persist in the absence of detectable preretinal membranes. One must be alert to the possibility of subretinal proliferation in such instances. Removal of PFO, in whole or in part, may be necessary to allow access to subretinal proliferation.

Pre-equatorial traction

The high specific gravity of PFO relative to saline is used to advantage to provide mechanical tamponade. The anteroposterior "counter-traction" renders the retina less mobile, minimizing the risk of retinal incarceration within the sclerotomies as well as the likelihood of creating an inadvertent retinal break. In addition, the vitreous base, which tends to progressively move anteriorly and peripherally as the dissection ensues, is drawn posteriorly. The pre-equatorial proliferation is thereby more easily visualized and accessible (Fig. 4). Furthermore, stabilization of the peripheral retina facilitates meticulous anterior dissection (Fig. 5). Air-fluid exchange is performed to remove the aqueous layer (infusate) lying on top of the PFO to re-attach the anterior retina and detached pars plana. The PFO is then removed following circumferential photocoagulation of pre-equatorial retina supported by the buckle including treatment of all retinal breaks (Figs. 6-10).

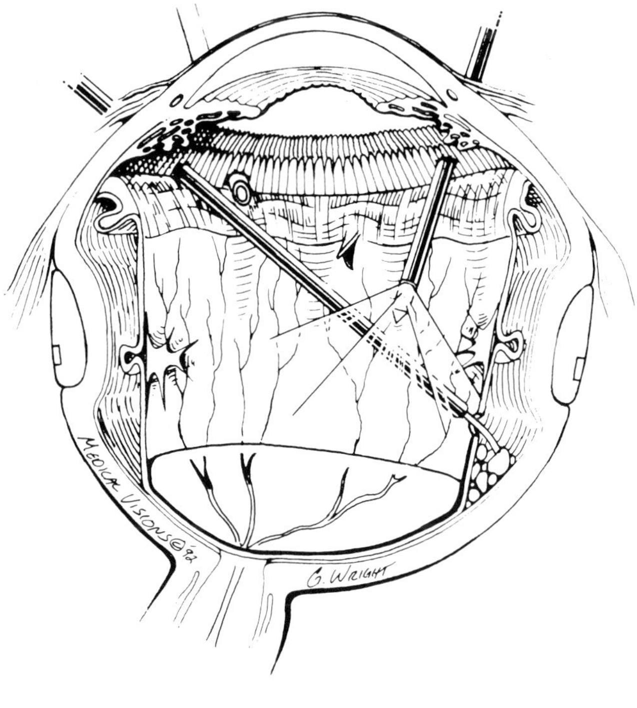

Fig. 11. Excursion of PFO into the subretinal space may occur through retinal breaks which are not free of traction. Once intravitreal PFO has been removed, a cannulated subretinal fluid aspirator is extended posteriorly to the peripapillary region, whereupon subretinal PFO is gently actively extruded.

Complications

Complications resulting from the intraocular use of PFO are minimal. Migration of PFO into the subretinal space is the most commonly encountered intraoperative complication (Fig. 11), and was discussed above. The most common complication encountered postoperatively is retained intraocular PFO[16,19,20], seen in nearly 25% (4/17) of eyes in one series[15]. As with intraoperative subretinal PFO, this complication occurs less often as the surgeon gains experience.

Retained intraocular PFO may be either intravitreal or subretinal. Small droplets of intravitreal PFO appear to be well tolerated clinically for at least 15 months[14]. In aphakic and many pseudophakic patients these small globules of PFO may be brought into the anterior chamber postoperatively (Fig. 12) by positioning the patient face down, whereupon they may be carefully aspirated with a 30-gauge needle through the limbus

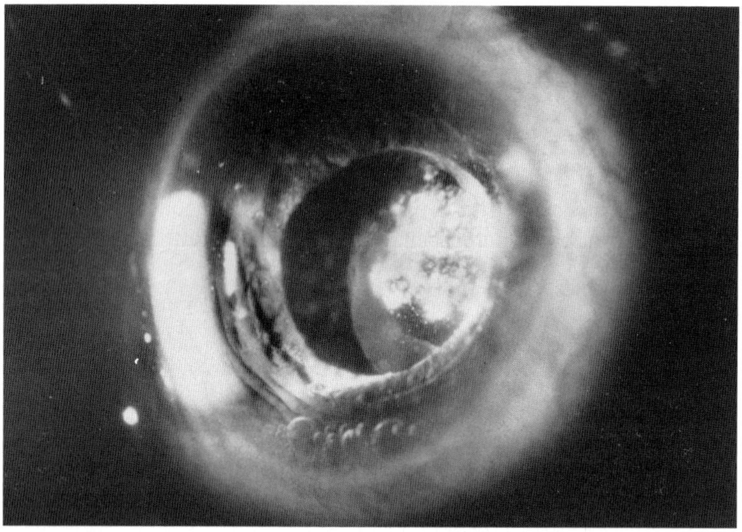

Fig. 12. Droplets of PFO brought into the inferior anterior chamber angle after patient positioning.

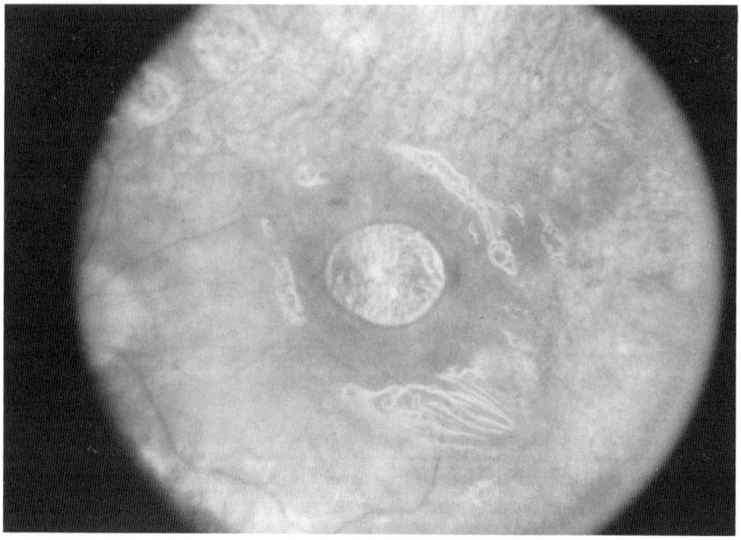

Fig. 13. Localized collection of submacular PFO in a silicone oil filled eye.

under topical anesthesia on an outpatient basis. If present in a silicone oil filled eye, PFO will gravitate inferiorly. Whether removed or retained, the globules of intravitreal PFO are generally of little visual consequence.

An exception to this statement is the case of retained subretinal PFO. Perfluorocarbon-related photoreceptor toxicity has been discussed above. If the collection of PFO is small and extramacular, observation is an acceptable management option. When small collections of subretinal PFO become trapped beneath the macula (Fig. 13) the patient will note a relative central scotoma. Prompt removal of PFO is necessary in order to prevent permanent compromise of central vision.

In vitro study has demonstrated that PFO of high purity is a poor substrate for fibroblast growth or proliferation[10]. It is thus unlikely that the use of PFO would exacerbate or promote the development of PVR.

References

1. Haidt SJ, Clark LC, Ginsberg J: Liquid perfluorocarbon replacement of the eye. Invest Ophthalmol Vis Sci (Suppl) 22:233, 1982
2. Chang S: Low viscosity liquid fluorochemicals in vitreous surgery. Am J Ophthalmol 103:38, 1987
3. Chang S, Ozmert E, Zimmernman NJ: Intraoperative perfluorocarbon liquids in the management of proliferative vitreoretinopathy. Am J Ophthalmol 106:668, 1988
4. Chang S, Lincoff H, Zimmerman NJ, Fuchs W: Giant retinal tears: surgical techniques and results using perfluorocarbon liquids. Arch Ophthalmol 107:761, 1989
5. Chang S, Reppucci V, Zimmerman NJ, Heinemann M, Coleman DJ: Perfluorocarbon liquids in the management of traumatic retinal detachments. Ophthalmology 96:785, 1989
6. Glaser BM, Carter JB, Kuppermann BD, Michels RG: Perfluorooctane in the treatment of giant retinal tears with proliferative vitreoretinopathy. Ophthalmology 98:1613, 1991
7. Le Mer Y, Haut J: Perfluorooctane liquid in the giant retinal tear with retinal inversion. J Fr Ophtalmol 13:247, 1990
8. Mathis A, Pagot V, David JL: The use of perfluorodecalin in diabetic vitrectomy. Fortschr Ophthalmol 88:148, 1991
9. Sargent JW, Seffl RJ: Properties of perfluorinated liquids. Fed Proc 29:1699, 1970
10. Sparrow JR, Ortiz R, MacLeish PR, Chang S: Fibroblast behaviour at aqueous interfaces with perfluorocarbon, silicone, and fluorosilicone liquids. Invest Ophthalmol Vis Sci 31:638, 1990
11. Eckardt C, Nicolai U, Winter M, Knop E: Experimental intraocular tolerance to liquid perfluorooctane and perfluoropolyether. Retina 11:375, 1991
12. Keese CR, Giaver I: Cell growth on liquid interfaces: role of surface active compounds. Proc Nat Acad Sci USA 80:5622, 1983
13. Rosenberg MD: The culture of cells and tissues at the saline-fluorocarbon interface. In: Ramakrishnan CV (ed) Tissue Culture, p 63. The Hague: W Junk 1965
14. Nabih M, Peyman GA, Clark LC et al: Experimental evaluation of perfluorophenanthrene as a high specific gravity vitreous substitute: a preliminary report. Ophthalmic Surg 20:286, 1990
16. Chang S, Sparrow J, Iwamoto T, Gershbein A, Ross R, Ortiz R: Experimental studies of tolerance to intravitreal perfluoro-n-octane liquid. Retina 11:367, 1991
16. Gonvers M, Horning JP, De Courten C: The effect of liquid silicone on the rabbit retina: histologic and ultrastructural study. Arch Ophthalmol 104:1057, 1986
17. Chang S, Zimmerman NJ, Iwamoto T et al: Experimental vitreous replacement with perfluorotributylamine. Am J Ophthalmol 103:29, 1987
18. Flynn HW, Blumenkranz MS, Parel JM, Lee WG: Cannulated subretinal fluid aspirator for vitreoretinal microsurgery. Am J Ophthalmol 103:106, 1987
19. McDonald HM, Lewis H, Aaberg TM, Abrams GW: Complications of endodrainage retinotomies created during vitreous surgery for complicated retinal detachment. Ophthalmology 96:358, 1989
20. Blinder KJ, Peyman GA, Paris CL, Dailey JP, Alturki W, Lui KR, Gremillion CM, Clark LC: Vitreon, a new perfluorocarbon. Br J Ophthalmol 75:240, 1991
21. Machemer PM, Aaberg TM, Freeman MH, Irvine AR, Leas JS, Michels RM: An updated classification of retinal detachment with proliferative vitreoretinopathy. Am J Ophthalmol 112:159, 1991

22. Han DP, Abrams GW, Aaberg TM: Surgical excision of the attached posterior hyaloid. Arch Ophthalmol 106:998, 1988
23. Kelly NE, Wendel RT: Vitreous surgery for idiopathic macular holes. Arch Ophthalmol 109:654, 1991
24. Sternberg P, Machemer R: Subretinal proliferation. Am J Ophthalmol 98:456, 1984
25. Lewis H, Aaberg TM, Abrams GW, McDonald HR, Williams GA, Mieler WF: Subretinal membranes in proliferative vitreoretinopathy. Ophthalmology 96:1403, 1989

ADVANCES IN VITREOUS SURGERY: PERFLUOROCARBON LIQUIDS

Gary W. Abrams, Everton L. Arrindell, Mitchell D. Wolf, William F. Mieler and Dennis P. Han

Department of Ophthalmology, Medical College of Wisconsin, Milwaukee, WI, USA

Abstract

The perfluorocarbon liquids (PFCLs) are a class of heavier than water liquids useful as an intraoperative tool in vitreoretinal surgery. Injected posteriorly over the detached retina during vitrectomy, PFCL will re-attach the retina from posteriorly to anteriorly, making a drainage retinotomy unnecessary. PFCLs are used to unfold and re-attach the flap of a giant tear or retinotomy, to intraoperatively fixate bullous posterior retina during anterior vitrectomy and membrane peeling, to open folds of retina to reveal membranes, and to displace subretinal blood anteriorly to facilitate removal. In addition, PFCL can be used to float a dislocated lens or pseudophakos away from the retina to aid in management. Clinical reports are summarized and show favorable early results. Major complications, usually preventable, are corneal damage if PFCL is left in contact with the corneal endothelium and subretinal PFCL.

Introduction

Since the initial descriptions of vitreous surgery by Machemer *et al.* [1-4], there have been many advances. While there has been steady progress in both instrumentation and technique, several advances have had major impact on the practice of vitreoretinal surgery. During the history of vitreoretinal surgery, the management of some diseases was transformed in a short period of time by the introduction of a new method or technique. An example is the marked improvement in the management of retinal detachment with proliferative vitreoretinopathy (PVR) following the introduction of air pumps[5,6] and laser endophotocoagulation[7] and the description of the use of these modalities in the management of PVR. Further improvements came with the introduction of long-acting gases[8], postoperative fluid-gas exchange[9], retinotomy and retinectomy[10-12], and the use of silicone oil in vitreous surgery[13]. Within a relatively short period of time, results improved from approximately 35%[14] success to currently reported success in 70-90%[15]. A recent advance which may have a similar influence on the practice of vitreoretinal surgery is the use of perfluorocarbon liquids (PFCLs). In this paper, we will describe the characteristics of perfluorocarbon liquids, the types currently available, and the clinical use of the compounds.

Supported in part by Core Grant EY01931-15 from the National Eye Institute/NIH, Bethesda, MD, and an unrestricted grant from Research to Prevent Blindness, Inc., New York, NY

Address for correspondence: Gary W. Abrams, MD, Department of Ophthalmology, Medical College of Wisconsin, 8700 W. Wisconsin Avenue, Milwaukee, WI 53226, USA

Retina and Vitreous, pp. 237-247
Proceedings of the Symposium on Retina and Vitreous,
organized by the New Orleans Academy of Ophthalmology
New Orleans, LA, USA, March 12-15, 1992
edited by Rudolph M. Franklin

Perfluorocarbon liquids

The PCFLs are a class of heavier than water liquids useful for vitreoretinal surgery. These stable, inert man-made substances are fully saturated compounds which contain carbon and fluoride only and have been investigated as blood replacement vehicles because of the high solubility of oxygen in the compounds[16]. Three principal PFCLs have been used clinically: perfluoro-N-octane, perfluorodecalin, and perfluorophenanthrene. The differential characteristics of these PFCLs are listed in Table 1[17,18]. The PFCLs are clear and immiscible with water and silicone oil. They have high specific gravities and the only heavier liquid is mercury. When placed in saline or silicone oil, the PFCL displaces either substance and accumulates in the bottom of the vessel (Fig. 1). There is a sharp interface between the PFCL and the saline or silicone oil (Fig. 1), and the visibility of the interface varies with the refractive index of the PFCL. A PFCL with a low refractive index different from saline such as perfluoro-N-octane is more easily seen than one with a higher refractive index near that of saline. The compounds have a low viscosity near that of water.

The physical characteristics of the PFCLs make them useful for vitreoretinal surgery. They have been used intraoperatively to reattach the retina, to unfold and reattach flaps of retina following giant tear or retinotomy, to stabilize the retina during membrane dissection, to displace subretinal blood, and to assist in the removal of a posteriorly dislocated crystalline lens or pseudophakos. In addition PFCLs have been investigated as long-term vitreous replacement substances.

Table 1. Physical characteristics of perfluorocarbon liquids

	Perfluoro-N-octane C_8F_{18}	*Perfluoro-decalin* $C_{10}F_{18}$	*Perfluoro-phenanthrene* $C_{14}F_{24}$
Specific gravity	1.76	1.94	2.03
Refractive index	1.27	1.31	1.33
Viscosity	0.80	1.31	8.03
Vapor pressure (mm Hg 37°C)	50	13.5	<1.0

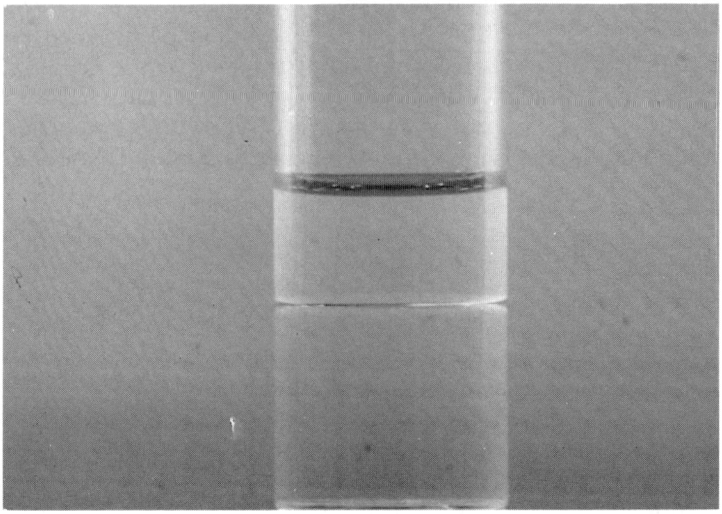

Fig. 1. Perfluoro-N-octane (PFO) and saline in a test tube. Heavier PFO displaces saline and occupies bottom of vessel. Note sharp interface between PFO and saline.

PFCLs are currently used as intraoperative tools, and are not left in the eye after surgery. Early studies of perfluoroether, a hetero-atom-containing fluorocarbon, in the rabbit eye revealed vacuolization of the retina, retinal gliosis, and retinal disorganization and detachment[19]. Perfluorotributylamine, a nitrogen containing perfluorochemical, has also been investigated as a vitreous substitute. Chang and co-workers showed that perfluorotributylamine was initially tolerated well, but after two weeks, photoreceptor damage was found[20]. Perfluorochemicals which contain an oxygen or nitrogen hetero-atom may be more biologically reactive[21]. PFCLs which contain only fluorine and carbon atoms appear to be much better tolerated[21]. Intraocular proteins and other substances act to reduce an already low interfacial surface tension to cause emulsification of all currently used PFCLs. Nabih, Peyman, and associates showed that perfluorophenanthrene was relatively well tolerated in the rabbit vitreous cavity without histopathologic or electrophysiologic evidence of retinal toxicity for up to six weeks[18]. However, all the PFCLs damage the corneal endothelium when left in contact for an extended period of time[18,20,22]. There is evidence that perfluoro-N-octane is toxic after 24 hours of corneal exposure[20,22]. It is thought that the corneal toxicity is due to obstruction of nutrients to the corneal endothelium, rather than a true chemical toxicity. Though clinical trials of postoperative retention of perfluorophenanthrene are underway, current use is otherwise restricted to intraoperative use.

Clinical use of perfluorocarbon liquids

Giant tear or retinotomy

The major current indication for PCFLs in vitreoretinal surgery is in the management of retinal detachment when there is a giant retinal tear or an extensive retinotomy. Prior to the availability of PFCLs, management of giant tears and retinotomies was often problematic. A fluid-air exchange with the patient in a supine position often caused slippage and folding of the flap of the retina. While techniques existed for supine fluid-air exchange to unfold the flap of a giant tear or retinotomy, visibility was sometimes compromised by the air or due to corneal striae or pupillary miosis during fluid-air exchange. In addition there was risk of retinal or choroidal hemorrhage during the exchange as the retina was manipulated beneath the air. The patient could be placed in a prone position for fluid-air exchange, but this was a difficult procedure often hampered by poor visibility. Fluid-silicone oil exchange could be used in the supine patient, but there was risk of retinal damage and retinal or choroidal hemorrhage as the retina was manipulated during the procedure. PFCLs offer an easier, less traumatic alternative to the above methods.

A scleral buckle is used for most giant tears less than 270° in extent. While the scleral buckle is not necessary to support the flap of the giant tear in most cases, it is often helpful to support non-torn retina and the ends of the giant tear where recurrent anterior traction often recurs. Except for 360° tears, a scleral buckle is necessary for all cases with proliferative vitreoretinopathy. There is little rationale for a scleral buckle for a 360° tear if all traction on the edges is relieved. Tears near 360° should usually be converted to a 360° tear to reduce the likelihood that traction will occur at the edge of non-torn retina.

Prior to PFCL injection the retina should be mobile and free of membranes. It is important to excise peripheral vitreous and scleral depression is recommended to facilitate vitrectomy in the vitreous base region. Membranes on the inner and outer retinal surfaces should be removed. A particularly important area is each end of the giant tear. Vitreous and membranes in this area can contract postoperatively to elevate the edge of the tear to re-detach the retina. In order adequately to remove peripheral vitreous to prevent ante-

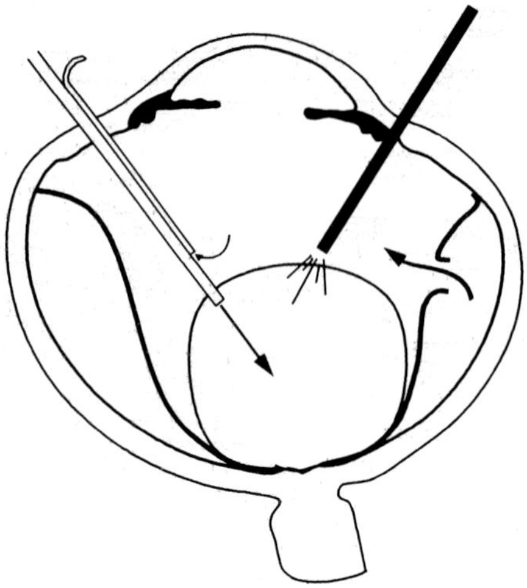

Fig. 2. Injection of PFCL to re-attach retina. Expanding PFCL bubble re-attaches retina from posteriorly to anteriorly. Subretinal fluid extruded through anterior retinal break into vitreous cavity. Fluid in vitreous cavity extruded through drainage needle out of eye. Special PFCL injection needle available through Infinitech, Inc., St Louis, MO.

rior proliferation and contraction, the lens should be removed in most cases. The lens should be removed in all eyes with proliferative vitreoretinopathy, and in most cases with tears greater than 180° in extent. It is preferable to remove the lens capsule which can be involved in anterior membrane formation.

The PFCL is injected over the optic disc and reattaches the retina from posteriorly to anteriorly (Fig. 2). During injection of the PFCL, fluid must be vented from the eye or the intraocular pressure will become elevated. This can be accomplished in two ways: a small gauge, blunt needle can be used which allows fluid to escape from the sclerotomy site during PFCL injection, or a special 20-gauge needle designed for PFCL injection (Infinitech, Inc., St. Louis, MO) which has an attached cannula vented to the outside of the eye can be used (Fig. 2). After posterior membranes are removed, a small amount of PFCL can be injected over the posterior pole to stabilize the retina as anterior membranes are removed. This maneuver is particularly helpful when the flap of the giant tear is fixed and folded. As the PFCL holds the posterior retina in place, the anterior flap can be mobilized with membrane peeling techniques. If the flap is still fixed after membrane removal, then it is best to apply diathermy for hemostasis and excise the fixed part of the flap. As the PFCL opens folds, sometimes membranes obscured by the folds can be seen. Membranes can be stripped beneath the PFCL. The PFCL holds the retina back during membrane peeling, and to some degree facilitates the peeling process. However, fine membranes may be more difficult to visualize under the PFCL when the retina is reattached, and it may be more difficult to engage the membrane when the retina is flattened. In most cases it is preferable to remove membranes prior to injection of PFCL over an area of retina.

PFCLs can be injected in the presence of posterior tears in the retina as long as all traction has been released from the retina. If traction distorts or elevates the edge of a tear, then there is a significant risk that PFCL will go beneath the retina. When peripheral membranes are stripped with PFCL stabilizing the posterior retina, traction is often applied to the retina which can elevate posterior tears. This traction, as well, can cause PFCL to go beneath the retina. Therefore, in the presence of retinal breaks, it is important that all traction be removed prior to PFCL injection.

The anterior edge of the retina should be carefully monitored during PFCL injection. If the retina is completely mobile, then the level of the PFCL can be safely brought anterior to the edge of the torn retina. However, just as described for posterior breaks, if traction remains on the anterior retina, the PFCL may go posterior to the retina. Therefore, if traction remains, the anterior edge of the flap should usually be excised prior to further PFCL injection. With traction relieved, PFCL can be safely injected anterior to the flap of the tear to completely re-attach the retina. The PFCL interface should not be brought in contact with the infusion cannula because small bubbles of PFCL will be created which can migrate under the edge of the retina if the edge is still elevated. Therefore, a shorter infusion cannula is preferred in cases in which PFCL is to be used.

Laser photocoagulation can be applied to the edge of the retina either before or after exchanging the perfluorocarbon for air or silicone oil. If the anterior edge of the giant tear or retinotomy has been completely flattened by PFCL, it is easier to apply laser through the PFCL than through air or silicone oil. The view is usually superior through PFCL than through air or silicone oil. While the fluid anterior to the PFCL maintains good corneal clarity and pupillary dilatation, air sometimes causes striate keratopathy and pupillary miosis, as well as a minified view. Small bubbles suspended in silicone oil can sometimes interfere with treatment through silicone oil. However, if it was not possible to completely flatten the edge of the tear with PFCL, then treatment should be delayed until after exchanging the PFCL for air or silicone oil.

Exchange of the PFCL for air or silicone oil is an important step which can lead to problems if not performed correctly. There is often a small amount of subretinal fluid beneath the anterior edge of the retina, and unless this subretinal fluid is removed, it will be forced posteriorly during the exchange, and can lead to posterior slippage of the retina or subretinal PFCL. During PFCL-air exchange, the fluid anterior to the PFCL is first replaced with air. Before removing PFCL, fluid beneath the anterior aspect of the retina should be removed. This "drying" of the anterior edge of the retina is accomplished with either a backflush brush or other soft-tipped extrusion or suction cannula placed just anterior to the retinal flap. After all subretinal fluid is removed and the anterior edge is thoroughly "dried", then the exchange is completed. The PFCL is easily removed with the suction or extrusion cannula. It is important that small bubbles of PFCL be removed from the retinal surface. The perfluoro-N-octane-air or -silicone oil interface is more easily seen than the interface with other available PFCLs. In addition, the high vapor pressure of perfluoro-N-octane causes vaporization and disappearance of small bubbles of PFCL in air at body temperature. Small bubbles of PFCL may become suspended in silicone oil or trapped against the retinal surface outside of the posterior pole. Suspended bubbles will slowly sink posteriorly so they can be differentiated from air or other fluid bubbles which will float to the anterior surface of the silicone oil. These bubbles of PFCL should be identified and removed.

If there is retinal slippage during exchange of PFCL for air, this usually indicates inadequate "drying" of the anterior edge of the retina. Sometimes it is possible to manipulate the anterior edge of the retina with the backflush brush to pull the retina to its proper position. However, if the retina cannot be brought to its normal position, then the air should be removed and the retina once more flattened with PFCL. Further retinal slippage is usually prevented by thorough "drying" of the anterior edge of the retina during exchange, and repeat exchange with silicone oil rather than air may less likely cause slippage of the retina.

Chang and associates reported 17 patients with giant retinal tears of whom 11 had tears of 180° or more. Seven eyes also had PVR[23]. Intraoperative re-attachment was accomplished in all patients and 16 (94%) of 17 retinas were attached after at least six months of follow-up. The lens was preserved in five of eight phakic patients because of easier anterior retinal manipulation facilitated by the perfluoro-N-octane. Twenty-nine percent were re-attached without a scleral buckle. Visual acuity results were extremely encouraging with 15 of 17 eyes seeing 20/400 or better, ten eyes 20/80 or better and six eyes 20/40 or better.

Glaser and co-workers reported ten eyes with giant retinal tears and D-1 PVR or worse using perfluoro-N-octane and long-acting gas tamponade[24]. All eyes were re-attached intraoperatively and nine of ten remained attached after six months of follow-up. Visual acuity improved in eight of ten eyes. Final visual acuity was 20/200 or better in six (60%) eyes and 20/60 or better in three (30%) eyes. Five eyes required a total of six re-operations for epiretinal membrane formation without retinal detachment. In a series published five years earlier by the same authors, a group of 19 eyes with giant tears and PVR were operated on without PFCLs[25]. Intraoperative re-attachment occurred in 18 eyes. Intravitreal silicone oil was used in all cases and recurrent periretinal proliferation was identified in all eyes. Final visual acuity of 20/200 or better was present in two eyes (10%) only compared to 60% of the later Glaser series. Although the number of eyes are small in each study, the superior anatomic and visual results may be in part attributed to the intraoperative use of liquid perfluorocarbons, though the patient populations may have been different, and other changes in surgical technique might have occurred.

A series of ten consecutive patients with giant retinal tears have been managed with perfluoro-N-octane at our institution over the past 13 months. In our series, eight eyes had PVR with seven eyes having grade D-1 or worse. All eyes were re-attached intraoperatively. Intraoperatively, retinal slippage occurred in only one eye at the time of perfluorocarbon-air exchange which resulted in a small, extramacular retinal fold. No PFCL-related complications occurred. Three eyes with PVR required re-operation for recurrent retinal detachment with PVR. With a minimum follow-up of three months, nine of the eyes were attached with stable or improved visual acuities. Two eyes without PVR had final visual acuities of 20/25 and 20/30. The perfluorocarbon was a useful temporary surgical adjunct for re-attaching the retina in these patients.

Other types of retinal detachment

The general principles for use of PFCLs in eyes with other types of retinal detachment are similar to those presented for giant retinal tears and retinotomies. PFCLs are useful for retinal detachment associated with PVR, trauma, diabetic retinopathy, and other causes. PFCL is used to stabilize the posterior retina to facilitate anterior vitrectomy and membrane dissection. This is most useful when the retina is bullously detached and very mobile. There is risk of retinal break formation during peripheral vitrectomy when the retina is detached, and it is sometimes difficult to separate membranes from detached retina. Bullous retinal detachment may become excessively mobile, making visualization difficult, and there is risk of incarceration of bullous retina in the sclerotomy sites. After posterior membrane removal, PFCL is injected over the posterior pole to flatten the posterior retina. By holding the posterior retina in place, the PFCL facilitates anterior work and reduces the risks of complications while working with bullous, detached retina. In addition, the PFCL acts as a "second hand" to hold the retina back during vitrectomy and membranectomy.

A major advantage of PFCLs is that no posterior drainage retinotomy is necessary in order to re-attach the retina. Posterior retinotomies may be associated with intraoperative bleeding and are often sites of reproliferation. As the PFCL is injected posteriorly, the subretinal fluid is extruded through anterior breaks into the vitreous cavity. The PFCL is brought up to the level of the retinal breaks, then during PFCL-air exchange, anterior subretinal fluid is removed through the anterior breaks before the PFCL is removed. The same principles regarding posterior and anterior retinal breaks apply to all forms of retinal detachment. PFCL should not be injected over breaks until all traction has been relieved, and no traction should be placed on the retina when PFCL overlies a retinal break.

Chang and associates reported the outcome in management of 23 eyes with advanced proliferative vitreoretinopathy with PFCL[17]. In 21 eyes the retina could be re-attached intraoperatively without a posterior drainage retinotomy, and the PFCL helped stabilize the retina during peripheral membrane dissection. Results with 15 eyes maintaining long-term retinal re-attachment were similar to those previously reported[15].

We have used PFCL to manage 11 patients with retinal detachments with PVR not associated with trauma or giant retinal tears. All eyes were re-attached intraoperatively. At the last follow-up all 11 eyes were attached with six eyes attaining visual acuities of 5/200 or better.

Trauma

PFCLs are useful in the management of retinal detachment due to trauma. Methods previously described for management of giant tears, retinotomies, and other retinal detachments including those with proliferative vitreoretinopathy are useful in eyes following trauma. Another indication is subretinal hemorrhage. Subretinal hemorrhage following trauma often pools beneath the macula. After vitrectomy, PFCL is injected posteriorly and the unclotted blood is displaced towards the periphery where it can be removed safely through peripheral retinal breaks.

Chang and co-workers reported the results of management of 14 patients with retinal detachments following ocular trauma[26]. Indications for PFCL were giant tears or retinotomies in six eyes, subretinal hemorrhage in five eyes, and proliferative vitreoretinopathy in the majority of eyes. They were able to avoid posterior drainage retinotomies in all eyes, and were able to obtain retinal re-attachment at surgery in all eyes. Long-term retinal re-attachment was obtained in eight eyes, and seven had a final visual acuity of 5/200 or better. We have used PFCL in the management of four patients with extensive traumatic retinal incarceration in the scleral wound with retinal detachment. Two eyes required 360° retinotomies in order to separate the retina from the incarcerations and then PFCL was used to reattach the retina. In two eyes PFCL was used to stabilize the retina while a retinotomy was made to separate the retina from the incarceration. In one of these two eyes, subretinal blood was displaced from the posterior pole by the PFCL and removed through a peripheral break. The first two eyes were successfully re-attached at surgery, but both, with 360° retinotomies, became hypotonous with low vision. The third eye, with a 100° retinotomy, remained attached with 20/200 visual acuity. In the fourth eye the retina was attached intraoperatively, however, recurrent detachment with PVR occurred after three months, necessitating a second vitrectomy with silicone oil tamponade. Following subsequent removal of the silicone oil the retina remained attached with 5/200 visual acuity.

Dislocated crystalline lens or pseudophakos

The specific gravities of the PFCLs are greater than that of either the crystalline lens or an intraocular lens (IOL). PFCLs can help in the removal of both from the vitreous cavity.

When a crystalline lens is dislocated into the vitreous cavity, it may cause no problems and may not require surgical intervention. However, when a posteriorly dislocated lens causes complications such as glaucoma, retinal damage, inflammation, or macular edema, surgical intervention with removal may sometimes be indicated. Posterior dislocation of the lens nucleus may occur during phacoemulsification if there is inadvertent rupture of the posterior capsule of the lens. Complications of glaucoma, inflammation, and retinal detachment may follow, so the nucleus and lens cortical material should usually be removed.

The most commonly used techniques for removal of a dislocated lens or lens nucleus is vitrectomy and posterior phacofragmentation or removal through the limbus. The phacofragmentation procedure can occasionally lead to retinal damage if the ultrasound probe is activated near the retina. Also there is risk of retinal damage by manipulation of a hard nucleus on the retinal surface. The lens or the lens nucleus can be floated away from the retinal surface with PFCL and then fragmented and removed. The PFCL lies between the retina and the lens material, so there is less risk of retinal damage. The major problem with the technique is that the meniscus of the PFCL bubble is convex anteriorly. The lens and lens fragments during phacofragmentation tend to fall to the periphery of the bubble so they may be difficult to engage. If limbal removal of a hard nucleus is planned, then PFCL may be quite useful. The lens material can be floated to the level of the pupil, then the limbus opened and the lens or nucleus can be extracted with a cryoprobe or other instrument.

A posteriorly dislocated IOL may sometimes be well tolerated and can be left in place. However, complications of inflammation, cystoid macular edema, and retinal damage, or excessive mobility may necessitate repositioning or removal. If the IOL is not removed or replaced, then another method of dealing with aphakia will be necessary. If the patient cannot tolerate aphakic spectacles or a contact lens, then replacement or removal and exchange with another IOL is necessary. Occasionally the dislocated lens reduces visual acuity by lying in the visual axis and must be removed, repositioned, or exchanged.

The most common method for removal, repositioning, or exchange is to do a vitrectomy to free the dislocated IOL from posterior vitreous attachments, then to grasp with forceps. Various techniques have been developed to reposition a posterior chamber IOL in the ciliary sulcus with or without suture fixation to the iris or transsclerally. When the IOL is to be removed, with or without exchange for another IOL, it is usually brought forward into the anterior chamber, or held with forceps and passed out of a limbal wound. A problem common to any of the techniques is anterior fixation of the IOL during the repositioning, suturing, or removal. The IOL can fall back against the retina during the maneuvers. Campo and associates described a technique in which a needle is placed

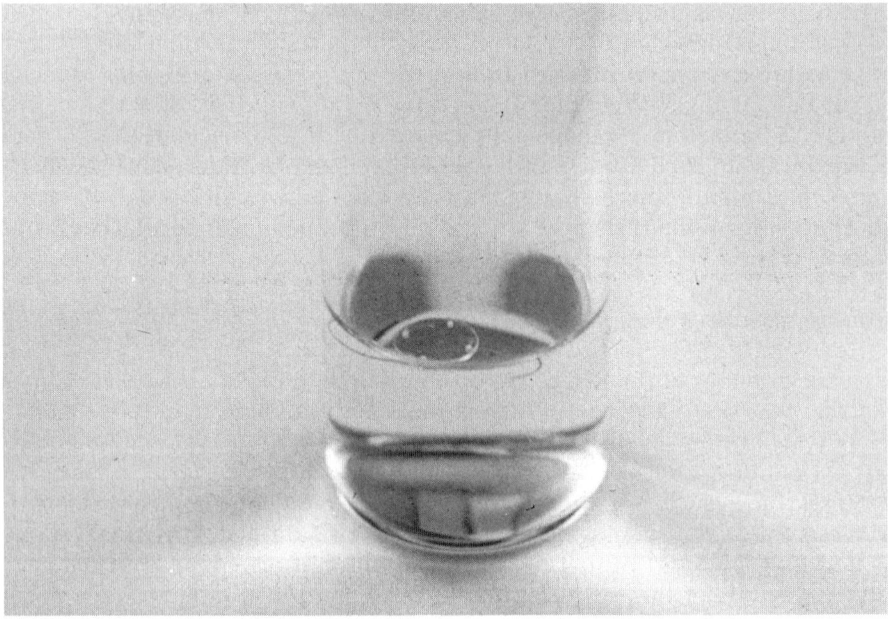

Fig. 3. Specific gravity of PFCL is greater than that of IOL seen floating on surface of PFCL.

transsclerally through the pars plana, passed across the vitreous cavity and brought out the sclera on the opposite side through the pars plana behind the IOL to fixate the IOL[27]. This technique may be effective, but has risks of hemorrhage or retinal damage. The IOL can be floated anteriorly to the level of the pupil or the anterior vitreous cavity with PFCL (Fig. 3). Then the IOL can be placed in the ciliary sulcus with or without sutures as indicated, or removed through the limbus with or without exchange for another IOL. Just as described for lens fragments, the IOL will initially be displaced toward the periphery of the convex bubble. However, as the PFCL bubble is enlarged and fills the vitreous cavity, the lens can be centered at or just posterior to the pupil.

Several authors have described the use of various high-density vitreous substitutes in the management of posteriorly dislocated crystalline or intraocular lenses. Liu *et al.* used fluorosilicone oil successfully to manage four posteriorly dislocated crystalline lenses[28]. In the same report, the use of perfluorophenanthrene in two patients with dislocated intraocular lenses and one patient with a dislocated crystalline lens was described. Shapiro *et al.* reported on their use of perfluoro-N-octane in the removal of a dislocated crystalline lens in one patient[29]. No complications related to the use of these agents were reported.

In these clinical situations major advantages of PFCLs over other high-density vitreous substitutes including fluorosilicone oil are their lower viscosities which make injection and removal easier, and superior visualization within these eyes which are often inflamed with media opacities.

We have likewise used perfluoro-N-octane to manage dislocated crystalline lenses in two patients. One patient developed glaucoma after dislocation of the whole lens following blunt trauma. The lens was removed through the limbus with a cryoprobe after vitrectomy and after floating the lens to the pupil with PFCL. The surgery was uneventful, but the patient developed a giant tear of 100° and retinal detachment ten days after surgery. The retinal detachment was successfully repaired using PFCL. A second patient had a dislocated lens nucleus after phacoemulsification. The nucleus was removed with phagofragmentation after vitrectomy and injection of PFCL to float the lens away from the retina. The nucleus was successfully removed, but it was noted that lens fragments tended to be displaced towards the periphery of the PFCL bubble.

Complications of perfluorocarbon liquids

Intraoperatively, the major complication of PFCL is subretinal extension. This usually results from injection of PFCL over a retinal break under traction, or manual traction on the retina (usually during membrane peeling) which elevates a retinal break covered by PFCL. Additionally, subretinal bubbles of PFCL can follow emulsification of the PFCL caused by bringing the level of the PFCL to the level of the infusion port, and mechanical dispersion of the PFCL by the fluid or air infusion. The small PFCL bubbles can go through open anterior retinal breaks into the subretinal space. Management of subretinal PFCL has been covered previously.

Small bubbles of PFCL may be inadvertently left in the eye following surgery. The small bubbles of those PFCLs with a refractive index similar to saline are difficult to visualize, and can be left behind. Perfluoro-N-octane, with a refractive index less than that of saline is more easily seen than other PFCLs used clinically, so it is less likely to be left behind. It may be useful to refill a small amount of infusion fluid over the posterior retina and repeat the posterior fluid-air exchange to remove residual bubbles of PFCL in eyes in which the PFCL is difficult to visualize. In addition, perfluoro-N-octane has a high vapor pressure and will vaporize in air at body temperature and will be vented out of the sclerotomy sites in an air-filled eye. The other PFCLs used clinically have low vapor pressures and will not similarly vaporize in air at body temperature.

There is no current evidence that PFCLs used only intraoperatively cause inflammation, cellular proliferation, corneal damage, retinal damage, cataract, or any other complications. PFCL left in contact with the cornea after surgery will lead to endothelial damage. Small bubbles of PFCL left in the eye, even when intermittently in the anterior chamber, have not caused retinal or corneal damage. Several eyes with small bubbles of PFCL beneath the retina have shown no progressive retinal damage, although a small scotoma which correlates with the subretinal PFCL has been reported[23].

References

1. Machemer R, Buettner H, Norton EWD, Parel JM: Vitrectomy: a pars plana approach. Trans Am Acad Ophthalmol Otolaryngol 75:813, 1971
2. Norton EWD, Machemer R: New approach to the treatment of selected retinal detachments secondary to vitreous loss at cataract surgery. Am J Ophthalmol 72:705, 1971
3. Machemer R, Parel JM, Buettner H: A new concept for vitreous surgery. 1. Instrumentation. Am J Ophthalmol 73:1, 1972
4. Machemer R: A new concept for vitreous surgery. 2. Surgical technique and complications. Am J Ophthalmol 74:1022, 1972
5. Brucker AJ, Hoffman ME, Nevyas HJ, Wule AE: New instrumentation for fluid-air exchange. Retina 3:135, 1983
6. Huenecke RL, Aaberg TM: Instrumentation for continuous fluid-air exchange during vitreous surgery. Am J Ophthalmol 96:547, 1983
7. Parke DW II, Aaberg TM: Intraocular argon laser photocoagulation in the management of severe proliferative vitreoretinopathy. Am J Ophthalmol 97:434, 1984
8. Chang S, Coleman DJ, Lincoff H et al: Perfluoropropane gas in the management of proliferative vitreoretinopathy. Am J Ophthalmol 98:180, 1984
9. Stern WH, Blumenkranz MS: Fluid-gas exchange after vitrectomy. Am J Ophthalmol 96:400-401, 1983
10. Charles S: Vitrectomy for retinal detachment. Trans Ophthalmol Soc UK 100:542-549, 1980
11. Charles S: Vitreous Microsurgery, p 81. Baltimore: Williams & Wilkins 1981
12. Gonvers M: Retinal perforator for internal drainage. Am J Ophthalmol 97:786-787, 1984
13. Zivojnovic R: Silicone Oil in Vitreoretinal Surgery. Dordrecht: Martinus Nijhoff/DW Junk 1987
14. Sternberg P Jr, Machemer R: Results of conventional vitreous surgery for proliferative vitreoretinopathy. Am J Ophthalmol 100:141-146, 1985
15. Lewis H, Aaberg TM, Abrams GW: Causes of failure after initial vitreoretinal surgery for severe proliferative vitreoretinopathy. Am J Ophthalmol 111:8-14, 1991
16. Biro GP, Blais P: Perfluorocarbon blood substitutes. CRC Crit Rev Oncol Hematol 6:311-374, 1987
17. Chang S, Ozmert E, Zimmerman NJ: Intraoperative perfluorocarbon liquids in the management of proliferative vitreoretinopathy. Am J Ophthalmol 106:668-674, 1988
18. Nabih M, Peyman GA, Clark LC, Hoffman RE, Miceli M, Abou-Steit M, Tawakol M, Liu K: Experimental evaluation of perfluorophenanthrene as a high specific gravity vitreous substitute: a preliminary report. Ophthalmic Surg 20:286-293, 1989
19. Miyamoto K, Refojo MF, Tolentino FI, Fournier GA, Albert DM: Perfluoroether liquid as a long-term vitreous substitute. Retina 4:264-268, 1984
20. Chang S, Zimmerman NJ, Iwamoto T, Ortiz R, Faris D: Experimental vitreous replacement with perfluorotributylamine. Am J Ophthalmol 103:29-37, 1987
21. Refojo MF: Biomedical materials to repair retinal detachments. Materials Research Society Symposium Proceedings 55:55-61, 1986
22. Hyndiuk RA, Murray TG, Palmer M, Boldt HC, Han DP, Mieler WF, Abrams GW: Perfluoro-n-octane: evaluation of anterior segment toxicity associated with intraocular use. Invest Ophthalmol Vis Sci (Suppl) 32:880, 1991
23. Chang S, Lincoff H, Zimmerman NJ, Fuchs W: Giant retinal tears. Surgical techniques and results using perfluorocarbon liquids. Arch Ophthalmol 107:761-766, 1989
24. Glaser BM, Carter JB, Kuppermann BD, Michels RG: Perfluoro-octane in the treatment of giant retinal tears with proliferative vitreoretinopathy. Ophthalmology 98:1613-1621, 1991
25. Glaser BM: Treatment of giant retinal tears combined with proliferative vitreoretinopathy. Ophthalmology 93:1193-1197, 1986

26. Chang S, Reppucci V, Zimmerman NJ, Heinemann MH, Coleman DJ: Perfluorocarbon liquids in the management of traumatic retinal detachments. Ophthalmology 96:785-792, 1989
27. Campo RV, Chung KD, Oyakawa RT: Pars plana vitrectomy in the management of dislocated posterior chamber lenses. Am J Ophthalmol 108:529-534, 1989
28. Liu K, Peyman GA, Chen M, Chang K: Use of high density vitreous substitute in the removal of posteriorly dislocated lenses or intraocular lenses. Ophthalmic Surg 22:503-507, 1991
29. Shapiro MJ, Resnick KI, Kim SH, Wernberg A: Management of the dislocated crystalline lens with a perfluorocarbon liquid. Am J Ophthalmol 112:401-405, 1991

ROUND TABLE: DRUG TREATMENT FOR VITREORETINAL DISEASE

Thomas M. Aaberg, Sr., moderator

Thomas M. Aaberg, Sr.: Discussion is certainly open to all the topics of the morning, but it was suggested that we initially direct the attention of the panel to drug treatment for vitreoretinal disease. Gary Abrams has spent much of his career on that subject, and I would like to ask him to start, if you would Gary, and give us an update.

Gary W. Abrams: Thanks Tom. We have been interested in drug therapy for retinal detachment and proliferative vitreoretinopathy (PVR) for many years. This dates back to really the early 1970s, and the original premise was that, and I think it still holds, if we could prevent reproliferation then we could reattach nearly 100% of retinas with severe PVR. Now, to begin, I must say that even though we have been working on this idea for over 15 years, all of the advances in management of PVR up to this point have been mechanical surgical advances. We have not accomplished our goal of being able to prevent reproliferation; however, as we have seen from Tom's presentation, we have made remarkable advances in our ability to surgically manage PVR. When surgery fails, it almost always fails due to reproliferation. There is a cycle that goes on in the reproliferative process which includes inflammatory reaction, exudation, cellular proliferation, cellular contraction, and redetachment, and we see it over and over again. We may reoperate these eyes several times because of this cycle of reproliferation and redetachment. There are several strategies to manage recurrent proliferation. The first major strategy is the management of inflammation with anti-inflammatory drugs; second is inhibition of cellular proliferation; and the third is prevention of attachment of proliferative cells to collagen. Of the anti-inflammatory medicines, the most commonly used are corticosteroids. Robert Machemer has pointed out that steroids have both anti-inflammatory effects and anti-mitotic effects. Machemer and co-workers have looked at the effect of triamcinolone acetonide, one of the more potent steroids, in reducing proliferation. They have done a number of experimental studies which clearly demonstrate that steroids will inhibit inflammation and proliferation. However, at this point there has been no demonstrated benefit of steroids in preventing reproliferation in clinical PVR. The second strategy, that of direct inhibition of the mitotic activity of cells, has involved the study of a number of drugs including the fluoropyrimidines, which include 5-fluorouracil (5-FU), by a number of authors including Mark Blumenkranz and Walter Stern. Peter Wiedeman, Steve Ryan, and others have looked at daunomycin, and it has shown some promise. Colchicine was investigated by Bert Glaser and colleagues. Mark Blumenkranz and his co-workers have studied lipophilic prodrug-linked 5-FU in silicone oil which slowly leeches out of the silicone oil over time to inhibit proliferation. That is one of the major problems: finding a sustained-release delivery system that will continue to affect the proliferative cycle during the first few weeks after surgery. Others have looked at liposomes as possible delivery mechanisms. Peyman and co-workers and Stern and associates have done work on liposomes. The third strategy to prevent reproliferation is to try to pre-

Retina and Vitreous, pp. 249-253
Proceedings of the Symposium on Retina and Vitreous,
organized by the New Orleans Academy of Ophthalmology
New Orleans, LA, USA, March 12-15, 1992
edited by Rudolph M. Franklin

vent attachment of proliferative cells to collagen. Proliferative cells secrete fibronectin, and fibronectin causes adherence of these cells to collagen. Glaser and associates have sought a way to prevent attachment of the cells to the collagen, and a number of strategies have been worked out. They have identified a tetrapeptide that can block cellular attachment with fibronectin. Blumenkranz and associates have looked at heparin, which also has some effects in blocking cellular attachment. Heparin also may prevent the formation of fibrin. In Milwaukee, we have studied tissue plasminogen activator (TPA), which is an enzyme that will lyse fibrin. Fibrin produced in the inflammatory cycle may contribute to the proliferative cycle, so lysis of fibrin by TPA may help to inhibit reproliferation. But once again, none of these strategies have fulfilled the promise of 15 years ago. And still at this point all of the major advances in management of PVR have been surgical. We have a long way to go, but I still believe that we have the potential to obtain almost 100% reattachment in these terrible retinal detachments. And it is going to happen, but I still think we have a long way to go.

Aaberg: Thank you, Gary. That was a very nice over-view of the whole subject. Don, do you have some questions that you could address?

J. Donald Gass: Well, one relates to therapy – do the non-steroidal anti-inflammatory agents have any role in the premacular hole therapy, I presume in the treatment of a patient who is in the impending macular hole stage? I really do not know. We have never used anti-inflammatory agents as a means of treatment of the patient who comes in with the impending macular hole. So I guess you could say, maybe it could somehow cause things to relax or to separate, but I just have had absolutely no experience with that. We see so few patients with impending macular holes. We do not have a lot of opportunity to try a lot of different things, and since there are no signs of any inflammation in the eye, there is no reason to really suspect inflammation. I think the thought has never occurred to us to try corticosteroids or other anti-inflammatory agents.

Aaberg: Thank you.

Abrams: Tom, I would like to ask Dick Green, I know that Jerdan, Pepose and co-workers in the United States and Baudouin and associates from France have identified surface antigens which implicate an immunologic component in proliferative membranes, in PVR, and I just wonder if you have any insight into the role of the immunologic system in the development of PVR? Also, would any sort of treatment, possibly early on, help prevent these proliferative problems?

W.R. Green: Well, that is a tough question. Theoretically, yes, I suppose that it is possible, but practically it is not possible at this time. Daunomycin should affect that system. It does *in vitro*, and perhaps *in vivo*, but it is such a short-lived beneficial effect. I think perhaps the concept of continuous delivery might play a role, and that may be the area where we can break through with a continuous effect until the proliferation settles down. But I do not have any great hopes for the immunologic aspect of PVR and thus doubt that intervention and prevention of immune mechanisms will be helpful.

Aaberg: Thank you Dick. Stuart, do you have a question that you can answer?

Stuart L. Fine: Yes. Two short questions. What is TGF-beta? First, it is very well known that I am not a cell biologist, so my answer will be brief. There are a number of growth factors that have been isolated from biologic tissues. These include epidermal growth factor, platelet derived growth factor, and nerve growth factor. Transforming growth factor-beta is one of those factors. In biologic systems, growth factors modulate cellular growth; sometimes they stimulate and sometimes they inhibit, depending upon existing conditions in the environment. Transforming growth factor-beta is currently being employed to stimulate attachment of the retina around the perimeter of the macular hole, to the RPE, in an effort to seal the macular hole. The TGF-beta is applied in low concentration after a core vitrectomy is performed. Preliminary results suggest some beneficial effects.

Green: Stuart, could I comment?

Fine: Certainly.

Green: Some of the experimental data to support the efficacy of this was provided by Smiddy. He created holes in the retina, gave TGF-beta intravitreally, and more often than not there was sealing of the holes with the TGF-beta and less without it. It was mainly stimulation of the glial cells which sealed off the hole.

Aaberg: I am sorry. Did you have another...

Fine: Maybe some other people would like to take their questions.

Aaberg: Gary, did you have one on visual acuity?

Abrams: The question is at what visual acuity do you recommend surgery to your patients with epiretinal membranes? I think the cut-off I have used and the one most people have used is 20/60. It is difficult to give a definite bottom line because each patient's visual needs are different. There is an occasional patient who is prevented from doing his or her job by a macular epiretinal membrane, who might have visual acuity in the range of 20/40 or 20/50 that I might consider operating upon, but in my experience that is very unusual. Once again, it gets down to the old risk-benefit ratio and you do not want to take the risk of having a problem in a patient who has fairly good visual acuity at that 20/40 level. So, we generally adhere to that 20/60 bottom line.

Aaberg: Thank you. We are probably running over just a tad, but Don, I think you had an appropriate question.

Gass: One question, what would you tell your patient with a unilateral macular hole about the risk of hole formation in the fellow eye? Let me preface that first by saying that probably the most important thing you can do for that patient is do a contact lens examination on the normal eye to see if you can determine whether or not there is a separation of the vitreous. The main thing you are looking for is the prepapillary (vitreous) ring. If the prepapillary ring is well in front of the optic disc and is bobbing around in there, you can be pretty certain it is also separated from the macula. If you do not see that, then the next thing to look for is the pseudomacular hole, and that is a little more difficult and takes a little more time of playing with the light. But if you can find that little opacity sitting just in front of the fovea, that is evidence that the vitreous is separated from the fovea, and I would tell that patient with either of those situations, that their chances are almost zero – I am sure not zero – that they will ever get a macular hole. Now if the patient does not have any evidence of a posterior vitreous separation, then I tell them they have got approximately a 10 percent or less chance that they will eventually have the same problem in the second eye, or at least will get an impending macular hole. If they get an impending macular hole, the best we can say is somewhere in the rough neighborhood, 50% chance, they will even get by that with maybe at the most an inner lamellar hole and still good visual function. There is another question here – what signs and symptoms differentiate impending idiopathic macular hole from vitreoretinal traction syndrome. Well they are quite different, and there is really no trouble distinguishing them. All you see in the patient with an impending macular hole is a yellow spot or ring and no evidence of vitreous separation. You may occasionally see a few little lines, in particular when it gets to this 1B level, a few little lines around the edge. But in the vitreoretinal traction syndrome, the vitreous is separated up above, it is hung up in the area of the macula. The macula is tented forward like a volcano and very often there is some cystic change. If you do an angiogram, you will usually even see some staining of the retina. That is a very unusual case. You see 40 of the other cases for one vitreoretinal traction syndrome, at least in my experience.

Aaberg: Don, why is it that if a person's vitreous separates out to the ora serrata they get photopsia and Moore's lightning streaks? Symptomatically, they will have problems, yet if this is vitreous traction on the macula, I do not recall patients complaining of photopsia, yet they are presumably both tractional. Why is that?

Gass: You are talking about in the vitreoretinal traction maculopathy situation?

Aaberg: Or an impending macular hole.

Gass: Well, in an impending macular hole, the traction is primarily tangential traction that gradually causes the retina to move forward, so I would think there is just less stimulation of the receptor cells, which I think is the genesis of the photopsia; whereas out in the periphery with the vitreous pulling on the retina, I can visualize how that may be exciting the visual cells.

Aaberg: Well, Dick showed this picture of a bursa with fluid moving in that bursa. Now I would think you would have photopsia then. Or am I wrong?

Gass: Not entirely.

Green: Our knowledge of the vitreous is not very advanced. Worst, Jaffe, Sebag, and Kishi and co-workers have all described the presence of a premacular bursa. Sebag says, there are some anterior posterior fibers that go through a hole in the cortical vitreous over the fovea and attach to the macula. Unfortunately our knowledge of the normal microanatomy of the vitreous as it relates to the macula is poor.

Gass: I think there is a good possibility that movement of the vitreous is somehow playing a role in what is going on in this contraction of the vitreous in front of the fovea. First of all, this bursa that is described in pictures – it is always drawn as a ring as if you could look in there with a slit lamp and see the borders of this bursa. It is not like that at all. With a slit lamp, you have a very difficult time finding the borders of "a bursa". It is an optically empty space with some strands of vitreous in there, and it is a very ill-defined area. It is not a sharply defined bag that is moving back and forth. If you watch the vitreous in motion, I think you would have a difficult time, I mean the shape of it would be constantly changing. But nevertheless, it is still a possibility that somehow it is transmitting some forces to the surface of the retina. It is still a little difficult to explain why the holes form in this can opener-like fashion based on this movement; but nevertheless that could be contributing to it. One way to put it to the test is to do a core vitrectomy. This should get rid of most of the movement of a body of fluid within the vitreous gel. It would be nice to know, because that is a much simpler technique to do compared with a vitrectomy *and* peeling a membrane off the surface of the retina (macula).

Aaberg: Thank you. One final question. Dr. Davis, could you move up to the microphone just a minute, because this is a question I think would best be answered by you. How often should general ophthalmologists see patients with gestational diabetes?

Matthew D. Davis: With gestational diabetes? I am not sure that we need to see patients with gestational diabetes. Patients with type I diabetes who happen to be pregnant, should be seen in the first trimester to see whether they have any retinopathy. If they have no retinopathy, I would not be very worried about them. Certainly, if they have severe non-proliferative or proliferative retinopathy, and it has not been diagnosed before, they may need to be treated. Certainly, if they have high risk characteristics they need to be treated. My threshold for treating someone approaching high risk would be lowered if they are pregnant. I would watch them more carefully. There was a paper given at the American Academy meeting* dealing with the macular edema that sometimes develops during pregnancy in these patients, and their observations were that it usually gets better following delivery. I think if mild non-proliferative retinopathy is present in the first trimester, I would want to see the patient again perhaps in another three or four months.

Aaberg: Thank you.

*Stoessel KM, Liao PM, Thompson JT, Reece AE: Diabetic retinopathy and macular edema in pregnancy. *Note:* It appears that this paper has not yet been published based on a medline search and review of the contents of *Ophthalmology*, January 1992 through May 1992.

VI

MANAGEMENT OF CONDITIONS POST CATARACT EXTRACTION

POSTOPERATIVE ENDOPHTHALMITIS

Louis A. Wilson and Thomas M. Aaberg, Sr.

Department of Ophthalmology, Emory University School of Medicine, Atlanta, Georgia, USA

Incidence and causes

Microbial endophthalmitis can be a devastating intraocular infection which may occur endogenously, follow penetrating injury of the globe or present as an early or delayed complication of intraocular surgery. In fact, 70% of cases of endophthalmitis have been reported to be the result of such surgery[1]. When one also considers that over one million cataract extractions are performed yearly in the United States[2], then the incidence of postoperative endophthalmitis (POE) following this procedure is of more than passing interest to American ophthalmologists. Unfortunately, national data concerning the incidence is not readily available since most reports reflect institutional or regional occurrences. In 1983, a Food and Drug Administration report on intraocular lens (IOL) use suggested a POE incidence of 0.1%[3]. While their data were nation wide, the study was over a four-year period, involved only closely monitored CORE study patients and did not address culture results or causative organisms. A more recent study analyzed a nation wide data base of over 300,000 medicare patients (65 years or older) admitted to hospital for cataract surgery during 1984[4]. The investigators noted that the likelihood of POE and their sampling was consistent with previously reported series. Additionally they observed that the risk of infection was higher among patients who had intracapsular surgery when compared to those who had undergone extracapsular or phacoemulsification (0.17% *versus* 0.12%). Vitreous loss with any technique increased the risk of rehospitalization for POE within one month of surgery to nearly 4.5 times (0.41%) that following uncomplicated cataract surgery.

Unfortunately no data on culture results, etiopathogens or visual outcome following treatment were reported. These are important since at least some of the prognostic factors in microbial endophthalmitis relate to the causative agent(s) and its virulence factor(s). In a series of reports on POE during the 1980s, the visual outcome was clearly related to whether the vitreous biopsy was culture positive or negative[5-7]. Positive cultures were most frequently associated with Gram-positive bacteria and of these coagulase negative staphylococci (CNS) were predominant. In instances where CNS were the etiopathogens, the best visual results were obtained following treatment[1,5-10]. In reviewing an institutional series of POE[11], it was conclusively shown that the aerobic periocular microbiota is the source of the infecting organism in 83% of cases, and that *Staphylococcus epidermidis* is the most common causative agent[11] It may well be that the periocular anaerobic micro-

Supported in part by an NIH Departmental Core grant P30 EY06360 and Research to Prevent Blindness, Inc.

Address for correspondence: Professor Louis A. Wilson, MD, Department of Ophthalmology, Emory University School of Medicine, 1327 Clifton Road NE, Atlanta, GA 30322, USA

Retina and Vitreous, pp. 257-269
Proceedings of the Symposium on Retina and Vitreous,
organized by the New Orleans Academy of Ophthalmology
New Orleans, LA, USA, March 12-15, 1992
edited by Rudolph M. Franklin

flora is the source of *Propionibacterium acnes* as a cause of POE, since this Gram-positive, non-spore-forming, pleomorphic diphtheroid is the most frequently isolated anaerobe from the normal conjunctival sac[12].

Diagnosis

Clinical

Microbial endophthalmitis following cataract surgery is generally considered a fulminating infection characterized by the symptoms of pain, decreased vision, increased redness, and ocular discharge. The clinical findings may well include: lid edema and chemo-

a

b

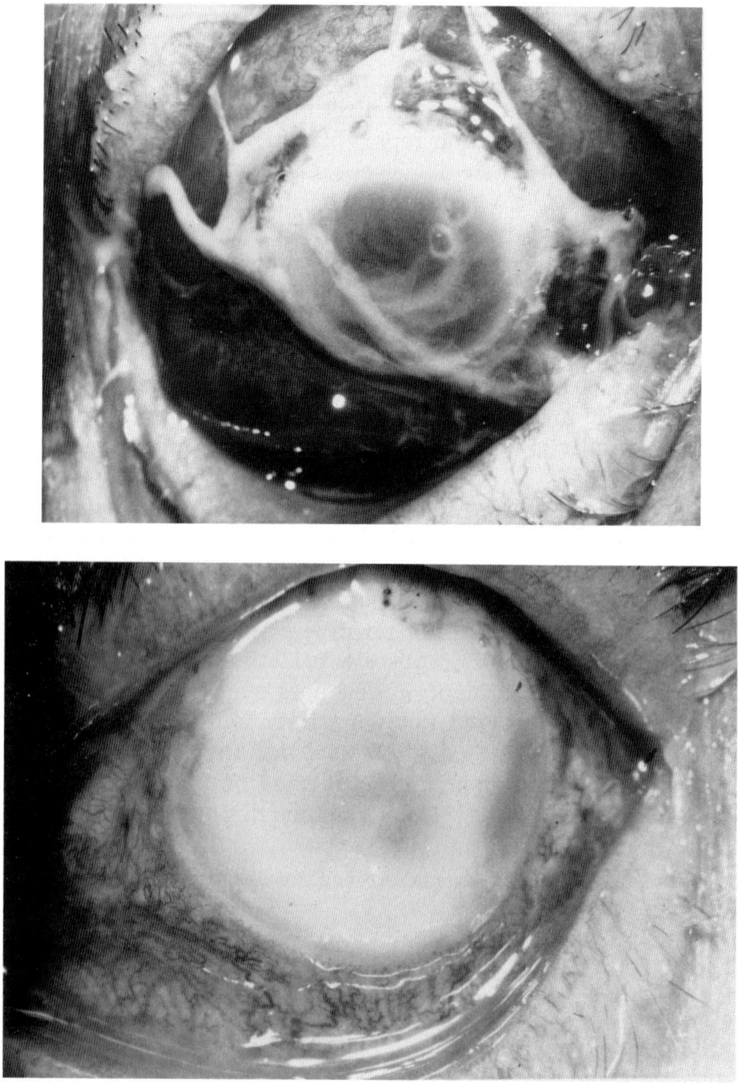

Fig. 1a. Gram-negative postoperative endophthalmitis caused by *Proteus mirabilis* – 24 hours postoperatively. *b.* Forty-eight hours post-cataract extraction: endophthalmitis caused by β-hemolytic streptococci.

sis, loss of anterior of chamber detail secondary to hypopyon, opacification of the cornea caused by inflammatory cell infiltrate and a vitritis or vitreous abscess as seen directly or acoustically. The time interval between surgery and the onset of POE is dependent in large measure on the attributes of pathogenicity which define the etiopathogen. Of these, virulence (small inoculum causes infections) and toxogenicity are best depicted in POE caused by a Gram-negative rod such as *Pseudomonas aeruginosa* or *Serratia marcescens*. In such a case, all the mentioned symptoms and signs may be evident within 24 hours of cataract surgery (Fig. 1a). Within 48 hours, Gram-positive bacteria such as *Streptococcus pneumoniae* or *Enterococcus faecalis* may cause a similar clinical picture (Fig. 1b).

Coagulase positive *Staphylococcus aureus* POE may also be clinically manifest within 48 hours. Coagulase negative staphylococci on the other hand are considerably less virulent and the onset of symptoms may not occur until several days following cataract extraction. Species and strain differences of CNS may result in varying severity of infection, but typically the cornea is not opacified and the anterior chamber while reactive, even with hypopyon, still permits visualization of some iris detail and in many cases also the vitreous (Fig. 2). The retina may be seen as a dull red reflex, or obscured, dependent on the severity of the vitreous infection. In its early stages, POE caused by CNS may be mistaken for a sterile postoperative inflammation which exacerbates with increased corticosteroid therapy. Perspicacious clinicians will be concerned about the possible occurrence of POE in any case exhibiting inflammatory findings greater than within the norm for their surgical technique. Such concern is justified since the interval between onset of POE and initial treatment is one of the major factors affecting visual outcome.

It must be noted that while cases of POE are clinically evident within four to six days of cataract surgery there are instances when the clinical symptoms and signs of infection have a delayed onset. One cause of such an infection is *P. acnes*. Typically, a granulomatous type uveitis occurs weeks or months following uneventful extracapsular cataract surgery. Associated findings include large keratitic precipitates on the posterior cornea and along fibrin strands in the anterior chamber, variable hypopyon and a white plaque on the posterior chamber IOL or posterior capsule (Fig. 3)[13].

The presence of *P. acnes* within the capsular bag, with some residual cortex, has led to speculation that the bacterium may act as an adjuvant stimulating an autoimmune re-

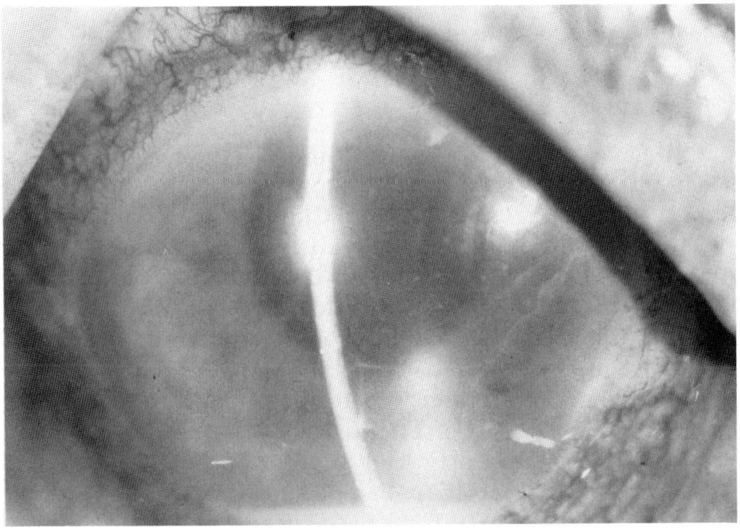

Fig. 2. Staphylococcus epidermidis postoperative endophthalmitis. Note that the cornea is relatively clear with visualization of the anterior chamber and anterior the vitreous.

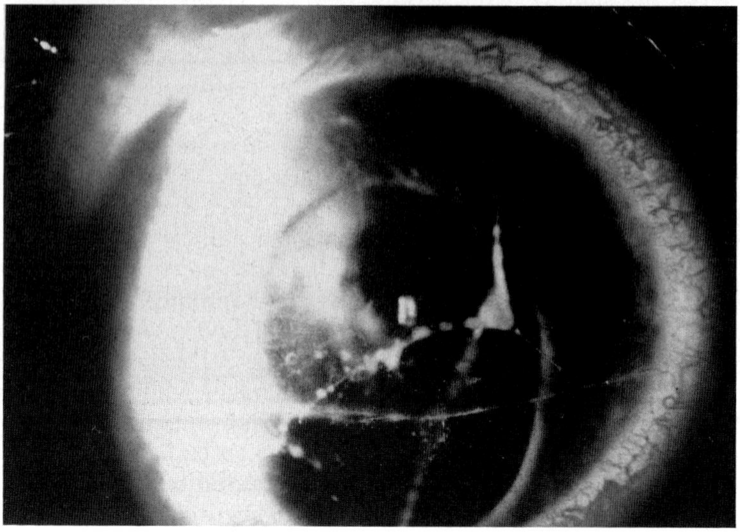

Fig. 3. Propionibacterium acnes postoperative endophthalmitis – several months post-cataract surgery. Note: fibrin strands in the anterior chamber with inflammatory cell infiltrate attached and large keratitic precipitates on the posterior cornea with a white plaque on posterior capsule. (Courtesy of R.D. Stulting, MD.)

sponse to lens protein[14]. A group of investigators[15] reviewed the fate of the fellow eye in 26 cases of culture proven *P. acnes* associated POE. They noted that none of the noninfected eyes became inflamed during the occurrence of *P. acnes* POE in the contralateral eye, suggesting that if an autoimmune inflammatory mechanism exists it is minimal.

Late onset POE has also been reported in association with other bacteria such as *S. epidermidis*, Achromobacter sp. and Cornynebacteria sp.[16,17]. While often indolent, these cases are clinically characterized by chronic uveitis, vitreous inflammation, decreasing vision and, in at least one case, by the presence of an endocapsular hypopyon[17]. Both yeast and mold fungi may also cause delayed onset POE[18-20], emphasizing the importance of not relying solely on clinical history and findings in making a rapid and specific diagnosis.

Laboratory diagnosis

Repeated studies have consistently demonstrated the diagnostic importance of culturing the contents of intraocular compartments (aqueous and vitreous) in cases of clinically suspected microbial endophthalmitis[1,6,7,21,22]. Cultures of the lid margins, conjunctiva and even the incisional wound are frequently misleading and do not give reliable information as to the causative organism. Therefore, dependable techniques are necessary for sampling the aqueous and vitreous in order to identify the etiopathogen(s), ascertain antimicrobial drug sensitivities and logically initiate or alter antimicrobial therapy.

Simplicity of culture technique combined with minimal media requirements will assist the surgeon in developing a compulsive, repetitive approach to each case. This is important because some common causes of POE represent periocular microbiota and media contamination with these bacteria may lead to an erroneous conclusion concerning the cause of the postoperative inflammation. Samples of both aqueous and vitreous should be cultured since in POE caused by CNS the aqueous cultures may often be negative while the vitreous culture is positive (Fig. 4).

It is better to use agar plates than slants for cultures because the surface can be marked

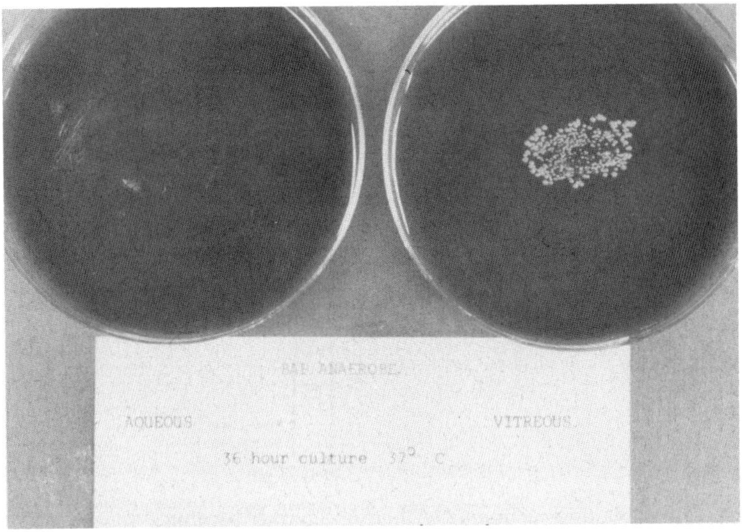

Fig. 4. Coagulase negative staphylococci from a case of postoperative endophthalmitis growing on anaerobic agar at 36 hours. Note: negative culture of the aspirate from the anterior chamber at 36 hours compared to positive vitreous culture with significant growth along the inoculation streaks.

with either an "A" or "V"indicating the precise point of inoculation on the center of the medium. Growth peripheral to these markings can be identified as contaminants and not legitimate isolates. The three media are:

1. Freshly reduced thioglycolate broth enriched with hemin and vitamin K is commercially available and used primarily for isolation of obligate anaerobes such as *P. acnes.* Since some aerobic and microaerophilic bacteria also replicate in this media, it can be used to confirm this growth on solid media.
2. Chocolate agar permits growth of more fastidious bacteria than does blood agar and also indicates to the microbiology laboratory that the sample should be incubated in a capnophilic environment. Bacteria which can be isolated on blood agar can also be isolated on chocolate agar although the converse is not necessarily true.
3. Sabouraud dextrose agar (without antimicrobial additives) permits growth of yeast and hyphomycete fungi. Alter inoculation the plates should be incubated aerobically at 25°C. Sometimes the fungal isolate may grow equally well at 35-37°C on both Sabouraud dextrose and chocolate agar.

To obtain dependable results, it is best to have the culture media available in the operating room for direct inoculation by the surgeon. Since both aqueous and vitreous samples must be cultured, two of each media are required.

Aqueous sampling

A non-penetrating, but deep, knife-needle incision is made tangential to the corneal limbus away from the cataract wound. Through this, the anterior chamber is entered with a 27-gauge needle, attached to a tuberculin syringe and 0.1-0.2 ml of fluid aspirated. A drop of this is placed centrally on each of the two agar plates. Using a blunt instrument "A" is inscribed on the agar service; thus, dispersing the inoculum along the mark (Fig. 5). A third drop is placed into the thioglycolate broth. Obligate anaerobes are more readily isolated if the sample is placed deep, into the bottom of the broth. To accomplish this, a disposable 22-gauge 3.5-inch spinal needle can be affixed to the syringe and in-

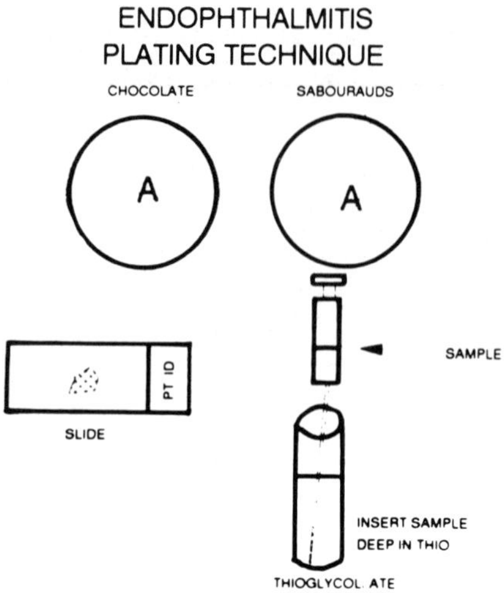

Fig. 5. Endophthalmitis platting technique. Anterior chamber aspirates are inscribed centrally onto the solid media (chocolate agar and Sabouraud dextrose agar) with a sterile, blunt instrument, forming an "A". A 3.5 -inch, 22-gauge spinal needle attached to the tuberculin syringe is inserted deep into the thioglycolate for inoculation. The broth may be pulled into the syringe and placed back into the tube, if necessary. A drop of specimen, if available, should be placed on a pre-cleaned slide and smeared thinly. The same procedure is used for the undiluted vitreous specimen inscribing a "V" in the central portion of the solid media to indicate the point of inoculation.

serted into the bottom of the tube containing the broth. If the aqueous specimen is exhausted after inoculation of the agar media, insert the sterile spinal needle deeply into the thioglycolate broth, aspirate into the syringe and then push back into the broth. This allows sufficient contact of the sample with the medium (Fig. 5).

If there is sufficient aqueous sample remaining, an additional drop is placed on a precleaned glass slide and smeared thin, using a blunt, sterile instrument. This smear is submitted for Gram stain.

Vitreous sampling

This may be accomplished by passing a 25- 27-gauge needle on a 3-ml syringe through the pars plana, 3 mm posterior to the limbus, into the anterior vitreous and gently aspirating 0.2-0.5 ml of fluid vitreous. In the event vitrectomy is to be performed or resistance to aspiration necessitates a vitreous biopsy, the vitrectomy instrument tip is passed through a sclerotomy incision 3 mm posterior to the limbus. A syringe attached to the suction line combined with the cutting action of the instrument facilitates removal of 0.3-0.5 mm of vitreous specimen. In the event of pars plana vitrectomy, the vitreous biopsy is obtained before infusion of balanced salt solution. The undiluted vitreous specimen is then inoculated using the same media and techniques described for culture of the anterior chamber fluid. With vitreous samples, however, a "V" is inscribed on the agar plates (Fig. 5). If possible, a drop of vitreous is reserved for smear and Gram stain.

As noted, it is preferable for the surgeon to inoculate the media directly upon removal from the anterior chamber and vitreous compartment. Lacking this, the respective syringe tip should be sealed with a sterile cap and submitted to the microbiology laboratory for culture and smear of its contents within 30 minutes of aspiration.

If a vitrectomy is performed, a cassette containing vitreous mixed with infusion fluid is capped in a sterile manner and sent to the microbiology laboratory as soon as possible.

The fluid from the cassette is aseptically suctioned through a 0.22 or 0.45 micron membrane filter. Under sterile conditions, the filter is then divided into three wedges, placing one each on a chocolate agar, Sabouraud dextrose agar and anaerobic blood agar enriched with hemin and vitamin K. The results of these cultures should confirm those of the undiluted aqueous and vitreous specimens.

If the vitrectomy cassette contents cannot be filtered and cultured immediately after arrival at the microbiology laboratory, the cassette can be held for 12 hours at room temperature or preferably at 37°C. Since the cell population may increase during this time, quantitation of colony forming units (CFU) is not meaningful from the vitrectomy filtrate.

If the amount of undiluted aqueous or vitreous is really inadequate for culture and smear, then prioritization is exercised based on the known causes of POE. Chocolate agar should be the first medium inoculated (CNS and some fungi), thioglycolate broth the second (*P. acnes*) and Sabouraud dextrose agar third. The smear for Gram stain is fourth in priority.

All culture media should be observed daily for at least ten days to ensure that slow growing organisms are not missed. The results should be interpreted as follows:

Positive

1. Growth of the same microorganism along "A" or "V" marks or along either one in combination with growth in the thioglycolate broth.
2. Confluent growth of more than 50 colony forming units (CFU) or semiconfluent growth (11-50 CFU) along the inoculation marks ("A" or "V") of one solid medium is also evidence of a positive culture.
3. Scant growth (>10 CFU) along an "A" or "V" mark or in liquid media only – confirmed by growth of the same organism from the vitrectomy cassette filtrate.
4. Growth, on any media, from aqueous, undiluted vitreous or cassette filtrate, corroborated a Gram stain observation of an organism of similar morphology from the aqueous or undiluted vitreous.

Equivocal

No Gram stain evidence of microorganisms from the aqueous or undiluted vitreous *and*:
1. Growth in thioglycolate broth only from the aqueous or undiluted vitreous.
2. Only scant growth along the "A" or "V" marks only one of the solid media.
3. Growth only from the vitrectomy cassette filtrate on any media.

Negative

Failure to isolate any microorganism on, or in, any of the media within 7-10 days constitutes a negative culture result, even if the stained smears suggest the presence of a microorganism.

Management

Numerous reports in the ophthalmic literature during the past decade have provided enough information for us to conclude that conventional, infectious disease treatment in cases of POE fails. This failure of topical, periocular and many oral or parenteral antimicrobics to penetrate the avascular vitreous in insufficient concentration to kill bacteria or even inhibit their growth, has led ophthalmologists to search for alternative forms of treatment. What has evolved is the direct injection of antibiotics into the vitreous cavity, either alone or in combination with the pars plana vitrectomy.

Intraocular antibiotics (IOAB)

For almost a decade, there has been near universal agreement that direct injection of antibiotics into the vitreous cavity is essential in the management of POE[23]. In considering today's choice of what, and how much, to inject into the vitreous cavity, the following must be considered:

1. Coagulase negative staphylococci are the most frequent cause of POE and of these *S. epidermidis* is the predominant etiopathogen. Methicillin and cephalosporin resistance strains of *S. epidermidis* are generally sensitive to vancomycin as are streptococci and enterococci.
2. Vancomycin is reported efficacious in experimental methicillin-resistant *S. epidermidis* endophthalmitis[24] and has been investigationally proven safe in treating such infections[25]. In 1 mg intravitreal doses, vancomycin has been effective and non-toxic in the management of human endophthalmitis caused by *S. epidermidis*, *P. acnes*, and Bacillus sp.[26]. Experimentally, its vitreal half life is rather long (22-38 hours) providing a cidal concentration over a relatively long time period[27]. When administered systemically, vancomycin can be nephrotoxic and even at unacceptably high serum levels penetrates the vitreous poorly, if at all[28].
3. Amikacin is an aminoglycoside antibiotic with a broad spectrum of activity against Gram-negative bacilli including some gentamicin-resistant organisms[29]. Some strains of *S. aureus* are also susceptible to amikacin. It is reportedly less toxic as an IOAB than gentamicin[31-32] and has been suggested as the aminoglycoside of choice for intravitreal injection at a dose of 0.4 mg in the management of bacterial endophthalmitis[33]. Retinal toxicity associated with intravitreal injection of aminoglycosides has been chiefly associated with injections of 0.4 mg of gentamicin in vitrectomized eyes[34,35]. A recent survey, however, incriminates intravitreal gentamicin at even lower doses and in four of five cases suggests that macular infraction was related to the intravitreal injection of amikacin[36].

Vancomycin hydrochloride (1 mg/0.1 ml) and amikacin sulfate (0.4 mg/0.1 ml) are the antibiotics used in all patients admitted to a multicenter, clinical study of treatment strategy for POE[37]. The same study is attempting to define the role of intravitreous antibiotics and the treatment of this infection. This is of some importance since systemic antibiotic treatment is not without potentially serious complications and, at least, some patients with culture-proven infection were managed successfully with one or more intravitreal injections alone[38]. However, experimental data suggest increasing intravitreal levels of antibiotics in the inflamed eye with sustained intravenous administration[39-41]. Ceftazidime, a third generation cephalosporin (1.5-2.0 grams) every 12 hours intravenously and amikacin sulfate (in dosage is weight dependent) are administered to endophthalmitis vitrectomy study patients who are randomized to intravenous treatment[37].

The use of oral or parenteral corticosteroids may assist greatly in retarding the host inflammatory response to POE. If one is comfortable in assuming from clinical features and Gram-stain cytology that CNS are the cause, then steroid therapy could be initiated with initial antibiotic management. Lacking this, it is probably best to await culture results and preliminary antimicrobial sensitivities.

Cycloplegia can be obtained with 1% atropine or 0.25% scopolamine applied topically as drops several times daily.

Periocular antibiotic injections and fortified solutions for drop application (gentamicin, vancomycin, cefazolin, etc.) have certainly been used in treating POE and may prove useful in the presence of wound infection. There are, however, no data to suggest their usefulness in treating infection within the vitreous compartment.

Vitrectomy surgery in the management of bacterial endophthalmitis

The multiple factors involved in the eventual visual outcome of an eye with POE perpetuates uncertainty as to the efficacy of vitrectomy alone, vitrectomy with IOAB, vitrectomy with IOAB and steroid treatment, systemic antibiotics without surgery or systemic, periocular and IOAB without vitrectomy. A number of reports have advocated the use of vitrectomy in the management of endophthalmitis[8,11-42]. Each paper has emphasized that the variability of results is due to differences in time of onset and initiating treatment because of delays in diagnosis, differences in antibiotic choice, dose and route of administration, use of concurrent steroid therapy, type of organism and size of the reported sample. There is general agreement, however, that vitrectomy is advisable for the more severe cases of endophthalmitis while milder forms, based on visual parameters, acoustic imaging and ophthalmoscopy may be initially managed by IOAB, topical and periocular, as well as intravenous antibiotics therapy, without vitrectomy. Many of the questions involving timing and choice of antibiotics for post-cataract extraction and endophthalmitis will, hopefully, be answered by the endophthalmitis study (EVS)[37].

Timing of vitrectomy

In general, the infecting organism correlates with the prognosis rather than the actual timing of vitrectomy. In a reported series[43], no statistically significant difference in visual results could be attributed to either early or late vitrectomy in the small series of 12 eyes undergoing pars plana vitrectomy. Two eyes in this series assigned to late vitrectomy, did lose all perception of light (both having streptococcal organisms as causative). In a similar series[42], it was noted that 13 of 15 eyes with poor visual results also had streptococcal endophthalmitis. Eyes with streptococcal endophthalmitis, which have late vitrectomy appear to have poor visual results due to the virulence and toxigenicity of the organism. Vitrectomy, in concept, has been likened to "lancing a boil", thus, removing a nidos of infecting organisms, removing the source of liberated toxins and allowing space for injection of antibiotics to eradicate residual organisms. This technique has been preferred by some to systemic administration of antibiotics[43,44].

Technique

Culture of the anterior chamber and vitreous should be performed, as previously described, before influx of infusion fluid. If vitrectomy is to be performed, the cutting instrument may be used without infusion to obtain a vitreous sample allowing the eye to soften. In aphakic or pseudophakic eyes, one does not have to worry about the crystalline lens and, thus, the eye may be allowed to soften slightly. In most situations, 1.0-1.5 ml of solution can easily be obtained prior to starting infusion. The specimen is immediately plated as previously described on chocolate agar, Sabouraud dextrose agar, and in thioglycolate broth. If the solutions are allowed to remain unplated for a period of time, the chance for positive culture results decreases markedly. The extend of vitrectomy varies depending on the amount of debris present. It is not considered critical to perform extensive vitrectomy. In many cases, the posterior hyaloid will not be detached. In such eyes, the removal of the posterior hyaloid with friable underlying retina, will cause extensive tears and destruction of the retina. Removal of a large amount of vitreous may enhance the possibility of retinal toxicity from injected intravitreal antibiotics, allowing the medication to gravitationally settle on the fovea. Upon removal of adequate vitreous debris, the antibiotics are then injected slowly into the vitreous cavity with a beveled position towards the anterior segments. The patient is immediately turned toward the nasal side upon completion of the vitrectomy to prevent, if possible, the localization of antibiotic upon the macular region.

Intraocular steroids

The inflammatory reaction resulting from bacterial endophthalmitis can be severe and may, in some situations, cause pathologic complications greater than the bacterial insult. Vitrectomy removes a portion of the necrotic tissue and bacterial toxins, thus, preventing the development of inflammatory membranes, which adhere to the collagen framework of the vitreous gel. Antibiotic sterilization of the intraocular vitreous cavity may not be enough to prevent these late complications in the severely inflamed eyes, necessitating corticosteroids to be started, usually within 48 hours of the installation of intravitreal antibiotics to reduce the risks of these secondary complications. Other authors have started corticosteroids simultaneously with the installation of antibiotics[43]. Investigational data in at least one report suggest that intraocular dexamethasone produces a harmful effect in the treatment of experimental endophthalmitis[45]. If only antibiotics are injected, the lysis of bacteria may provoke an increased release of endotoxins into the eye. A vitrectomy is necessary to try to "debulk" this quantity of inflammatory necrotizing toxins.

Management of intraocular lenses

The vast majority of eyes do not require removal of intraocular lenses. In some situations, fibrin may be so dense on the surface of the lens that visualization does not allow vitrectomy. In those eyes, injection of 3 μg of tissue plasminogen activator (tPA) will result in the dissolution of the fibrin, enough to permit vitrectomy. Injection of viscoelastic material on the surface of the lens may then clear the surface sufficiently to permit vitrectomy in those eyes where debris exists. In a reported series[7], intraocular lenses were removed in 28% of pseudophakic eyes with endophthalmitis to facilitate performance of the vitrectomy at a time prior to the use of tPA. More representative is a Scandinavian series[43] in which the intraocular lens was left in place in all cases. Actual removal of a posterior chamber lens from inflamed eye may, in fact, prove to be very dangerous and result in severe complication, such as hemorrhage, detached retina, etc. However, there are reports of bacterial contamination and adherence to the intraocular lens[46-48] and in cases of recurrent or chronic endophthalmitis, particularly when repeat cultures are positive, serious consideration should be given to the removal of the intraocular lens[49-51].

Prevention

Sufficient data now exist to point towards the periocular microbial flora (CNS) as the source of the most common causes of POE[11]. Additionally, there are studies indicating that these same bacteria are present in the anterior chamber fluid of some patients at completion of uneventful cataract surgery[51]. *Staphylococcus aureus* can often be isolated from the anterior nares and streptococci from the nasopharynx and from obstructed lacrimal drainage systems. Gram-negative bacilli may transiently colonize a quiet outer eye, gaining access to the aqueous and vitreous at the time of cataract surgery. Awareness of these facts will certainly help the cataract surgeon in minimizing the risk of POE.

Obtaining a careful history seems obvious; but, is often given insufficient preoperative attention. Is there a history of infections elsewhere (sinusitis, cystitis, etc)? Is the patient taking oral antibiotics? If so, why?

Be certain there are no clinical signs of chronic adnexal microbial infection (microbial blepharitis, chronic dacryocystitis, etc).

While there are no controlled studies on the value of preoperative topical antibiotics drops in preventing POE, their use is associated with minimal, if any, risk and a broad spectrum topical agent may, indeed, help in decreasing or eliminating bacteria colonizing the conjunctiva.

Since *S. epidermidis* and other CNS constitute normal lid and periocular skin microflora and are also a common cause of POE, meticulous attention to preoperative prepping and draping would seem prudent. One study observed a lower incidence of POE among patients having an application of topical, 5% povidone-iodine solution to the ocular surface compared to a group receiving silver protein solution topically[53].

Contamination of the optic or hyptics of the IOL at the time of implantation should be of major concern[45-47]. Electrostatic attraction of bacteria may be diminished by irrigating the IOL. Any IOL which has touched the lid margin or conjunctival surface, particularly if coated with viscoelastic material, should be copiously irrigated with balanced salt solution prior to insertion into the eye.

There are no useful data available on the effect of periocular antibiotics when employed as prophylaxis against POE. Cases have occurred with and without use of subconjunctival antibiotics at conclusion of surgery. It is better to depend on a reliable history, documented absence of adnexa infection, meticulous attention to preoperative preparation and draping and good surgical technique to minimize the risk of postoperative infection.

References

1. Forster RK: Management of infectious endophthalmitis. Ophthalmology 87:313-319, 1980
2. Stark WJ, Sommer A, Smith RE: Changing trends in intraocular lens implantation (editorial). Arch Ophthalmol 107:1441-1444, 1989
3. Stark WJ, Worthen DM, Holladay JT et al: The FDA report on intraocular lenses. Ophthalmology 90:311-317, 1983
4. Javitt JC, Vitale S, Canner JK et al: National outcomes of cataract extraction: endophthalmitis following inpatient surgery. Arch Ophthalmol 109:1085-1089, 1991
5. Rowsey JJ, Newson DC, Sexton DJ, Harms WK: Endophthalmitis: current approaches. Ophthalmology 89:1055-1066, 1982
6. Olson JC, Flynn HW, Forster RK, Culbertson WW: Results in the treatment of postoperative endophthalmitis. Ophthalmology 90:692-699, 1983
7. Driebe WT, Mandelbaum S, Forster RK et al: Pseudophakic endophthalmitis. Ophthalmology 93:442-448, 1986
8. Bohigian GM, Olk RJ: Factors associated with poor visual results in endophthalmitis. Am J Ophthalmol 101:332-334, 1986
9. Pulafito CA, Baker AS, Haaf J, Foster CS: Infectious endophthalmitis. Ophthalmology 89:921-929, 1982
10. Weber DJ, Hoffman KL, Thoft RA, Baker AS: Endophthalmitis following intraocular lens implantation: report of 30 cases and review of the literature. Rev Infect Dis 8:12-20, 1986
11. Speaker MG, Milch FA, Shah MK et al: Role of external bacterial flora in the pathogenesis of acute postoperative endophthalmitis. Ophthalmology 98:639-649, 1991
12. McNatt J, Allen S, Wilson LA, McDowell BR: Anaerobic flora of the normal human conjunctival sac. Arch Ophthalmol 96:1448-1450, 1978
13. Meisler DM, Mandelbaum S: Propionibacterium associated endophthalmitis after extracapsular cataract extraction: review of reported cases. Ophthalmology 96:54-60, 1989
14. Discussion of Meisler DN, Mandelbaum S: Propionibacterium associated endophthalmitis after cataract extraction: review of reported cases. Ophthalmology 96:60-61, 1989
15. Yang CM, Cousins SW: Fate of the fellow eye after *Propionibacterium acnes* endophthalmitis. Am J Ophthalmol 112:99-100, 1991
16. Ficker LA, Meredith TA, Wilson LA et al: Chronic bacterial endophthalmitis. Am J Ophthalmol 112:747-748, 1987
17. Stefansson E, Cobo LM, Carlson AN, Kesler JL: Endocapsular hypopyon: a clinical sign of localized endophthalmitis. Ophthalmic Surg 21:221-222, 1990

18. Stern WH, Tamura E, Jacobs RA et al: Epidemic postsurgical *Candida parapsilosis* endophthalmitis: clinical findings in management of 15 consecutive cases. Ophthalmology 92:1701-1709, 1985
19. Margo CE, Fitzgerald CR: Postoperative endophthalmitis caused by *Wangiella dermatitis*. Am J Ophthalmol 110:322-323, 1990
20. Rummelt V, Ruprecht KW, Boltze HJ, Naumann GOH: Chronic *Alternari alternata* endophthalmitis following intraocular lens implantation. Arch Ophthalmol 109:178, 1991
21. Katten NM, Flynn HW Jr, Pflugfelder SC et al: Nosocomial endophthalmitis survey: current incidence of infection after intraocular surgery. Ophthalmology 98:227-238, 1991
22. Verbraaken H, Geeroms B, Karemera A: Treatment of endophthalmitis by pars plana vitrectomy. Ophthalmologica 197:19-25, 1988
23. Baum J, Peyman GA, Barza M: Intravitreal administration of antibiotic in the treatment of endophthalmitis. III. Consensus. Surv Ophthalmol 26:204-206, 1982
24. Smith MR, Sorenson JA, Lowry FD et al: Treatment of methicillin-resistant *Staphylococcus epidermidis* endophthalmitis with intravitreal vancomycin. Ophthalmology 93:1328-1335, 1986
26. Homer P, Peyman GA, Koziol J, Sanders D: Intravitreal injections of vancomycin in experimental staphylococcal endophthalmitis. Acta Ophthalmol 53:311-320, 1975
26. Pavan PR, Brinser JH: Letter to the Editor. Ophthalmology 94:896, 1987
27. Barza M, Baum J, Sliwkowski M: Ocular pharmacokinetics of LY 146032 (LY), teicoplanin and vancomycin in a rabbit model. In: Program and Abstracts of the 27th Interscience Conference on Antimicrobial Agents and Chemotherapy of the American Society for Microbiology. October 4-7, 1987, New York. Abstr No. 152
28. Pryor J, Apt L, Leopold I: Intraocular penetration of vancomycin. Arch Ophthalmol 67:92-95, 1962
29. Gammon JA, Schwab I, Joseph P: Gentamicin-resistant *Serratia marcescens* endophthalmitis. Arch Ophthalmol 98:1221-1223, 1980
30. D'Amico DJ, Casper-Velu L, Liebert J et al: Comparative toxicity of intravitreal aminoglycoside antibiotics. Am L Ophthalmol 100:264-275, 1985
31. Talamo JH, D'Amico DJ, Hanninen LA et al: The influence of aphakia and vitrectomy in experimental retinal toxicity of aminoglycoside antibiotics. Am J Ophthalmol 100:840-847, 1985
32. Conway BP: Amikacin is less toxic than gentamicin in the primate retina. Invest Ophthalmol Vis Sci (Suppl) 29:404, 1988
33. Talamo JH, D'Amico DJ, Kenyon KR: Intravitreal amakacin in the treatment of bacterial endophthalmitis. Arch Ophthalmol 104:1483-1485, 1986
34. McDonald AR, Schantz H, Allen AW et al: Retinal toxicity secondary to intraocular gentamicin injection. Ophthalmology 93:871-877, 1986
35. Conway BP, Campochiaro PA: Macular infarction after endophthalmitis treated with vitrectomy and intravitreal gentamicin. Arch Ophthalmol 104:367-371, 1986
36. Campochiaro PA, Conway BP: Aminoglycoside toxicity: a survey of retinal specialists: indications for ocular use. Arch Ophthalmol 109:946-950, 1991
37. Doft BH: The endophthalmitis vitrectomy study (editorial). Arch Ophthalmol 109:487-488, 1991
38. Pavan PR, Brinser JH: Exogenous bacterial endophthalmitis treated without systemic antibiotics. Am J Ophthalmol 104:121-126, 1987
39. Barza M, Kane A, Baum J: Comparison of the effects of continuous and intermittent systemic administration on the penetration of gentamicin into the infected rabbit eye. J Infect Dis 147:144-148, 1983
40. Walstad R, Blika S, Nielsen E, Halvarsen T: The penetration of ceftazidime into the inflamed rabbit eye. Scand J Infect Dis 19:131-135, 1987
41. Martin DF, Ficker LA, Aquilar HE et al: Vitreous cefazolin levels after intravenous injection. Arch Ophthalmol 108:411-414, 1990
42. Bohigian GM, Olk RJ: Endophthalmitis. Acta Ophthalmol 24:573-576, 1983
43. Olk RJ, Bohigian GM: The management of endophthalmitis: diagnostic and therapeutic guidelines including the use of vitrectomy. Ophthalmic Surg 18:262-267, 1987
44. Laatinkien L, Tarkkanen A: Early vitrectomy in the treatment of postoperative purulent endophthalmitis. Acta Ophthalmol 65:455-460, 1987
45. Meredith TA, Aquilar HE, Drews CD et al: Intraocular dexamethasone produced a harmful effect in the treatment of experimental *Staphylococcus aureus* endophthalmitis. Invest Ophthalmol Vis Sci (Suppl) 31:140, 1990
46. Vafidis GC, Marsh RJ, Stacey AR: Bacterial contamination of intraocular lens surgery. Br J Ophthalmol 68:520-523, 1984.
47. Dilly PN, Holmes-Sellors PJ: Bacterial adhesion to intraocular lenses. J Cataract Refract Surg 15:317-330, 1989

48. Griffith PG, Elliott SJ, McTaggart L: Adherence of *Staphylococcus epidermidis* to intraocular lenses. Br J Ophthalmol 73:402-406, 1989
49. Nobe J, Fingold SM, Rife LL et al: Chronic anaerobic bacterial endophthalmitis in pseudophakic rabbit eyes. Invest Ophthalmol Vis Sci 28:259-263, 1987
50. Stern GA, Engle HM, Driebe WT Jr: Recurrent postoperative endophthalmitis. Cornea 9:102-107, 1990
51. Jansen B, Hartmann C, Schumacher-Perdreau F, Peters G: Late onset endophthalmitis with intraocular lens: a case of molecularly proven *S. epidermidis* aetiology. Br J Ophthalmol 75:440-441, 1991
52. Sherwood DR, Rich WJ, Jacob JS, Fairchild WY: Bacterial contamination of intraocular and extraocular fluids during extracapsular cataract extraction. Eye 3:308-312, 1989
53. Dickey JB, Thompson KD, Jay WM: Anterior chamber aspirate cultures after uncomplicated cataract surgery. Am J Ophthalmol 112:278-282, 1991
54. Speaker MG, Menikoff JA: Prophylaxis of endophthalmitis with topical povidone iodine. Ophthalmology 98:1769-1775, 1991

CONTEMPORARY VITREORETINAL SURGICAL MANAGEMENT OF POSTERIORLY DISLOCATED INTRAOCULAR LENSES

Antonio Capone, Jr., Barry A. Mandell, Thomas M. Aaberg, Sr., Paul Sternberg, Jr., H. Michael Lambert and Pedro F. Lopez

Retina Service, Department of Ophthalmology, Emory University, Atlanta, Georgia, USA

Introduction

Posterior chamber intraocular lens (PCIOL) subluxation and dislocation are infrequent complications of planned cataract extraction. The reported incidence of PCIOL decentration ranges from 0.2% to 1.2% in most series[1-8]. Posterior dislocation into the vitreous cavity is considerably less common. Lens malposition generally occurs intraoperatively, and is often apparent on the first postoperative day[9-11]. Zonular dialysis or loss of posterior capsular integrity, which occur in up to 4.8% of planned extracapsular surgical procedures, are the typical predisposing conditions[12]. Posterior luxation of anterior chamber implants is rare, with large basal iridectomies representing the most common route of anterior segment egress[9,13].

Some have suggested that the posteriorly dislocated intraocular lens (PDIOL) need not be surgically addressed *per se*, emphasizing instead correction of the functional aphakia with spectacles, contact lenses[14], or secondary lens implantation[15]. Ostensibly conservative, such approaches place the eye at considerable risk for chronic intraocular inflammation, cystoid macular edema, pupillary block, vitreous hemorrhage, and retinal contusion or detachment[9,16,17]. Such eyes are thus neither properly visually rehabilitated nor anatomically or physiologically stable. With rare exceptions, vitreoretinal surgical intervention is the appropriate management strategy.

Surgical options for handling luxated IOLs include removal[11,13,17-19], repositioning[9,11,13,16,18,20-32], and exchange[9,11,13,17], with or without suture fixation to surrounding ocular structures in the latter two instances. Herein we describe our philosophy and vitreoretinal surgical techniques for the management of posteriorly dislocated intraocular lenses (PDIOLs).

Surgical techniques

General considerations

The goal of surgical management of PDIOLs is a pseudophakic eye with stable, anatomically correct IOL fixation. This objective is best realized by:
1. recognition of IOL characteristics mitigating in favor of exchange *versus* repositioning;

Supported in part by a departmental grant from Research to Prevent Blindness, Inc.

Address for correspondence: Antonio Capone, Jr., MD, Retina Service, Department of Ophthalmology, Emory University, 1327 Clifton Road NE, 4th Floor, Atlanta, GA 30322, USA

Retina and Vitreous, pp. 271-281
Proceedings of the Symposium on Retina and Vitreous,
organized by the New Orleans Academy of Ophthalmology
New Orleans, LA, USA, March 12-15, 1992
edited by Rudolph M. Franklin

2. creation of scleral flaps to guard against transscleral suture erosion, placed so as to ensure lens centration;
3. removal of anterior vitreous and lens remnants;
4. meticulous release of vitreous attachments to the IOL;
5. uncomplicated retrieval of the luxated IOL from the posterior segment; and
6. ciliary sulcus fixation with a non-absorbable suture.

The determination of whether an IOL will be repositioned or exchanged is made preoperatively. Luxated ACIOLs are exchanged. Haptic configuration, mobility at the haptic-lens junction, and IOL production date are the factors which determine the fate of a luxated posterior chamber IOL as well as the selection of its replacement. We prefer non-cantilevered haptics designed such that the likelihood of suture slippage from the haptic end is minimized, such as J-loop haptics and C-loop designs with positioning eyelets, suture eyelets or bulb-shaped ends. IOLs manufactured after 1986 with the appropriate haptic design characteristics are repositioned. IOL chaffing complications (*i.e.*, mechanical damage to intraocular tissues with disruption of the blood-aqueous barrier and secondary uveitis, glaucoma, hyphema, corneal decompensation and cystoid macular edema) may occur with IOLs which are not smooth-edged and finely polished, as was often the case prior to the late 1980s[33]. Industry manufacturing standards were modified subsequent to the recognition of this syndrome.

IOL mobilization and preparation for fixation

A 360-degree limbal peritomy is performed. The limbus-based scleral flaps are created prior to entering the eye, as lamellar scleral dissection is performed with greater ease when the globe is formed. The flaps are placed in the horizontal meridian, oriented 180 degrees apart for optimal IOL centration within the pupillary space, and measuring 1.5 mm in both base length and height.

The eye is prepared for standard three-port, closed pars plana vitrectomy. A 4-mm infusion cannula is sewn into the inferotemporal quadrant, and two additional sclerotomies

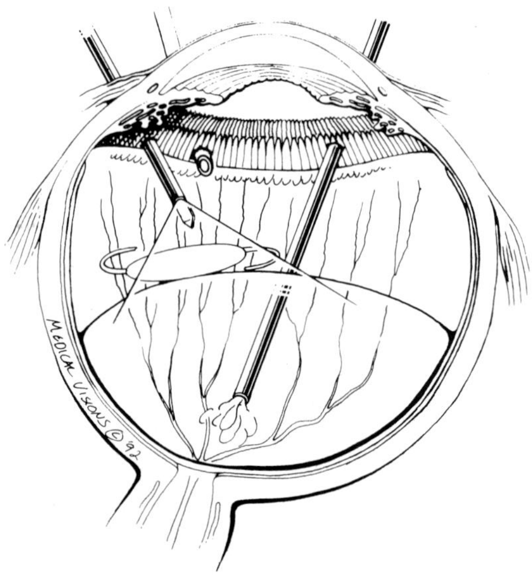

Fig. 1. Cross-sectional view of the eye following evacuation of vitreous from the anterior segment, total posterior vitrectomy, and removal of lens remnants. PFO is injected over the optic nerve to float the mobilized PDIOL off of the retinal surface.

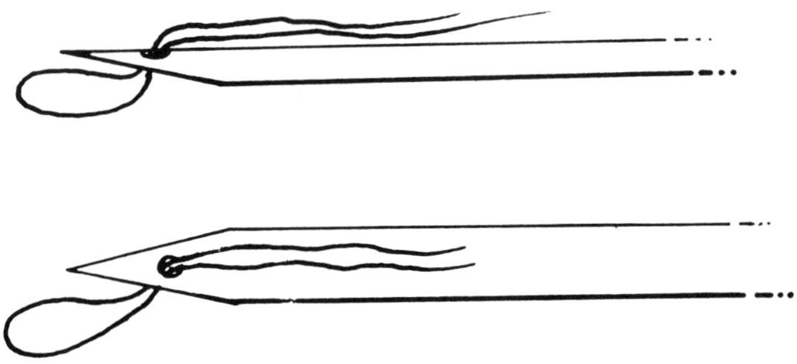

Fig. 2. For IOL repositioning, the prolene fixation suture is folded in half, with the midportion passed through the eyelet of the 27-gauge TREK needle prior to entering the eye

made superiorly at the 2:30 and 9:30 o'clock meridians. All sclerotomies are placed 3 mm posterior to the limbus. The vitrectomy probe is used to remove vitreous from the anterior segment as well as residual lens cortex. Residual lens capsule is either removed using alpha chymotrypsin[34], or with the vitrectomy probe using scleral indentation.

Attention is next directed posteriorly. The PDIOL is generally found either embedded in the inferior vitreous base or lying flatly over the posterior pole. Care is exercised in freeing the PDIOL haptics of all vitreous attachment to avoid iatrogenic vitreous base dialysis, retinal dialysis, or peripheral retinal breaks. After completion of the vitrectomy, perfluoro-N-octane (PFO) is instilled into the vitreous cavity (Fig. 1) to float the luxated IOL off of the retinal surface into the mid-vitreous cavity for either suture fixation or translimbal exchange[19]. The technique for PFO instillation is described in detail in another chapter. PFO is left in the eye until fixation is complete in the event that purchase on the lens is not maintained during execution of the surgical maneuvers described below. The entry position for transscleral suture passage is measured externally for both flaps in repositioning and exchange procedures alike at 0.5 mm posterior to the surgical limbus to ensure IOL fixation in the ciliary sulcus[35]. A non-absorbable suture (10-0 prolene) is utilized for long-term anatomic stability[36,37].

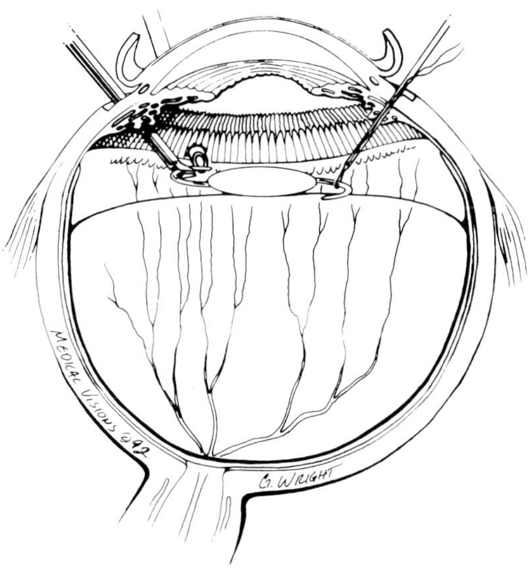

Fig. 3. The dislocated posterior chamber IOL is lifted off of the PFO with a vitreoretinal microforceps for stabilization. The IOL haptic is engaged with the prolene loop.

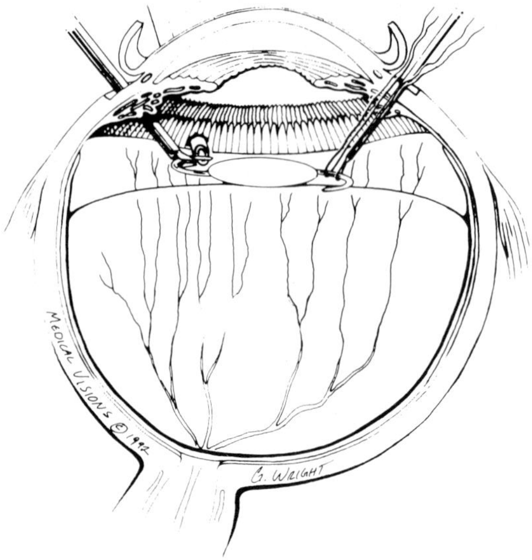

Fig. 4. A second prolene loop is similarly used to provide two-point haptic fixation, and the two suture pairs loosely tied for stabilization.

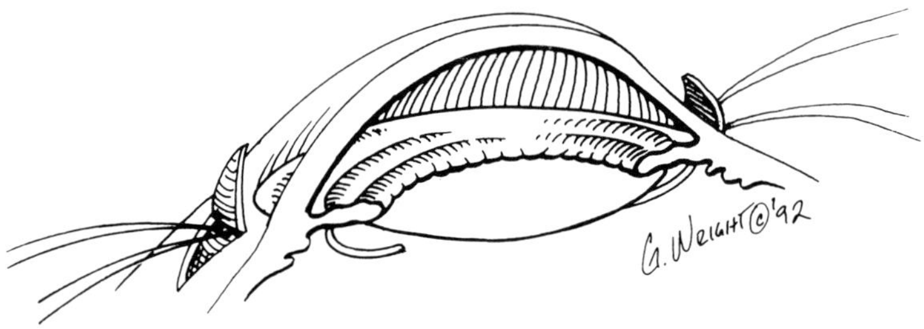

Fig. 5. Both haptics have been engaged and drawn into the ciliary sulcus. The suture pairs are snugly tied flush to the sclera. The IOL is internally fixated at four-points.

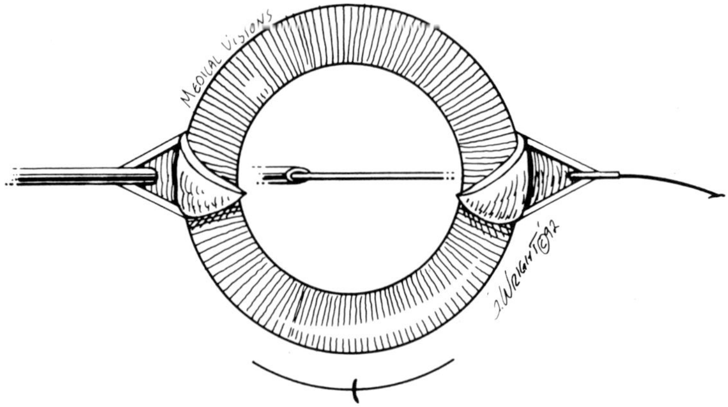

Fig. 6. Overhead view of the eye following translimbal removal of the PDIOL. Sclerotomies and the infusion port have not been included in the drawing for schematic simplicity. A straight needle bearing the 10-0 prolene has been passed through the temporal scleral flap bed 0.5 mm posterior to the surgical limbus and mated with the bore of the 28-gauge needle passed nasally.

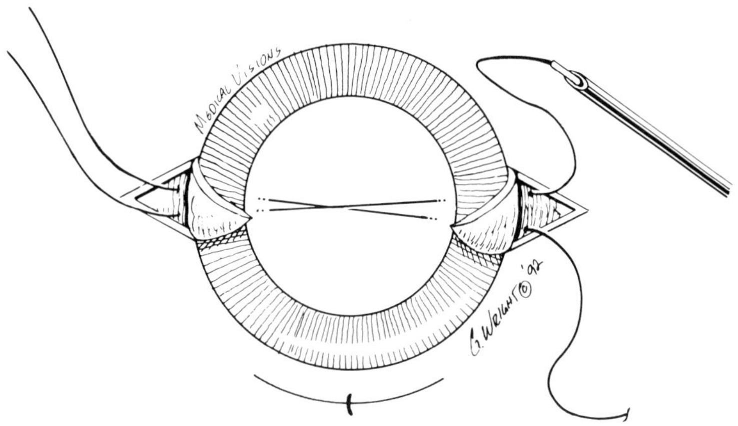

Fig. 7. The second pass has been completed, resulting in two transscleral sutures. Note the straight needle attached to the prolene and mated to the 28-gauge needle.

PDIOL repositioning

A 27-gauge needle originally designed for the placement of iris fixation sutures is used in all repositioning procedures[27]. This instrument, manufactured by TREK Medical Products, has a 7/1000-inch drill hole centered in the midportion of the needle bevel to accommodate suture material. A 10-0 prolene suture is folded at its midpoint, and the folded midpoint in turn passed through the drill hole to produce a loop approximately 2 mm in diameter (Fig. 2). The TREK needle is then passed transsclerally within the superior corner of the temporal flap bed at the level of the ciliary sulcus. The needle trajectory is perpendicular to the sclera. The IOL is grasped from the surface of the PFO with an intraocular microforceps inserted in the superonasal sclerotomy. The haptic of the stabilized IOL is engaged by the prolene loop (Fig. 3), and the TREK needle withdrawn from the eye. The prolene suture is disengaged from the TREK needle, and second transscleral prolene loop advanced to engage again the same haptic (Fig. 4). The two sutures are slowly pulled, drawing the haptic to its fixation point. The nasal haptic is similarly en-

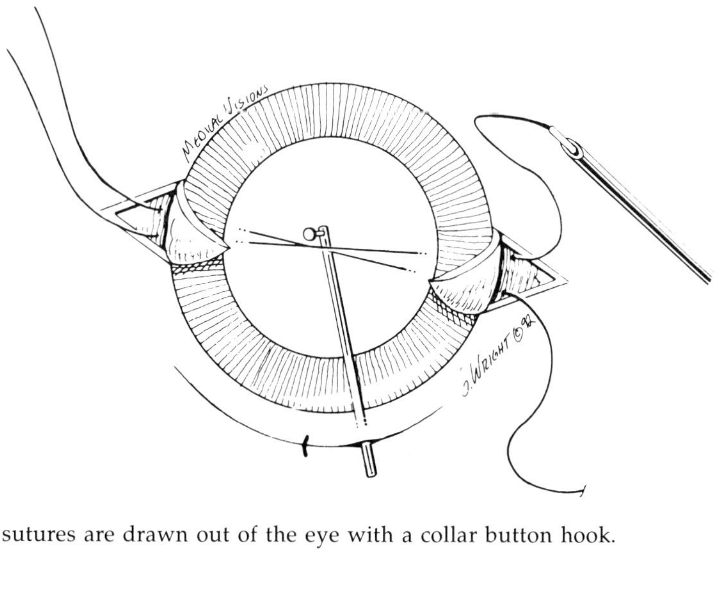

Fig. 8. The two sutures are drawn out of the eye with a collar button hook.

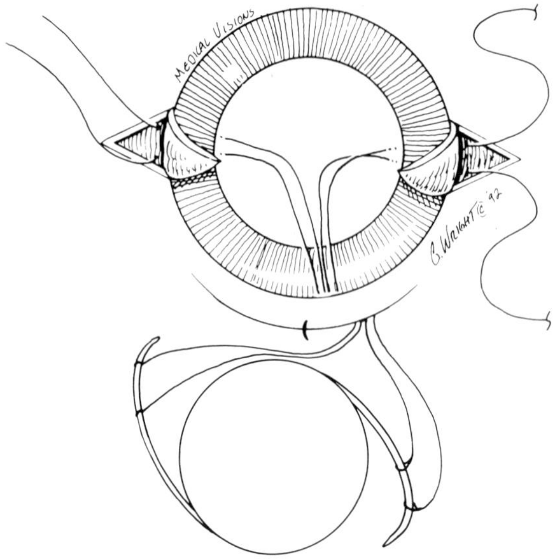

Fig. 9. The sutures have been cut, and each one tied to its respective haptic.

gaged and stabilized, ultimately resulting in four-point transscleral fixation of the IOL. The two suture pairs are tied to each other (Fig. 5). PFO is removed from the eye. The tip of the flap is sutured to the sclera with 10-0 nylon, and the knot buried.

PDIOL exchange

A scleral groove and an 8-mm chord length tunnel incision are made centered about the 12 o'clock meridian in anticipation of removal of a PCIOL with a 7-mm diameter optic. The pars plana infusion to the eye is momentarily clamped, and viscoelastic instilled into the anterior chamber. Intraocular microforceps are inserted into the eye via

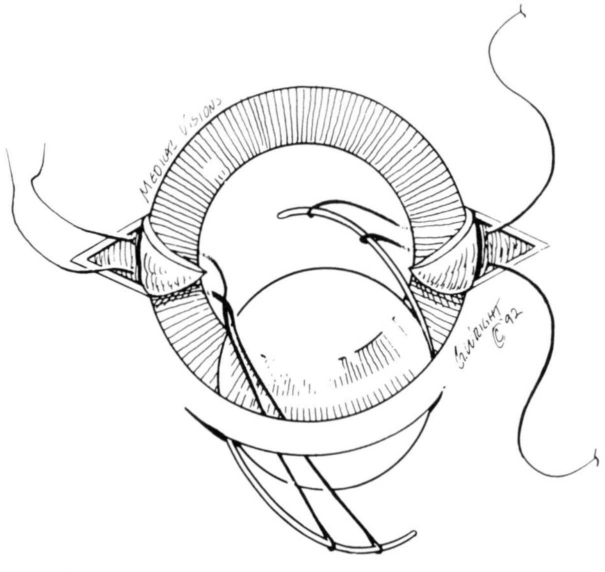

Fig. 10. The IOL is inserted into the eye with the haptics oriented towards 6 and 12 o'clock.

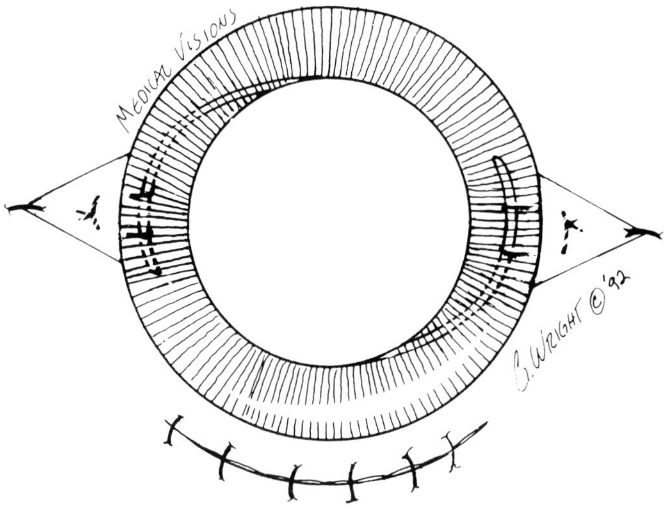

Fig. 11. The IOL has been rotated into position, the prolene sutures tied, and the scleral flap and corneal wound closed with 10-0 nylon.

the sclerotomies, the center of the optic is grasped, and the IOL is manipulated bimanually until the haptics are oriented in the 6 to 12 o'clock meridian. One pair of microforceps is then removed from the eye and exchanged for Kelman-Macpherson forceps. The superior IOL haptic is brought anterior to the iris to the internal aspect of the limbal incision. The superior scleral flap is elevated with the Kelman-Macpherson forceps, and the IOL haptic gently presented through the limbal incision. Infusion to the eye is resumed, and the IOL gently wrested from within the eye. A 10-0 nylon suture is placed at 12 o'clock and tied temporarily.

A straight needle bearing 10-0 prolene suture is inserted in the bed of the temporal scleral flap at the level of the ciliary sulcus with a needle holder. The needle trajectory is perpendicular to the sclera until the needle tip is within the eye, whereupon it is redirected parallel to the posterior iris plane. A 28-gauge needle is similarly passed from the nasal scleral flap bed. The proline bearing needle is mated to the 28-gauge needle and advanced as far as possible (Fig. 6). As the threaded 28-gauge needle is withdrawn from the eye, the proline suture will follow. This procedure is repeated, resulting in a double transscleral suture spanning the retropupillary space in the plane of the ciliary sulcus (Fig. 7).

Both proline strands are engaged from within the eye with a collar button hook, drawn out through the temporal aspect of the scleral tunnel (Fig. 8), and cut in half. The cut ends are each tied to their respective haptics, such that each haptic has two-point internal fixation to the eye wall (Fig. 9). Torsional IOL rotation about the axis of fixation is thereby minimized.

The temporary corneal suture is untied and drawn nasally. The IOL is inserted into the eye, with the haptic intended for the temporal ciliary sulcus entering first. Once both haptics are in the eye, oriented towards 6 and 12 o'clock (Fig. 10), the proline sutures are gently pulled through the sclera until the haptics are seated as desired. The proline sutures are tied. The temporary corneal suture is tied permanently. PFO is removed from the eye. Closure of the corneoscleral wound is completed with interrupted 10-0 nylon sutures. The tip of the flap is sutured to the sclera with 10-0 nylon, and the knot buried (Fig. 11).

We use posteriorly vaulted PCIOLs for exchange procedures to minimize posterior iris chaffing: either the Alcon CZ70BD (A-constant 118.9) or IOLAB FORMFLEX (A-constant

118.8). The former lens has a suture eyelet on each haptic, and is used by those who prefer single-point per haptic transscleral fixation. In such cases, a 10-0 prolene suture on a spatulated needle is passed through the base of the flap and tied to itself. The short end is tied to one end of the suture supporting the lens. The suture is rotated first in and then out of the eye, and the knot-bearing end cut. The resultant continuous prolene strand is then tied to itself.

Discussion

The most important decisions in the management of PDIOLs relate to issues regarding whether to exchange or reposit the IOL, lens choice for secondary placement, and selection of both the intended fixation plane and method of fixation.

Some authors have opted to replaced dislocated PCIOLs with anterior chamber lenses[11]. The relative advantages of posterior chamber intraocular lens implantation have been well documented[8]. While newer, open-loop multiflex style ACIOLs appear to be better tolerated than their closed-loop predecessors, the theoretical threat to the corneal endothelium over the long term renders their use in younger patients undesirable. Alternatively, luxated PCIOLs have been reposited in the anterior chamber[38]. Although reportedly well tolerated, the use of IOLs sized for retropupillary placement within the anterior chamber may be expected to result in iris chaffing and/or erosion into the anterior chamber angle structures.

When remaining capsular remnants are sufficient to support a posterior chamber lens, the implant can be reposited within the ciliary sulcus[16,32]. Some authors have suggested waiting two weeks postoperatively before repositioning to allow for the development of posterior capsular fibrosis[11].

When capsular support is felt to be inadequate for secure lens positioning, the implant may be affixed to surrounding ocular structures. Stark *et al.*[39] and Sternberg *et al.*[32] used modified McCannel iris fixation sutures[40] to support iris clip lenses and posterior chamber lenses, respectively. Problems inherent with these methods include difficulties in capturing the haptic and the iris in a transcorneal pass using a large needle, and in diametrically opposing the two fixation sutures. Furthermore, suturing the haptic to the iris can lead to persistent iris chaffing, cystoid macular edema, inflammation, bleeding, and problems with dilation[30]. Iris fixation is not a physiologically stable method of IOL suture fixation.

Transscleral suture fixation is currently the most widely employed technique for IOL repositioning and exchange procedures. The creation of scleral flaps[23,29] to minimize the risk of transconjunctival suture erosion and the development of endophthalmitis[41] has become a standard feature of such procedures. The lens haptic is selected for IOL fixation, although the use of lens optic position holes has been reported[28].

Various methods for securing the suture to the repositioned lens haptic have been described. We, and others[20,26], snare the haptic with an open loop of suture. Difficulty in engaging the lens haptic and suture slippage are potential complications of this technique. Hu *et al.*[23] and Chan[22] recommend externalization of the lens haptic to form a clubbed deformity at its distal end with cautery, whereupon the suture is tied to the implant under direct visualization.

There has been considerable debate in the literature as to whether transsclerally sutured IOLs are best fixated in the ciliary sulcus[16,19,20,22,28-30], pars plicata[25,26], or pars plana[4,24]. Ciliary sulcus fixation restores the PCIOL to its intended position, and offers the advantage of IOL stabilization in the event that the integrity of the prolene suture is compromised. Haptic placement at the pars plicata and pars plana confers no such advantage. Histopathologic studies have demonstrated that minimal fibrosis develops around transsclerally sutured IOL haptics, and that the fixation suture represents the primary means of lens support[36,37]. This observation underscores the importance of avoiding non-absorbable sutures, such as hydrolytically degradable nylon[18], for suture fixation procedures.

Multiple needle passes and complicated intraocular maneuvers characterize many of the procedures reported previously[16,20,21,30]. The risk to intraocular structures from *ab interno* transscleral needle passage include corneal endothelial touch, hemorrhage from ciliary body or iris trauma, and iatrogenic retinal tears and detachment[30]. Measured external fixation provides the best method, short of direct visualization, for precise, minimally traumatic suture and implant localization. Our choice of 0.5 mm posterior to the surgical limbus for suture placement is based on data from cadaver eyes localizing the ciliary sulcus at 0.46 mm in the horizontal meridian[11].

Conclusions

The ultimate goal in managing the patient with a posteriorly dislocated intraocular lens is a surgical result which is without complication, anatomically correct, and stable over time. We have presented above the techniques which we employ to this end. IOL repositioning, when feasible, is preferred over exchange. A lens anticipated to be either anatomically unstable or otherwise harmful to the eye over the long term is exchanged. Atraumatic IOL retrieval from the retinal surface is achieved using the liquid perfluorocarbon PFO. Maintenance of the IOL in the anterior vitreous cavity with PFO facilitates the execution of surgical maneuvers necessary for repositioning/exchange and protects the macula from contusive damage in the event that purchase on the IOL is not maintained. Scleral flaps and four-point IOL fixation with prolene sutures serve to minimize long-term postoperative complications such as suture erosion, endophthalmitis, and recurrent luxation. Posteriorly vaulted PCIOLs are utilized in exchange procedures to minimize iris chaffing. The ciliary sulcus is the preferred site of IOL haptic fixation.

References

1. Jaffe NS, Clayman HM, Jaffe MS, Light DS: The results of extracapsular cataract extraction with a shearing anterior chamber lens implant 34 to 40 months after surgery. Ophthalmic Surg 13:47, 1982
2. Kraff MC, Sanders DR, Lieberman HL: The results of posterior chamber lens implantation. J Am Intraocular Implant Soc 9:148, 1983
3. Kratz RP: Symposium: intraocular lenses: complications associated with posterior chamber lenses. Ophthalmology 86:659, 1979
4. Kratz RP, Mazzocco TR, Davidson B et al: The Shearing intraocular lens: a report of 1000 cases. J Am Intraocular Implant Soc 7:55, 1981
5. Southwick PC, Olson RJ: Shearing posterior chamber lenses: five-year postoperative results. J Am Intraocular Implant Soc 10:318, 1984
6. Stark WJ, Worthen DM, Holladay JT et al: The FDA report on intraocular lenses. Ophthalmology 90:311, 1983
7. Taylor DM, Dalburg LA, Consentino RT, Khalig A: Intraocular lenses: 500 consecutive intracapsular cataract extractions with lens implantation compared with 500 intracapsular extractions-observations and comments. Ophthalmic Surg 9:29, 1978
8. Worthen DM, Boucher JA, Buxton JN et al: Interim FDA report on intraocular lenses. Ophthalmology 87:267, 1980
9. Flynn HW: Pars plana vitrectomy in the management of subluxed and posteriorly dislocated intraocular lenses. Graefe's Arch Clin Exp Ophthalmol 225:169, 1987
10. Murphy GE: Traumatic dislocation of a Shearing lens 31 months after implantation. Ophthalmic Surg 14:53, 1983

11. Smiddy WE, Flynn HW: Management of dislocated posterior chamber intraocular lenses. Ophthalmology 98:889, 1991
12. O'Donnel FE, Santos B: Posterior capsular-zonular disruption in planned extracapsular surgery. Arch Ophthalmol 103:652, 1985
13. Flynn HW, Buus D, Culbertson WW: Management of subluxated and posteriorly dislocated intraocular lenses using pars plana vitrectomy instrumentation. J Cataract Refract Surg 16:51, 1990
14. Jakobi KW, Drey H: Surgical management of intraocular lens dislocation into the vitreous. J Am Intraocular Implant Soc 9:58, 1983
15. Balent A, Civerchia L, Mohamadi P: The double implant: alternative management for intraocular lens dislocation. J Cataract Refract Surg 12:79, 1986
16. Campo RV, Chung KD, Oyakawa RT: Pars plana vitrectomy in the management of dislocated posterior chamber lenses. Am J Ophthalmol 108:529, 1989
17. Flynn HW: Management and repositioning of posteriorly dislocated intraocular lenses. In: Stark WJ (ed) Anterior Segment Surgery: IOLs, Laser and Refractive Keratoplasty, Vol 15, pp 321-329. Baltimore: Williams and Wilkins 1986
18. Brod RD, Flynn HW, Clarkson JG, Blankenship GW: Management options for retinal detachment in the presence of a posteriorly dislocated intraocular lens. Retina 10:50, 1990
19. Liu KR, Peyman GA, Chen MS, Chang KB: Use of high density vitreous substitutes in the removal of posteriorly dislocated lenses or intraocular lenses. Ophthalmic Surg 22:503, 1991
20. Anand R, Bowman RW: Simplified technique for suturing dislocated posterior chamber intraocular lens to the ciliary sulcus. Arch Ophthalmol 108:1205, 1990
21. Bloom SM, Wyszynski RE, Brucker AJ: Scleral fixation suture for dislocated posterior chamber intraocular lens. Ophthalmic Surg 21:851, 1990
22. Chan CK: An improved technique for management of dislocated posterior chamber implants. Ophthalmology 99:51, 1992
23. Hu BV, Shin DH, Gibbs KA, Hong YJ: Implantation of posterior chamber lens in the absence of capsular and zonular support. Arch Ophthalmol 106:416, 1988
24. Insler MS, Mani H, Peyman GA: A new surgical technique for dislocated posterior chamber intraocular lenses. Ophthalmic Surg 19:480, 1988
25. Lyons CJ, Steele ADM: Report of a repositioned posteriorly dislocated intraocular lens via pars plicata sclerotomy. J Cataract Refract Surg 16:509, 1990
26. Maguire AM, Blumenkranz MS, Ward TG, Winkelman JZ: Scleral loop fixation for posteriorly dislocated intraocular lenses: operative technique and long-term results. Arch Ophthalmol 109:1754, 1991
27. Murray TG, Abrams GW, Stanley J: Pars plana vitrectomy in the management of dislocated posterior chamber lenses. Am J Ophthalmol 15:362, 1990
28. Nabors G, Varley MP, Charles S: Ciliary sulcus suturing of a posterior chamber intraocular lens. Ophthalmic Surg 21:263, 1990
29. Shin DH: Dislocated posterior chamber intraocular lens: a new technique of management. Arch Ophthalmol 108:777, 1990
30. Smiddy WE: Dislocated posterior chamber intraocular lens: a new technique of management. Arch Ophthalmol 107:1678, 1989
31. Stark WJ, Michels RG, Bruner WE: Management of posteriorly dislocated intraocular lenses. Ophthalmic Surg 11:495, 1980
32. Sternberg P, Michels RG: Treatment of dislocated posterior chamber intraocular lenses. Arch Ophthalmol 104:1391, 1986
33. Apple DJ: Intraocular Lenses: Evolution, Designs, Complications and Pathology. Baltimore: Williams & Wilkins 1989
34. Lewis H, Aaberg TM, Abrams GW, Han DP, Kreiger AE: Management of the lens capsule during pars plana lensectomy. Am J Ophthalmol 103:109, 1987
35. Duffey RJ, Holland EJ, Agapitos PJ, Lindstron RL: Anatomic study of transsclerally sutured intraocular lens implantation. Am J Ophthalmol 108:300, 1989
36. Apple DJ, Price FW, Gwin T, Imkamp E, Daun M, Casanova R, Hansen S, Carlson AN: Sutured retropupillary posterior chamber intraocular lenses for exchange or secondary implantation: The 12th Annual Binkhorst Lecture 1988. Ophthalmology 96:1241, 1989
37. Lubniewski AJ, Holland EJ, Van Meter WS, Gussler D, Parelman J, Smith ME: Histologic study of eyes with transsclerally sutured posterior chamber intraocular lenses. Am J Ophthalmol 110:237, 1990
38. Allara RD, Weinstein GW: A new surgical technique for managing sunset syndrome. Ophthalmic Surg 18:811, 1987

39. Stark WJ, Goodman G, Goodman D, Gottsch J: Posterior chamber intraocular lens implantation in the absence of posterior capsular support. Ophthalmic Surg 19:240, 1988
40. McCannel MA: A retrievable suture idea for anterior uveal problems. Ophthalmic Surg 7:98, 1976
41. Heilskov T, Joondeph BC, Olsen KR, Blankenship GW: Late endophthalmitis after transscleral fixation of a posterior chamber intraocular lens. Arch Ophthalmol 107:1427, 1989
42. Girard LJ: Pars plana phacoprosthesis (aphakic intraocular implant): a preliminary report. Ophthalmic Surg 12:19, 1981

VITRECTOMY IN CYSTOID MACULAR EDEMA

Mitchell D. Wolf and Gary W. Abrams

Department of Ophthalmology, Medical College of Wisconsin, Milwaukee, WI, USA

Abstract

Cystoid macular edema is a visually important disorder with a wide variety of specific causes. Fortunately, the vast majority of cases resolves either spontaneously or with medical therapy. Pars plana vitrectomy may be an effective treatment for CME after cataract surgery complicated by vitreous incarceration into the corneoscleral wound, chronic uveitis, diabetic macular edema due to traction by a thickened, attached posterior hyaloid, and in cases of subluxated or dislocated IOLs.

Introduction

Cystoid macular edema (CME) is a common cause of visual loss and occurs when perifoveal capillaries become abnormally permeable with resultant exudation and loss of visual function[1-7]. Common causes of CME include cataract extraction[1-7], diabetic retinopathy[8,9], uveitis[10-19] and subluxated or dislocated intraocular lenses (IOLs)[20,21]. These causes of CME have all been proven under specific circumstances to benefit from pars plana vitrectomy. Other causes of CME including retinal venous obstruction, retinal detachment, choroidal melanoma, tapetoretinal dystrophies, congenital juxtafoveal capillary telangiectasis, choroidal neovascularization, topical epinephrine, oral nicotinic acid, as well as familial, infantile, or idiopathic cases, have not been treated with vitreous surgery[7]. This paper will discuss the role of vitreous surgery in CME associated with cataract surgery, diabetic macular edema, chronic uveitis, and subluxated or dislocated IOLs.

Cataract surgery and cystoid macular edema

Postoperative CME may occur after all types of cataract surgery, when an IOL is placed or not[1-7]. Because 50-70% of patients following uneventful intracapsular cataract surgery have fluorescein angiographic evidence of perifoveal capillary leakage, some consider this a normal physiologic response to surgery[6]. More than 90% of those eyes have no biomicroscopic evidence of CME[6]. Approximately 5-15% of those with fluorescein angiographic leakage will develop visual loss secondary to CME following uncomplicated intracapsular cataract surgery[7]. Clinically significant CME most commonly occurs between

Supported in part by Core Grant EY01931-15 from the National Eye Institute/NIH, Bethesda, MD, and by an unrestricted grant from Research to Prevent Blindness, Inc., New York, NY

Address for correspondence: Gary W. Abrams, MD, 3535 West Thirteen Mile Road, Suite 632, Royal Oak, Michigan 48073, USA

Retina and Vitreous, pp. 283-291
Proceedings of the Symposium on Retina and Vitreous,
organized by the New Orleans Academy of Ophthalmology
New Orleans, LA, USA, March 12-15, 1992
edited by Rudolph M. Franklin

four and 12 weeks postoperatively, with reduction in visual acuity to the 20/30-20/70 level[6,7,22]. Mild symptoms of irritation or signs of anterior and posterior inflammation may be present. Circumlimbal conjunctival injection may also be present.

The incidence of clinically significant CME after intracapsular surgery without an IOL is 2%[23]. If similar surgery is performed and an iris-supported IOL is placed, the incidence rises to 9.9%, while following extracapsular cataract surgery with posterior chamber IOL implantation, the incidence is 1.3%[23]. The incidence of CME is greater in eyes with an anterior *versus* a posterior chamber IOL[24]. The incidence of clinically significant CME following phacoemulsification and "in-the-bag" posterior chamber IOL implantation is 0.5%, when pupillary distortion is absent[25]. In eyes with extracapsular cataract surgery with posterior chamber lens implantation, eyes with a primary posterior capsulotomy had a significantly greater incidence of fluorescein angiographic CME than those without a primary capsulotomy, although short-term visual acuity was not significantly different[26].

The mechanism of CME formation is not completely understood, although chronic anterior uveal irritation may produce a low-grade intraocular inflammation with subsequent perifoveal capillary leakage[27-29]. Vitreous aspirates show acute and chronic inflammatory cells in eyes with CME[28]. Intraocular inflammation on histopathologic examination, including iritis, cyclitis, vitritis, and retinal phlebitis has been found to correlate with the presence of macular edema[29]. Iridovitreal synechiae have been found strongly to correlate with CME. Almost all eyes with vitreous adherent to the wound have iridovitreal synechiae with subsequent pupillary distortion and chronic inflammatory cell infiltrates[29]. The histopathology of eyes with CME suggests that relief of iridovitreal traction is critical to resolution of inflammation and CME.

An anterior chamber IOL may trigger inflammation by pressing against the anterior surface of the iris or the ciliary body. Iris-supported IOLs can elicit chronic uveal inflammation by iris irritation and traction. Posterior chamber IOLs placed in the ciliary sulcus may also produce a low-grade ciliary body irritation and subsequent CME formation[25]. Pupillary distortion from a malpositioned IOL or from vitreous incarceration may be an additional source of chronic low-grade intraocular inflammation. Synechiae between remnants of the anterior lens capsule and the posterior surface of the IOL may also be associated with CME. It is likely that vitreous incarcerated into the corneoscleral surgical wound may induce CME by the resultant pupillary distortion and uveal inflammation rather than the vitreous incarceration *per se*. However, the exact nature of CME associated with vitreous incarceration is unknown. Retinal traction may play a role in some cases.

The indication for surgical treatment of aphakic or pseudophakic CME is failure of medical therapy in eyes with vitreous incarcerated into the corneoscleral wound, pupillary distortion secondary to a subluxated or dislocated IOL, or vitreous prolapse into the anterior chamber with specific vitreomacular traction. The latter situation in which vitreous traction on the macula can be identified biomicroscopically with a fundus contact lens is unusual. In all eyes, particularly those with a posterior chamber IOL "in-the-bag" and normal pupils, other causes of CME should be sought.

The vast majority of cases of aphakic CME are subclinical and visual acuity is minimally affected. Most patients are comfortable and spontaneous recovery usually occurs by the third postoperative month. In a small percentage of cases, the clinical course is more chronic and severe. These eyes may be photophobic, irritable, injected, and suffer central visual loss. Inflammatory cells may be present in the anterior and posterior vitreous. Typical CME can be identified clinically and by fluorescein angiography. The presence of vitreous incarceration in the corneoscleral wound and pupillary distortion are commonly found in this important subset of patients. Treatment of vitreous adherent to the corneoscleral wound has consisted of neodymium:YAG laser vitreolysis, and vitrectomy both by an anterior and a pars plana approach.

Neodymium:YAG laser vitreolysis

An alternative for the treatment of aphakic or pseudophakic CME as a consequence of vitreous incarceration into the corneoscleral surgical wound is incision of the vitreous strand with the Nd:YAG laser[30-34]. The laser is capable of photodisruption of non-pigmented structures and has been used both in the treatment of CME from vitreous incarceration and also as prophylaxis against CME in eyes with vitreous incarceration in the corneoscleral wound. Visual acuity has reportedly improved two lines or more in 40-100% of cases[30-34]. The larger series report an improvement in visual acuity of two lines or more in 83-89% of eyes[30-32]. Complete transection of the vitreous strand cannot always be achieved, although resolution of CME has been documented despite incomplete lysis[34]. Pupil abnormalities may resolve immediately following vitreolysis.

Complications occurring after YAG vitreolysis have included elevated intraocular pressure, transient corneal edema, and retinal detachment (in a previously traumatized eye)[30-35]. Prophylactic treatment with apraclonidine has been effective in preventing postoperative pressure elevation in argon laser trabeculoplasty, laser peripheral iridotomy, and Nd:YAG capsulotomy procedures. Use of this agent prior to and after Nd:YAG vitreolysis may also reduce the risk of postoperative pressure elevation[36,37].

The major advantage of Nd:YAG vitreolysis is the non-invasive nature of the procedure and the protection it offers from subsequent endophthalmitis and other complications of vitrectomy. It has less systemic risks than vitrectomy and can always be carried out as an outpatient procedure. Complete lysis of vitreous strands cannot always be achieved by the Nd:YAG laser. However, cases have also been reported of persistent vitreous strands following anterior or pars plana vitrectomy. Nd:YAG vitreolysis is ideally suited for those cases in which vitreous strands bridge from the margin of the pupil to the undersurface of the cataract wound without adherence to the surface of the iris. When vitreous membranes are adherent to the anterior surface of the iris, hemorrhage from the iris during treatment may obscure focus. Posterior iridovitreal adhesions are frequently involved in the etiology of CME after cataract surgery[29]. These adhesions cannot be addressed with the Nd:YAG laser and may require a vitrectomy procedure.

Anterior vitrectomy

Anterior or limbal vitrectomy has been demonstrated to relieve vitreous incarceration and improve visual acuity[22,27,38,39]. An early study which relied on anterior vitrectomy to remove incarcerated and anterior vitreous and to restore the pupil to a normal configuration produced visual improvement and relief of pain and photophobic symptoms in nine of 13 patients examined[27]. In a study of 15 eyes with chronic aphakic CME and vitreous adherent to the cataract incision with pupillary distortion or adherence of vitreous strands to the iris, an anterior vitrectomy was performed. Visual improvement of two lines or more occurred in 12 of 15 eyes[38]. Postoperative fluorescein angiography demonstrated improvement, but not complete resolution of CME. Other series have demonstrated improvement in visual acuity, macular edema, perifoveal capillary leakage, and symptoms of irritation and photophobia after anterior vitrectomy[22,39]. Visual acuity sometimes showed continued improvement for six months postoperatively.

Advocates of an anterior vitrectomy approach *versus* a pars plana approach suggest that the risk of retinal breaks and detachment may be less when entering through the limbus[22,27,38,39], although one postoperative retinal detachment has been reported following an anterior vitrectomy for vitreous incarceration and CME[40]. In addition, anterior vitrectomy is within the competence of many anterior segment surgeons, while the posterior approach usually is not. The ability to sweep along the anterior iris surface without distorting the pupil is enhanced with an anterior approach.

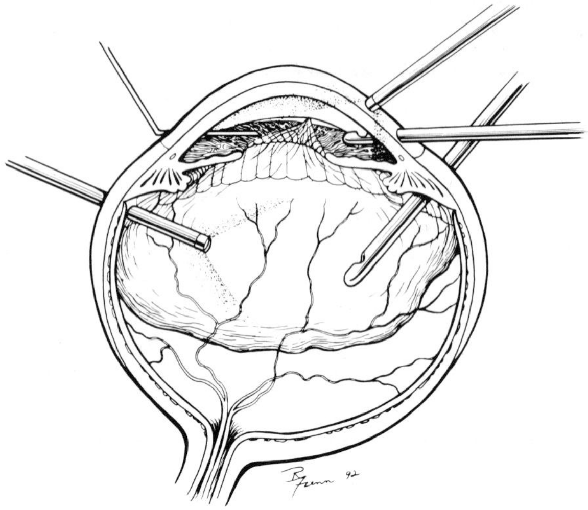

Fig. 1. Diagram of anterior (limbal) and posterior (pars plana) approaches for vitrectomy for vitreous incarcerated in cataract wound. The pars plana approach also has pars plana infusion (not shown). The posterior approach has endoillumination which improves visualization of vitreous and iridovitreal adhesions. The anterior approach includes limbal infusion with a 20-gauge needle. Visualization of vitreous is enhanced by holding an external fiberoptic light probe against the cornea.

There are several methods of anterior vitrectomy. A useful approach when using 20-gauge instrumentation is a bimanual technique with a 20-gauge infusion needle held in one hand, and a vitreous cutting instrument in the other. Visualization of the vitreous strands is enhanced by an external fiberoptic light pipe held near the cornea by the assistant (Fig. 1).

Pars plana vitrectomy

Pars plana vitrectomy has been proven to be of benefit in the treatment of CME, either alone or combined with anterior vitrectomy[22,39,39,41]. The major advantages of a pars plana approach include better visualization of vitreous strands by endoillumination, and the ability to lyse iridovitreal adhesions that may be involved in the pathogenesis of CME (Fig. 1). Disengagement of vitreous strands and sheets to the corneoscleral wound may be accomplished with either an anterior or posterior approach. When an IOL is in place, a separate limbal incision may be needed to transect the adherent vitreous to the corneoscleral wound. A study of 17 eyes using the pars plana approach demonstrated fluorescein angiographic and clinical improvement in 15 eyes. Visual improvement of two lines or more occurred in 13 eyes and of one line in another[41].

The Vitrectomy-Aphakic Cystoid Macular Edema (ACME) Study Group examined the natural history of ACME and compared translimbal vitrectomy, pars plana vitrectomy, and observation alone in 115 eyes in a multicenter, randomized, controlled clinical trial[22]. Each patient was initially followed for three months after a clinical and fluorescein angiographic diagnosis of ACME was made. Patients could be treated with topical corticosteroids or oral non-steroidal anti-inflammatory agents in a non-randomized fashion for a three-week period at least three months prior to randomization. Patients whose visual acuity was 20/70 or better or whose visual acuity had improved three lines or more at the end of this initial three-month period, were not randomized and were treated medically as the treating physician desired (observed group). Patients whose visual acuity was 20/80 or worse and who did not achieve a three-line improvement were randomized to control (no vitrectomy or medical therapy, one-third of patients) or vitrectomy (two-thirds of patients). Surgery consisted of a limbal vitrectomy, pars plana vitrectomy, or both.

Twenty-one percent of observed eyes with initial visual acuity of 20/70 or better achieved a final visual acuity of 20/40 or better, while only 4% of control eyes with initial visual acuity of less than 20/70 spontaneously improved to 20/40 or better. Of 43 eyes randomized to vitrectomy, 29 (67%) had a two-line improvement in visual acuity while only eight of 24 (33%) control eyes had a similar visual improvement.

The Vitrectomy-ACME Study Group demonstrated that a pars plana approach was more effective than a limbal approach ($p = 0.05$). The patients receiving an anterior vitrectomy improved by a mean of 0.47 lines *versus* 2.3 lines in the pars plana vitrectomy group. Although an equal number of eyes was randomized to each surgical group, six of eight eyes with the most dramatic visual recovery underwent pars plana vitrectomy. The reason that a posterior approach may be superior is unclear. Only five of 136 (3.6%) eyes initially evaluated had evidence of vitreous attachment to the macula on repeated contact lens examination. In fact, the posterior vitreous appeared to be detached in 88% of eyes. Therefore, vitreomacular traction did not appear to play a significant role in the pathogenesis of aphakic CME. It is possible that the pars plana approach may decrease chronic anterior inflammation more than the anterior approach because of more complete removal of vitreous adherent to the posterior surface of the iris, or because this method is more effective in removing intraocular substances which may be responsible for ACME. The Vitrectomy-ACME Study demonstrated the effectiveness of both anterior and posterior vitrectomy in the treatment of CME. Nearly 75% of control eyes received no medical therapy throughout the clinical trial. This study, therefore, compared surgical treatment *versus* observation, rather than surgical *versus* medical treatment. However, the natural history of ACME secondary to vitreous incarceration undergoing medical therapy alone is frequently poor over long periods of follow-up. Finally, the results of vitrectomy were not compared with the newer technique of Nd:YAG vitreolysis.

Eyes with varying durations of CME undergoing either anterior or posterior vitrectomy obtained visual improvement of a similar degree. Although significant visual improvement may occur despite chronic CME, atrophic macular pigmentary changes may limit visual recovery and explain the lack of visual improvement in some surgical failures.

Vitrectomy for diabetic macular edema due to vitreomacular traction

The Early Treatment Diabetic Retinopathy Study has demonstrated that focal macular photocoagulation is effective in the treatment of clinically significant macular edema[8]. Vitreous traction may have a role in the production or exacerbation of diabetic macular edema[42,43]. In a study comparing the prevalence of posterior vitreous separation between eyes with diabetic retinopathy with and without macular edema, the vitreous was detached in 11 of 20 eyes (55%) without macular edema, compared to 21 of 105 eyes (20%) with macular edema[42]. The finding of a significantly lower rate of posterior vitreous detachment in eyes with macular edema suggests that a posterior vitreous detachment may be somewhat protective.

An uncommon subset of eyes with diabetic macular edema possesses an intact, taut, unseparated premacular posterior hyaloid with resultant macular traction. Fluorescein angiography demonstrates intact perifoveal capillaries and a deep and diffuse pattern of macular leakage. A report of ten patients treated with pars plana vitrectomy and posterior hyaloidal separation showed visual improvement in nine eyes[9]. Nine of the ten eyes had previous macular photocoagulation and five had previous panretinal photocoagulation for proliferative diabetic retinopathy. It was noted intraoperatively that the posterior hyaloid was completely attached in eight eyes and there was partial posterior vitreous attachment, including attachment over the macula and optic nerve head, in the other two eyes. Following vitrectomy, the macular traction and edema resolved in eight eyes and decreased in the other two. Preoperative visual acuity ranged from 20/60 to 20/400 with seven eyes having a visual acuity of 20/100 or worse. Postoperative visual acuity was 20/60 or better in six eyes and 20/30 or better in three eyes. Postoperative complications included an epiretinal membrane, a rhegmatogenous retinal detachment and a vitreous hemorrhage, found in one eye each. Six eyes had mild progression of nuclear sclerosis which did not affect visual acuity, and two had moderate progression. One of the latter two underwent extracapsular cataract extraction with posterior chamber IOL implantation. Pars plana vitrectomy and posterior hyaloid separation may be beneficial in this distinct subset of patients with an attached and taut posterior hyaloid and diffuse macular edema.

Vitrectomy in uveitis

Cystoid macular edema commonly complicates either acute or chronic intraocular inflammation and is often the cause of long-term visual loss in these patients[10-19]. Nonspecific uveitis treatment consisting primarily of topical, periocular or systemic corticosteroids may result in improvement of both intraocular inflammation and CME. Eyes with failure of medical management of uveitis and complications of uveitis may be treated with pars plana vitrectomy. Conditions which may benefit from vitrectomy include cataract formation, cyclitic membrane formation, persistent vitreous opacification or hemorrhage, rhegmatogenous or tractional retinal detachment, and epiretinal membrane formation.

The relationship between pars plana vitrectomy and CME is unclear. Pars plana vitrectomy in the management of uveitis has most frequently been performed in intermediate uveitis. In a series of 42 eyes undergoing pars plana vitrectomy, 17 had CME at the time of surgery[17]. In 37 (88%) eyes, chronic inflammation quieted and episodes of exacerbation occurred less frequently and were less severe than prior to surgery. Regression of edema occurred in 14 of the 17 eyes with CME, and only one of the remaining 27 eyes without preoperative CME developed it in the postoperative period. In another series of 11 uveitis patients with intermediate uveitis with decreased vision from CME and no opacity of the visual axis, seven eyes experienced visual improvement and resolution of CME after vitrectomy[19]. Additional small series have documented reduction in CME and improvement in visual acuity in intermediate uveitis and other types of chronic uveitis[10-16,18]. Because media opacification is common, accurate preoperative assessment of CME may be difficult. In juvenile rheumatoid arthritis, both combined lensectomy and vitrectomy, as well as extracapsular cataract surgery with vitrectomy, have resulted in improvement of visual acuity[10,13,16]. Both modalities will clear media opacities due to cataract.

It is unclear whether the course of CME is altered differentially based on whether or not vitreous surgery is performed. Meticulous pre- and postoperative control of inflammation is mandatory in these patients. Although these studies of vitrectomy and chronic uveitis cannot prove a definite beneficial effect of vitreous surgery on CME, they all suggest an overall amelioration of the chronic inflammatory response after vitreous surgery. This diminution of chronic inflammation may explain the improvement in CME over the long term.

In vitrectomy for uveitis, care must be taken to avoid complications. Inflammation should be controlled perioperatively. Topical, periocular, or systemic corticosteroids are necessary in most cases. In eyes with chronic uveitis, especially those with intermediate uveitis, there may be peripheral fibrosis at the vitreous base with anterior retinal displacement. Creation of sclerotomy sites and instrument placement during vitrectomy can cause retinal breaks and detachment. Avoidance of areas of fibrosis when making sclerotomies and more anterior placement of the sclerotomies in some cases may help to minimize potential complications.

Vitrectomy for dislocated intraocular lenses

Dislocation of an IOL is an uncommon complication of cataract surgery. Most patients who experience dislocation of an IOL into the vitreous cavity retain good vision with the appropriate aphakic spectacle or contact lens. Complications of a dislocated IOL include CME, chronic inflammation, and retinal detachment.

Indications for surgical intervention include persistent CME with significant visual loss, or anterior segment inflammation caused by retained cortical lens material, by the malpositioned IOL, or by vitreous adherent to the cataract wound. Lens repositioning is also indicated when visual distortion is created by the posteriorly dislocated IOL in the visual axis, and with intolerance to alternative means of visual correction. In a series of nine eyes with posteriorly dislocated IOLs or anterior chamber IOLs subluxated into large basal peripheral iridectomies, four eyes had significant CME of 20/60 or worse. After pars plana vitrectomy and IOL repositioning or replacement, visual acuity improved to 20/40 or better in all cases. In addition, fluorescein angiography confirmed improvement of CME postoperatively compared to preoperatively[21].

The mechanism of CME formation in eyes with dislocated or subluxated IOLs is uncertain[44-46]. Some eyes had disruption of the anterior hyaloid and vitreous adherent to the inner aspect of the cataract incision. Chronic anterior segment inflammation may result from retained cortical lens material and a disrupted anterior hyaloid face following complicated cataract extraction. Simple excision of the inflammatory material independent of IOL repositioning may be the reason for improvement of CME in some cases.

A pars plana vitrectomy is performed with delivery of the IOL into the anterior or posterior chamber with an intraocular forceps[44-46]. Perfluorocarbon liquids may be useful for floating the IOL anteriorly and stabilizing it at the pupil during surgery[47,48]. The lens may be either repositioned or a limbal incision created and the IOL exchanged. Additional stabilization of a posterior chamber IOL may be obtained with a suture to fixate the lens to the iris, or with a transscleral suture to fixate the lens to the ciliary sulcus[44-46].

References

1. Irvine SR: A newly defined vitreous syndrome following cataract surgery, interpreted according to recent concepts regarding the vitreous. Am J Ophthalmol 36:599-619, 1953
2. Iliff CE: Treatment of vitreous-tug syndrome. Am J Ophthalmol 73:665-682, 1966
3. Gass JDM, Norton EWD: Follow-up study of cystoid macular edema following cataract extraction. Trans Am Acad Ophthalmol Otolaryngol 73:665-682, 1969
4. Wilkinson CP: A long-term follow-up study of cystoid macular edema in aphakic and pseudophakic eyes. Trans Am Ophthalmol Soc 79:810-839, 1981
5. Sternberg P Jr, Fitzke F, Finkelstein D: Cyclic macular edema. Am J Ophthalmol 94:664-669, 1982
6. Irvine AR, Bresky R, Crowder BM, Forster RK, Hunter DM, Kulvin SM: Macular edema after cataract extraction. Ann Ophthalmol 3:1234-1240, 1971
7. Gass JDM (ed): Stereoscopic Atlas of Macular Diseases: Diagnosis and Treatment, 3rd edn, pp 368-383. St Louis: CV Mosby 1987
8. Early Treatment Diabetic Retinopathy Study Research Group: Photocoagulation for diabetic macular edema: Early Treatment Diabetic Retinopathy Study Report No. 1. Arch Ophthalmol 103:1796-1806, 1985

9. Lewis H, Abrams GW, Blumenkranz MS, Campo RV: Vitrectomy for diabetic macular traction and edema associated with posterior hyaloidal traction. Ophthalmology 1992 (in press)
10. Diamond JG, Kaplan HJ: Lensectomy and vitrectomy for complicated cataract secondary to uveitis. Arch Ophthalmol 96:1798-1804, 1978
11. Diamond JG, Kaplan HJ: Uveitis: effect of vitrectomy combined with lensectomy. Ophthalmology 86:1320-1327, 1979
12. Smith RE, Kokoris N: Lensectomy-vitrectomy in chronic uveitis. Trans Am Ophthalmol Soc 81:261-275, 1983
13. Flynn HW, Davis JL, Culbertson WW: Pars plana lensectomy and vitrectomy for complicated cataracts in juvenile rheumatoid arthritis. Ophthalmology 95:1114-1119, 1988
14. Mieler WF, Will BR, Lewis H, Aaberg TM: Vitrectomy in the management of peripheral uveitis. Ophthalmology 95:958-864, 1988
15. Mieler WF: Closed vitrectomy and chronic uveitis. Sem Ophthalmol 4:1-7, 1989
16. Foster CS, Fong LP, Singh G: Cataract surgery and intraocular lens implantation in patients with uveitis. Ophthalmology 96:281-288, 1989
17. Eckhardt C, Bacskulin A: Vitrectomy in intermediate uveitis. In: Böke WRF, Manthey KF, Nussenblatt RB (eds) Developmental Ophthalmology, Vol 23, pp 232-238. Basel: Karger 1992
18. Heiman K, Schmanke L, Brunner R, Amerian B: Pars plana vitrectomy in the treatment of chronic uveitis. In: Böke WRF, Manthey KF, Nussenblatt RB (eds) Developmental Ophthalmology, Vol 23, pp 196-203. Basel: Karger 1992
19. Kaplan HJ: Surgical treatment of intermediate uveitis. In: Böke WRF, Manthey KF, Nussenblatt RB (eds) Developmental Ophthalmology, Vol 23, pp 185-189. Basel: Karger 1992
20. Sternberg P Jr, Michels RG: Treatment of dislocated posterior chamber intraocular lenses. Arch Ophthalmol 104:1391-1393, 1986
21. Flynn HW: Pars plana vitrectomy in the management of subluxed and posteriorly dislocated intraocular lenses. Graefe's Arch Clin Exp Ophthalmol 225:169-172, 1987
22. Fung WE: Vitrectomy for chronic aphakic cystoid macular edema: result of a national, collaborative, prospective, randomized investigation. Ophthalmology 92:1102-1111, 1985
23. Taylor DM, Sachs SW, Stern AL: Aphakic cystoid macular edema: long-term clinical observations. Surv Ophthalmol 28:437-441, 1984
24. Stark WJ Jr, Maumenee AE, Fagadau W, Dariles M, Baker CC, Worthen D, Klein P, Auer C: Cystoid macular edema in pseudophakia. Surv Ophthalmol 28:442-451, 1984
25. Fung WE: Aphakic cystoid macular edema. In: Ryan SJ (ed) Retina, Vol 2, pp 767-779. St Louis: CV Mosby 1989
26. Kraff MC, Sanders DR, Jampol LM, Peyman GA, Lieberman HL: Effect of primary capsulotomy with extracapsular cataract surgery on the incidence of pseudophakic cystoid macular edema. Am J Ophthalmol 98:166-170, 1984
27. Robinson D, Landers MB, Hahn DK: An anterior approach to aphakic cystoid macular edema. Am J Ophthalmol 95:811-817, 1983
28. Martin NF, Green WR, Martin LW: Retinal phlebitis in the Irvine-Gass syndrome. Am J Ophthalmol 83:377-386, 1977
29. McDonnell PJ, De la Cruz ZC, Green WR: Vitreous incarceration complicated cataract surgery. Ophthalmology 93:247-253, 1986
30. Katzen LE, Fleischman JA, Trokel S: YAG laser treatment of cystoid macular edema. Am J Ophthalmol 95:589-592, 1983
31. Katzen LE, Lapinsky PT, Fleischman JA, Trokel S: YAG laser treatment of cystoid macular edema: clinical update. Cataract 1:27-29, 1984
32. Steinert RF, Puliafito CA: In: Steinert RF, Puliafito CA (eds) The Nd:YAG Laser in Ophthalmology: Principles and Clinical Applications of Photodisruption, pp 115-123. Philadelphia: WB Saunders 1985
33. Levy JH, Pisacano AM: Clinical experience with Nd:YAG laser vitreolysis in anterior segment. J Cat Refract Surg 13:548-550, 1987
34. Tchach H, Rosenberg M, Larson RS, Lindstrom RL: Neodymium:YAG laser vitreolysis for treatment and prophylaxis of cystoid macular edema. Aust NZ J Ophthalmol 17:179-183, 1989
35. Nirankari VS, Richards RD: Complications associated with the use of the neodymium:YAG laser. Ophthalmology 93:1371-1375, 1985
36. Coleman AL, Robin AL, Pollack IP: Apraclonidine hydrochloride. Ophthalmol Clin North Am 2:97-108, 1989
37. Robin AL, Pollack IP, De Faller JM: Effects of topical ALO 2145 (p-aminoclonidine hydrochloride) on the acute IOP rise after laser iridotomy. Arch Ophthalmol 105:1208-1211, 1987

38. Federman JL, Annesley WH, Sarinik LK, Remer P: Vitrectomy and cystoid macular edema. Ophthalmology 87:622-628, 1980
39. Young PW, Shea MB: Pars plana vitrectomy in the management of the Irvine-Gass syndrome. Can J Ophthalmol 15:172-175, 1980
40. Fung WE: Anterior vitrectomy for chronic aphakic cystoid macular edema. Ophthalmology 87:189-193, 1980
41. Patel A, De Bustros S, Michels RG: Pars plana vitrectomy for aphakic cystoid macular edema. Retina 5:11-15, 1985
42. Nasrallah FP, Jalkh AE, Van Coppenolle F, Kado M, Trempe CL, McMeel JW, Schepens CL: The role of the vitreous in diabetic macular edema. Ophthalmology 95:1335-1339, 1988
43. Packer A: Vitrectomy for progressive macular traction associated with proliferative diabetic retinopathy. Arch Ophthalmol 105:1679-1682, 1987
44. Flynn HW: Management and repositioning of posteriorly dislocated intraocular lenses. In: Stark WJ (ed) Anterior Segment Surgery: IOLs, Laser, and Refractive Keratoplasty, Vol 15, pp 321-329. Baltimore: Williams & Wilkins 1986
45. Stark WJ, Michels RG, Bruner WE: Management of posteriorly dislocated intraocular lenses. Ophthalmic Surg 11:495-497, 1980
46. Stark WJ, Bruner WE, Martin NF: Management of subluxed posterior chamber intraocular lenses. Ophthalmic Surg 13:130-133, 1982
47. Shapiro MJ, Resnick KI, Kim SH, Weinberg A: Management of the dislocated crystalline lens with a perfluorocarbon liquid. Am J Ophthalmol 112:401-405, 1991
48. Liu K, Peyman GA, Chen M, Chang K: Use of high density vitreous substitute in the removal of posterior dislocated lenses or intraocular lenses. Ophthalmic Surg 22:503-507, 1991

VII

CURRENT CONCEPTS IN RETINAL DISEASES

CURRENT CONCEPTS CONCERNING CYSTOID MACULAR EDEMA

J. Donald M. Gass

Bascom Palmer Eye Institute, University of Miami School of Medicine, Miami, Florida, USA

There is a constant movement of water and electrolytes from the vitreous across the retina and choroid. In spite of this movement the retina is maintained in a relative state of deturgescence by physiologic pumps within the retinal capillary endothelium (inner blood-retinal barrier) and the retinal pigment epithelium (outer blood-retinal barrier) which prevents the accumulation of extracellular fluid within the sensory retina and the subretinal space[1b]. A breakdown in the endothelium results in accumulation of fluid in the extracellular spaces within the retina, particularly in the outer plexiform and inner nuclear layers. When this occurs in the macular area, it results in a characteristic polycystic swelling of the central macular area. The large central cysts in the nerve fiber layer of Henle are surrounded by progressively smaller cysts extending outward from the central foveolar area. The large central cysts compress the intervening nerve fibers which in the foveola area contain a heavy concentration of xanthophyll. If the retinal capillary leak is marked the flow of fluid outward may occasionally overload the RPE's ability to remove the fluid and a small localized serous retinal detachment may occur. An outer retinal yellow spot frequently seen posterior to the large central cysts biomicroscopically may be caused by increased visibility of the xanthophyll, either as the result of a small retinal separation or central displacement of the nerve fibers by the large cysts[1b,c]. If the RPE pump is damaged and the endothelium is intact, fluid begins to accumulate in the subretinal space. If both pumps are damaged, both CME and retinal detachment may result. While an ailing RPE may contribute to the maintenance of CME caused by endothelial dysfunction, there is little evidence to suggest that RPE dysfunction alone can cause CME.

The degree of endothelial dysfunction determines the nature of the extracellular exudation pooling within the retina. If the capillary leak is low grade, for example in aphakic CME, a clear serous exudation expands the extracellular spaces of the retina. If a high grade leak is present, such as often occurs in the congenital type of juxtafoveolar telangiectasis, a slightly cloudy exudate containing large lipids and proteins escapes into the retina. The protein is transported across the choroid and sclera. In the area of relatively normal retina surrounding the leaking capillaries the intraretinal and subretinal exudation is dehydrated as fluid is pumped back into the retinal vessels and into the choroid. As a result the lipids precipitate as yellow intraretinal and subretinal exudate often in a ring configuration. In rare conditions, such as CME caused by megadose ingestion of niacin, or in some patients with retinitis pigmentosa, there may be no angiographic evidence of capillary or RPE incompetence. It is uncertain whether this accumulation of extracellular fluid is caused by a low grade capillary leak, in which the fluorescein molecule is too large to permit it to escape through the endothelium, or is the result of osmotic forces caused by accumulation of extracellar products liberated by disturbed retinal cells.

Address for correspondence: J. Donald M. Gass, MD, Bascom Palmer Eye Institute, University of Miami School of Medicine, Miami, FL 33101, USA

Retina and Vitreous, pp. 295-297
Proceedings of the Symposium on Retina and Vitreous,
organized by the New Orleans Academy of Ophthalmology
New Orleans, LA, USA, March 12-15, 1992
edited by Rudolph M. Franklin

Whatever the cause, the CME disappears and function returns usually to normal after its discontinuance in the case of miacin maculopathy[2].

The biomicroscopic and stereoangiographic appearance of CME correlates closely to the histopathological findings, and it has been assumed that it was caused by extracellular fluid derived from incompetent retinal capillaries. Several years ago Fine and Brucker, as a result of electron microscopic study of formal in fixed eyes with CME, suggested that swollen Müller cells rather than extracellular fluid were responsible for the light microscopic and fluorescein angiographic picture of CME[3]. Gass and co-workers subsequently presented evidence to the contrary[4]. They examined electron microscopically an eye observed clinically and angiographically with CME just prior to its enucleation and fixation in glutaraldehyde in the operating room. They found that the cystic spaces were caused by extracellar fluid and not by swollen Müller cells.

The observations of Fine *et al.* suggest the possibility that in some cases intraretinal staining with fluorescein, particularly when it fails to show a polycystic appearance, may be caused by staining by ailing retinal cells. Such may be the case in some patients with diabetic retinopathy, retinitis pigmentosa, and the acquired form of bilateral juxtafoveal telangiectasis. This latter disorder is characterized by subtle biomicroscopic evidence of capillary telangiectasis, absence of CME, minimal lipid exudation and fluorescein staining of primarily the outer retina[1d]. Visual loss typically occurs slowly and is accompanied by progressive atrophy of the foveolar and central retina in the absence of cystoid swelling. Casswell *et al.* have suggested that the staining is at the level of the RPE[5]. These authors do not believe that stereoangiography is reliable in distinguishing staining at the level of the RPE from that occurring at the outer plexiform layer level. Other evidence that the staining is occurring within the retina is failure of the staining to occur in the foveolar area, the frequent development of prominent right-angle-venules draining the outer retinal capillaries, and the histopathologic and electronmicroscopic findings of Green *et al.*[6]. They examined the eyes removed from a patient with this disorder and found retinal capillary changes similar to that in diabetes, multiple small cystic expansions of the extracellar space in the sensory retina and no evidence of RPE changes.

In addition to niacin maculopathy there are other occasions where CME develops in the absence of evidence of retinal capillary permeability alterations. CME often develops in patients as choroidal neovascular membranes encroach upon the capillary-free zone. Although the explanation for this is unclear, it is probable that the progressive damage to the overlying RPE and loss of receptor cells accompanying choroidal neovascularization are important factors[1e]. Loss of receptor cells breaks the integrity of the outer limiting membrane that is composed of a system of tight junctions joining the receptor cells and Müller cells. Damage to this membrane, which is probably a mechanical barrier to passive movement of subretinal fluid into the retina, may be the primary cause of CME, not only in patients with subretinal neovascularization, but that which occurs occasionally in patients with chronic retinal detachment from other causes, *e.g.*, idiopathic central serous chorioretinopathy and choroidal hemangioma.

In summary, CME is a clinicopathologic name for thickening of the central retina caused by the expansion of the extracellular spaces of the retina by fluid. Although it is primarily caused by permeability changes in the retinal capillaries, in some patients it may occur in the absence of evidence of capillary abnormality. In such cases, it is postulated that it may be caused either by osmotically induced accumulation of fluid caused by extracellular materials released by diseased retinal cells, or by damage to the outer limiting membrane of the retina. While RPE dysfunction may contribute to the severity of CME, it probably rarely is the sole cause of CME.

The treatment of CME caused by leakage of retinal capillaries depends upon the cause of the leakage as well as the distribution of the affected capillaries. Anti-inflammatory agents are used in patients with CME caused by inflammatory disorders such as aphakic

CME and pars planitis. In the former patients, removal of vitreous incarcerated in the cataract wound, or removal of a malpositioned intraocular lens causing inflammation, may alleviate CME. Laser photocoagulation may be effective in reducing the edema and improving visual acuity in patients with CME caused by segmental parafoveal areas of capillary leakage, such as congenital retinal telangiectasis or secondary telangiectasis caused by branch retinal vein occlusion. Cox and co-workers have recently reported success in treating CME with oral acetazolamide, particularly those associated with tapetoretinal dystrophies and intraocular inflammation[7]. Chronic CME which occurs in 1% or less of patients with pseudophakia, and which occurs frequently in elder patients with senile vitritis, and bird-shot (vitiliginous) chorioretinitis, is often poorly responsive to treatment with anti-inflammatory agents.

References

1. Gass JDM: Stereoscopic Atlas of Macular Diseases. Vol 1, pp. (a)36-39, (b)368-373, (c)374-393, (d)384-397, (e)34-35. St Louis: CV Mosby Co 1987
2. Gass JDM: Nicotinic acid maculopathy. Am J Ophthalmol 76:500, 1973
3. Fine BS, Brucker AJ: Macular edema and cystoid macular edema. Am J Ophthalmol 92:466, 1981
4. Gass JDM, Anderson DR, Davis EB: A clinical fluorescein angiographic and electron microscopic correlation of cystoid macular edema. Am J Ophthalmol 100:82, 1985
5. Caswell AG, Chaine G, Rush P, Bird AC: Paramacular telangiectasis. Trans Ophthalmol Soc UK 105:683,1986
6. Green WR, Quigley HA, De La Cruz Z, Cohen B: Parafoveal telangiectasis. Trans Ophthalmol Soc UK 100:162, 1980
7. Cox SN, Hay E, Bird AC: Treatment of chronic macular edema with acetazolamide. Arch Ophthalmol 106:1190-1195, 1988

INVESTIGATION OF DISEASE MECHANISMS IN RETINITIS PIGMENTOSA

A.C. Bird

Department of Clinical Ophthalmology, Institute of Ophthalmology, Moorfields Eye Hospital, London, UK

Retinitis pigmentosa (RP) is the sole clinical manifestation of many genetically determined disorders. The degeneration is characterized by loss of dark adaptation and progressive loss of mid-peripheral visual fields early in disease, and may lead eventually to impairment of central vision. Although the disorders have different fundamental metabolic defects and there are both qualitative and quantitative differences between and within the genetic categories, there is also considerable similarity of behavior in RP as a group. Most patients have contiguous disease centered at 20-25° from the fovea, and more surprising is the report by Massof and Finkelstein that the time constant of visual loss as measured by Goldmann perimetry is identical in all forms of RP[1].

Over the last two decades there has been increasing investigative activity in the field of RP. Clinical studies have continued alongside research in retinal physiology and molecular biology undertaken in many centers; close contact has been maintained between clinicians, and pure and applied scientists. The early clinical work was directed towards identifying single nosological entities within RP or at least subdividing it into purer sample of disease. It is well recognised that there is variation of phenotype within a family. This implies that differences in functional deficit between two subjects cannot be assumed to be due to the effect of different genetic abnormalities but may be explained by the observations being made at different stages of the same disease or different phenotypic expression of the same genetic defect. In order to detect genetic heterogeneity, it was necessary to identify any characteristic which was common to all members of a family. If this attribute was absent in another family, it was reasonable to assume that the families had different genetic abnormalities responsible for their disease. It was also hoped that the nature of the deficit would give some clue as to the basic pathogenic defect or at least indicate the target cell of disease. However, this approach limits clinical research effectively to autosomal dominant and X-linked RP.

The advances in molecular biology whereby specific genomic defects have been identified, and in cell biology which demonstrate the influence of genomic defects on cell function, render the findings of clinical investigation much more significant. In the past the functional deficits in RP were of value in distinguishing one disorder from another or at least identifying categories of disease. It is now possible to relate these characteristics to putative disease mechanisms, and to generate hypotheses which are testable in the

A manuscript similar to this has been accepted for publication in *Ophthalmic Paediatrics and Genetics*, edited by M. Warburg

Address for correspondence: A.C. Bird, MD, FRCS, FCOphth, Department of Clinical Ophthalmology, Institute of Ophthalmology, Moorfields Eye Hospital, City Road, London EC1V 2PD, UK

Retina and Vitreous, pp. 299-307
Proceedings of the Symposium on Retina and Vitreous,
organized by the New Orleans Academy of Ophthalmology
New Orleans, LA, USA, March 12-15, 1992
edited by Rudolph M. Franklin

laboratory. It is also the case that observations are possible in man, particularly with respect to detailed recording of functional loss, which cannot be made in retinal degenerations in animals. Thus, the results of clinical and laboratory studies are relevant one to the other.

Clinical research

Genetic studies

The initial subdivision of RP was achieved on the basis of its inheritance. RP may be inherited as an autosomal dominant, autosomal recessive, or X-linked disorder, and there is good evidence from clinical and molecular biological studies of heterogeneity within each genetic subtype[2-13]. Autosomal dominant disease accounts for about 25% of the total number of patients with RP, X-linked disease 10-18% and the remainder is believed to be autosomal recessive.

Functional studies

By careful studies of visual function, considerable success has been achieved in that a basis for subdivision of RP has been established. In some disorders, the target cells have been identified, and the characteristics of functional loss indicate the nature of the disease mechanism.

Two broad categories of RP have been identified which are designated as class I or "diffuse" and class II or "regional" forms[10-12]. The functional characteristics are consistent within families indicating genetic heterogeneity. In diffuse-RP families, members show widespread loss of rod function with relatively well preserved cone function at some stage in the evolution of their disease. Regional RP shows variation in the state of rod and cone function with severe losses of both systems in some regions and near normal function in others. In regional RP, loss of rhodopsin accounts for the reduction of sensitivity, but in diffuse RP there is more rhodopsin than would be predicted if reduced light absorption by visual pigment were responsible for sensitivity loss[10]. These findings imply that in regional RP loss of rod function is due to photoreceptor cell death, short outer segments or a combination of the two, while in diffuse disease RP this cannot be the case.

Additional variants have been identified in autosomal dominant disease. Sector RP, is characterized by retinal atrophy restricted to part of the fundus, and gross field loss is confined to the area of visual field corresponding to the involved retina. The rod and cone ERGs show mild reduction in amplitude with normal cone implicit times[3,7,14]. This pattern of disease is common to all affected members within a family irrespective of age suggesting that the disease, in contrast to other forms of autosomal dominant RP, is non-progressive or progresses very slowly.

In some families there is slow recovery from bleach[15,16]. Cone adaptation and the early part of the recovery of rod sensitivity follow the normal time course, but the later phase of rod adaptation is markedly prolonged.

The expressivity in some families is highly variable such that about 70% of members with the abnormal genotype have moderate to severe disease while the remainder are destined to be asymptomatic, mild fundus abnormalities and electrophysiological changes indicating the presence of the abnormal gene[17]. There appears to be bimodal expression of disease though the factors which modulate the gene expression are unknown.

Specific clinical subtypes of RP have also been recognised with autosomal recessive disease. RP has been described with preservation of the retinal pigment epithelium adjacent to the retinal arterioles, and unlike many patients with RP they are consistently hypermetropic[18,19].

A further variant comprises restricted pigmentation in the ocular fundus, cystoid macular changes resembling macular schisis, and distinctive electroretinographic abnormalities[20]. The rod ERG is unrecordable, maximal stimulus evokes a large response with very prolonged implicit time of the B-wave, photopic and scotopic responses are of similar magnitude, and the response is much larger when produced by short than by long wavelength. The last attribute was known as the enhanced S-cone response.

Attempts have been made to subdivide X-linked retinitis pigmentosa on the basis of differential affection of heterozygotes. Only a few of the early reports described retinal degeneration in females of families with X-linked disease[21,22], but profound visual loss in heterozygotes was reported by McKenzie in New Zealand[23]. In 1960 Kobayashi described a family with even more severe involvement of the female members, five heterozygous females having retinitis pigmentosa, 11 having some stigmata of the disease and at least four being normal[24]. No accurate comparative analysis was made of the severity of the disease between affected men and women, although it was stated that the females were more mildly affected that the males. From this information, it was concluded that there are three separate X-linked conditions: X-linked recessive, X-linked intermediate and X-linked dominant retinitis pigmentosa. However, subsequent experience indicates that there is considerable intrafamilial variation in the severity of the disease in heterozygotes, and that there is no justification for separating X-linked retinitis pigmentosa into different categories on the basis of the severity of the disease in women[25,26].

It does appear that the presence of a tapetal reflex in women heterozygous for the abnormal gene characterizes some families but not others[27], such that this sign appears to segregate X-linked RP into two categories on clinical grounds.

Genomic studies

The first gene transmitting RP to be localized is one for X-linked RP using a probe L1.28[4] which is on the short arm near the centromere. Subsequent studies have supported the original observation[28-30]. The first indication of an alternative locus was derived from the identification of a deletion at Xp21 in a child with retinitis pigmentosa, Duchenne's muscular dystrophy and X-chromosome linked granulomatous disease[31]; this is some distance more telemeric on the short arm than the locus for L1.28. Localization of a gene linked with retinitis pigmentosa to this higher site was supported by other studies[32,33]. The most likely interpretation of these results is that at least two loci exist for X-linked retinitis pigmentosa. There is no universal agreement concerning clinical differences between disease transmitted at the two loci although all families in which a tapetal reflex is seen in the heterozygotes belong to those in which the gene is at the more telemetric locus. The possibility of more than one abnormal allele at each locus has not been excluded; that not all families with disease transmitted at the telemetric site have a tapetal reflex would support this view.

In 1989 a locus for autosomal dominant retinitis pigmentosa was identified on the long arm of chromosome 3[34]. Three candidate genes exist close to the proposed site, and within a short time a proline/histidine mutation was detected at codon 23 of the rhodopsin molecule[5]. Since then, more than 30 genomic defects have been detected on the rhodopsin gene and it appears that this gene accounts for about 25% of autosomal dominant RP[6,35-37]. Most of the substitutions appear to be peculiar to a single family, although some, notably the mutation at codon 347, have been found in many parts of the world. The proline/histidine mutation at codon 23 was identified in a large proportion of subjects in the United States but not in other countries. There is now some evidence that RP patients with this mutation may form part of one large pedigree.

In several families with autosomal dominant RP, there is no linkage with markers in the long arm of chromosome 3[38], confirming heterogeneity of dominant disease, and it has now been shown that genes other than that for rhodopsin may be responsible for autosomal dominant disease[39-43]. One of these is the gene for peripherin which is of particular interest since it is this gene which is responsible for the retinal degeneration in the rds mouse.

Functional consequences of genomic mutations

In the families with autosomal dominant RP showing mutations of the rod opsin gene on chromosome 3, different patterns of retinal dysfunction have been demonstrated with different mutations[9,16,44-47].

In three mutations (proline to leucine at codon 347, lysine to glutamic acid at codon 296 which is the binding site for retinal, an isoleucine deletion at codon 255 or 256 in which rod and cone function has been tested), functional loss compatible with diffuse (Type I) autosomal dominant RP was identified. With all three mutations, poor night vision was consistently identified in early life and rod ERGs were severely reduced or unmeasurable. In those with measurable visual function, psychophysical testing showed rod function to be severely affected throughout the retina (with threshold elevations of more than 3 log units) even in younger individuals, while loss of cone function varied widely between families, and was less widespread and less severe than loss of rod function. In the most severely affected family (lys296glu), there was little visual function after the age of 30 years in most members. With the isoleucine deletion at codon 256 cone function was limited to the central 10° by the age of 25 years but little further loss occurred thereafter. Cone function was retained over most of the visual field until middle life in the 347 mutation despite widespread and severe early rod losses.

The functional abnormality in families with mutations threonine to arginine at codon 17, proline to histidine at codon 23, threonine to arginine at codon 58 and glycine to arginine at codon 106 is qualitatively similar with altitudinal distribution of disease and this attribute appears to be constant with the families[16,46,47]. This characteristic of disease is in marked contrast with that seen in patients with other rhodopsin mutations examined to date. Rod function is severely depressed in the superior field but is nearly normal in the inferior field. Cone sensitivity losses closely follow the rod losses. In this respect the pattern of disease resembles regional (Type II) RP.

An additional striking finding in these families with sectorial type RP is a characteristic abnormality in one component of the kinetics of dark adaptation following exposure to a bright light. Prior to bleaching, measurements made in the relatively intact portion of the visual field show mild threshold elevations of approximately one log unit. Following light adaptation there is a marked delay in the recovery of sensitivity. The initial portion of recovery mediated by cones and rods is normal. However by one hour, when in the normal subjects recovery of sensitivity is complete, these patients showed residual threshold elevations of 1-2 log units from the prebleach values. Even after nearly two hours thresholds are still elevated by more than 1.0 log unit. In two subjects it was found that the time course of this slow recovery of sensitivity was of the order at least 80-120 hours[16].

Using a model based upon primate data of rod outer segment length and turnover, it has been calculated that the delayed phase of the recovery of rod sensitivity following strong light adaptation could be due in part to formation of new disc membrane with its normal concentration of rhodopsin rather than *in situ* regeneration of photopigment[16]. The model requires that the outer segments are short as a result of RP, and that a major portion of the outer segment is shed following strong light adaptation.

These observations show that there are both quantitative and qualitative differences in the RP consequent upon different mutations on the rhodopsin gene.

Also important is that it has been shown for the first time that some forms of RP are due to defects of metabolic systems which are limited to the rod photoreceptor, and yet it is evident that loss of photopic function is consistently found in these disorders. No explanation exists to account for cone cell death. It is possible that cone loss occurs as a result of either a release of endotoxins by dying rods or the cones being metabolically dependent upon the presence of rods. It follows that loss of cone function, although important to the patient, is a secondary effect.

Comparison with biochemical findings from site directed mutagenesis

The mechanism by which alteration of the amino-acid sequence of the rod opsin molecule may influence rod photoreceptor function is unclear. Some observations on the behavior of the abnormal protein made in the laboratory allow predictions to be made concerning possible effects of the mutation on metabolic systems. For example, it has been shown that rhodopsin with a mutation at the 296 amino acid, which is the binding site for retinal, fails to form a complex with 11-cis-retinal and reacts constantly with transducin (D. Oprian, personal communication). It would be predicted from this observation that the retina may act as if it were in constant lighting and would not dark adapt.

More general concepts can be formulated on the basis of recently identified mechanisms of protein formation and the cellular handling of abnormal proteins produced by mutant genes. It is known that abnormal proteins may or may not pass from the rough endoplasmic reticulum to the Golgi apparatus and that this depends on the influence of the mutation upon molecular folding[48]. Those proteins that do not pass on may be destroyed or may accumulate in the rough endoplasmic reticulum which in turn may interfere with cell function[49-52].

From these considerations, it is predictable that the nature of cell dysfunction would depend upon the site of expression of the abnormal protein. If it is incorporated into the photoreceptor outer disc membrane, it may generate physical instability of the membrane if glycolysation on the N-terminal or the disulphide bond between the cysteine residues 110 and 187 were abnormal[53,54]. Transduction efficiency may be reduced by mutations near the c-terminal causing a reduction of sensitivity be due to a reduced signal. Abnormal association with 11-cis-retinal may destabilize rhodopsin and such that down-regulation of transduction may be negated causing an increase of background noise. These two possibilities could be distinguished one from another by clinical testing. The interaction of the abnormal with the normal protein may also influence function.

The fate of rhodopsin produced by rhodopsin genes with mutations found in human RP has been investigated[55,56]. COS and 293S cells transfected with various mutant rhodopsin genes may express rhodopsin on the plasma membrane, which is appropriate to the normal protein, or the abnormal protein may remain bound to intracellular membrane complexes depending upon the mutation. It was also found that some mutant forms of rhodopsin bind to 11-cis-retinal readily to produce chromophores whereas others did not. The abnormal proteins could be divided into distinct classes according to their behavior when compared to normal[56]. In class I mutations rhodopsin was expressed normally on the plasma membrane and bound 11-cis-retinal, creating a chromophore with an absorbance spectrum similar to that of rhodopsin. Biochemical class II showed little if any ability to form a pigment when exposed to 11-cis-retinal, inefficient transport to the plasma membrane, and low levels of cell surface localization. It was suggested that the pathogenic mechanism for biochemical class I mutants was interference with rhodopsin carboxyl terminal function while for biochemical class II mutants misfolded or unstable opsin was degraded in the endoplasmic reticulum before incorporation into the plasma membrane.

Several of the experimental mutations were identical to those found in forms of RP in which the functional deficit has been characterized. Of the mutations described above, Pro-347-Leu was designated as biochemical class I and the same mutation in man causes diffuse RP. The mutations Pro-23-His, Thr-58-Arg and Gly-106-Trp were designated as biochemical class II and in man are associated with regional RP, and all have latitudinal distribution of disease with slow recovery from strong light adaptation. The information to date shows striking confirmation of the fundamental differences in mechanism for the RP types which may be confirmed by functional studies in the other mutations.

It is clear that these studies are incomplete and that further work will produce more information. There are also many other questions which are amenable to investigation. In autosomal dominant disease the abnormality is produced in the heterozygous state. It is not known whether the disease is due to the product of the abnormal gene or shortage of product from the normal gene; both situations may exist. That mice transfected with a mutant rhodopsin gene develop retinal degeneration indicate that the first mechanism exist. The second possibility is illustrated in the rds mouse which has an abnormality on the peripherin gene[57,58]. Transgenic rescue has been achieved by insertion of a normal peripherin gene on a rhodopsin promoter implying that lack of normal copy is the cause of disease[59]. Retinal changes in the heterozygous rds mouse are compatible with this concept[60]. The relevance of this model to human disease is illustrated by the finding of mutations on the peripherin gene in ADRP[42,43].

Although there are both quantitative and qualitative differences in functional loss between families, the severity of disease varies considerably within families. We have the impression that there is more concordance of affection within sibships than might be expected by chance alone at least in some families. If this is shown to be the case, it would have implications as to the determination of the phenotype in autosomal dominant RP in which disease appears in the heterozygous state, and it would allow investigation of the potential influence of mechanisms such as genomic imprinting and allelic competition on phenotypic expression[61,62].

Conclusions

Although there has been a very rapid advance in the understanding of disease mechanisms in RP and there is every prospect that the expansion of knowledge will accelerate in the next few years, it is evident to the clinician and patients that these have not yet brought any great advance in therapy. Nevertheless some effects on clinical management are already evident. Genetic counselling in a family is undoubtedly simplified if the genomic abnormality is known. Advice as to visual prognosis may be made on a firmer basis if single nosological entities are recognizable by genomic studies. It is to be hoped that the knowledge which will result from extension of the current studies will give clues as to how more direct intervention may be possible for the patient who is diagnosed as having this disease.

References

1. Massof RW, Dagnelie G, Benzschawel T, Palmer RW, Finkelstein D: First order dynamics of visual field loss in retinitis pigmentosa. Clin Vision Sci Res 5:1-26, 1990
2. Arden GB, Carter RM, Hogg CR, Powell DJ, Ernst WJK, Clover GM, Lyness AL, Quinlan MP: Rod and cone activity in patients with dominantly inherited retinitis pigmentosa: comparisons between psychophysical and electroretinographic measurements. Br J Ophthalmol 67:405-418, 1983

3. Berson EL, Howard J: Temporal aspects of the electroretinogram in sector retinitis pigmentosa. Arch Ophthalmol 48:653-665, 1971
4. Bhattacharya SS, Wright AF, Clayton JF, Price WH, Phillips CT, McKneown CME et al: Close genetic linkage between X-linked retinitis pigmentosa and a restriction fragments length polymorphism identified by recombinant DNA probe L1.28. Nature 309:253-255, 1984
5. Dryja TP, McGee TL, Reichel E, Hahn IB, Cowley GS, Yandel DW et al: A point mutation of the rhodopsin gene in one form of retinitis pigmentosa. Nature 343:364-366, 1990
6. Dryja TP, McGee TL, Hahn LB, Cowley CG, Olsson JE, Reichel E et al: Mutations within the rhodopsin gene in patients with autosomal dominant retinitis pigmentosa. New Engl J Med 323:1302-1307, 1990
7. Fulton AB, Hansen RM: The relationship of rhodopsin and scotopic retinal sensitivity in sector retinitis pigmentosa. Am J Ophthalmol 105:132-140, 1988
8. Inglehearn CF, Jay M, Lester DH, Bashir R, Jay B, Bird AC et al: No evidence for linkage between late onset autosomal dominant retinitis pigmentosa and chromosome 3 locus D3S47 (C17): evidence for genetic heterogeneity. Genomics 6:168-173, 1990
9. Jacobson SG, Kemp CM, Sung CH, Nathans J: Retinal function and rhodopsin levels in autosomal dominant retinitis pigmentosa with rhodopsin mutations. Am J Ophthalmol 112:256-271, 1991
10. Kemp CM, Faulkner DJ, Jacobson SG: Rhodopsin levels in autosomal dominant retinitis pigmentosa. Invest Ophthalmol Vis Sci 29:1235-1241, 1988
11. Lyness L, Ernst W, Quinlan MP, Clover GM, Arden GB, Carter R, Bird AC: A clinical, psychophysical and electroretinographic survey of patients with autosomal dominant retinitis pigmentosa. Br J Ophthalmol 69:326-339, 1985
12. Massof RW, Finkelstein D: Two forms of autosomal dominant retinitis pigmentosa. Doc Ophthalmol 51:289-346, 1981
13. Ott J, Bhattacharya S, Chen JD, Denton MJ, Donald J, Dubay C et al: Localizing multiple X chromosome-linked retinitis pigmentosa loci using multilocus homogeneity tests. Proc Nat Acad Sci USA 87:701-704, 1990
14. Massof RW, Finkelstein D: Vision threshold profiles in sector retinitis pigmentosa. Arch Ophthalmol 97:1899-1904, 1979
15. Alexander KR, Fishman GA: Prolonged rod adaptation in retinitis pigmentosa. Br J Ophthalmol 68:561-569, 1984
16. Moore AT, Fitzke FW, Kemp CM, Arden GB, Keen TJ, Inglehearn CF, Bhattacharya SS, Bird AC: Dark adaptation kinetics in autosomal dominant sector retinitis pigmentosa due to rod opsin mutation. Br J Ophthalmol 76:465-469, 1992
17. Ernst W, Moore AT: Heterogeneity, anomalous adaptation and incomplete penetrance in autosomal dominant retinitis pigmentosa. In: Zrenner E, Krastel H, Goebel HH (eds) Research in Retinitis Pigmentosa, pp 115-120. Oxford: Pergamon Press 1988
18. Heckenlively JR: Preserved para-arteriole retinal pigment epithelium (PPRPE) in retinitis pigmentosa. Br J Ophthalmol 66:26-31, 1982
19. Porta A, Pierrottet C, Aschero M, Orzalesi N: Preserved para-arteriole retinal pigment epithelium retinitis pigmentosa. Am J Ophthalmol 113:161-164, 1992
20. Marmor MF, Jacobson SG, Foerster MH, Kellner U, Weleber RG: Diagnostic findings of a new syndrome with night blindness, maculopathy, and enhanced S-cone sensitivity. Am J Ophthalmol 110:124-134, 1990
21. Jassen O: Zur Erbbiologie der Retinitis Pigmentosa. Inaugural Dissertation, Munster in Westfalen, 1938
22. McQuarrie MD: Two pedigrees of heredity blindness in man. J Genet 30:147-153, 1935
23. McKenzie DS: The inheritance of retinitis pigmentosa in one family. Trans Ophthalmol Soc NZ 79-82, 1951
24. Kobayashi VA: Genetic study on retinitis pigmentosa. Jpn J Ophthalmol 7:82-88, 1960
25. Berson EL, Gouras P, Gunkel RD, Myrianthopoulos NC: Rod and cone responses in sex-linked retinitis pigmentosa. Arch Ophthalmol 81:215-225, 1969
26. Bird AC: X-linked retinitis pigmentosa. Br J Ophthalmol 59:177-199, 1975
27. Schappert-Kimmijser J: Les dégenerescences tapéto-rétiniennes du type X chromosomal aux Pay-Bas. Bull Soc Fr Ophtalmol 76:122-129, 1963
28. Friedrich U, Warburg M, Wieacker P, Wienker TF, Gal A, Ropers HH: X-linked retinitis pigmentosa; linkage with the centromere and a cloned DNA sequence from the proximal short arm of the X chromosome. Hum Genet 71:93-99, 1985
29. Mukai S, Dryja TP, Bruns GAP, Alridge JF, Berson EL: Linkage between the X-linked retinitis pigmentosa locus and the L1.28 locus. Am J Ophthalmol 100:225-229, 1985

30. Wright AF, Bhattacharya SS, Clayton JF, Dempster M, Tippett P, McKeown CME, Jay M, Jay B, Bird AC: Linkage relationships between X-linked retinitis pigmentosa and six short arm markers: exclusion of the disease locus from Xp21. Am J Hum Genet 41:635-644, 1987
31. Francke U, Ochs HD, DeMartinville B, Giacalone J, Lindergren V, Disteche C et al: Minor Xp21 chromosome deletion in a male associated with expression of Duchenne muscular dystrophy and McLeod syndrome. Am J Hum Genet 37:250-267, 1985
32. Nussbaum RL, Lewis RA, Lesko JG, Ferrel R: Mapping ophthalmological disease. II. Linkage of relationship of X-linked retinitis pigmentosa to X chromosome short arm markers. Hum Genet 70:45-50, 1985
33. Denton MJ, Chen JD, Serravalle S, Colley P, Halliday FB, Donal J: Analysis of linkage relationships of X-linked retinitis pigmentosa with the following Xp loci. L1.28, OTC, XJ-1.1, pERT87 and C7. Hum Genet 78:60-64, 1988
34. McWilliam P, Farrar GJ, Kenna P, Bradley DG, Humphries MM, Sharp EM, McConnell DJ, Lawler M, Sheils D, Ryan C, Stevens K, Daiger SP, Humphries P: Autosomal dominant retinitis pigmentosa (ADRP): localization of an ADRP gene to the long arm of chromosome 3. Genomics 5:619-622, 1989
35. Sung CH, Davenport CM, Hennessey JC, Maumenee IH, Jacobson SG, Heckenlively JR et al: Rhodopsin mutations in autosomal dominant retinitis pigmentosa. Proc Nat Acad Sci USA 88:6481-6485, 1991
36. Keen TJ, Inglehearn CF, Lester DH, Bashir R, Jay M. Bird AC, Jay B, Bhattacharya SS: Autosomal dominant retinitis pigmentosa: four new mutations in rhodopsin, one of them at the retinal attachment site. Genomics 11:199-205, 1991
37. Ingelhearn CF, Keen TJ, Bashir R, Jay M, Fitzke F, Bird AC, Crombie A: A complete screen for mutations on the rhodopsin gene in a panel of patients with autosomal dominant retinitis pigmentosa. Hum Biol Genet 1:41-45, 1992
38. Lester DH, Inglehearn CF, Bashir R, Ackford H, Esakowitz L, Jay M et al: Linkage to D3S47 (C17) in one large dominant retinitis family and exclusion in another: confirmation of genetic heterogeneity. Am J Hum Genet 47:536-541, 1990
39. Blanton SH, Heckenlively JR, Cottingham AW et al: Linkage mapping of autosomal dominant retinitis pigmentosa (RP1) to the pericentric region of human chromosome 8. Genomics 11:857-869, 1991
40. Farrar GJ, Jordan SA, Kenna P et al: Autosomal dominant retinitis pigmentosa; localization of a disease gene (RP6) to the short arm of chromosome 6. Genomics 11:870-874, 1991
41. Blanton SH, Heckenlively JR, Cottingham AW et al: Linkage mapping of autosomal dominant retinitis pigmentosa (RP1) to the pericentric region of human chromosome 8. Genomics 11:857-869, 1991
42. Farrar GJ, Kenna P, Jordan SA, Kumar-Singh R, Humphries MM, Sharp EM, Sheils DM, Humphries P: A three-base-pair deletion in the peripherin-RDS gene in one form of retinitis pigmentosa. Nature 354:478-480, 1991
43. Kajiwara K, Hahn LB, Mukai S, Travis GH, Berson EL, Dryja TP: Mutations in the human retinal degeneration slow gene in autosomal dominant retinitis pigmentosa. Nature 354:480-483, 1991
44. Fishman GA, Stone EM, Gilbert LD, Kenna P, Sheffield VC: Ocular findings associated with a rhodopsin gene transversion mutation in autosomal dominant retinitis pigmentosa. Arch Ophthalmol 109:1387-1393, 1991
45. Heckenlively JR, Rodrigues JA, Daiger SP: Autosomal dominant sectoral retinitis pigmentosa, two families with transversion mutation in codon 23 of rhodopsin. Arch Ophthalmol 109:84-91, 1991
46. Kemp CM, Jacobson SG, Faulkner DJ: Two types of visual disfunction in autosomal dominant retinitis pigmentosa. Invest Ophthalmol Vis Sci 29:1235-1241, 1988
47. Kemp CM, Jacobson SG, Roman AJ, Sung CH, Nathans J: Abnormal rod adaptation in autosomal dominant retinitis pigmentosa with Pro-23-His rhodopsin mutation. Am J Ophthalmol 113:165-174, 1992
48. Lodish HF: Transport of secretory and membrane glycoproteins form the rough endoplasmic reticulum to the Golgi. J Biol Chem 263:2107-2110, 1988
49. Carlson JA, Rogers BB, Sifers RN, Hawkins HK, Finegold MJ, Woo SL: Multiple tissues express alpha 1-antitrypsin in transgenic mice and man. J Clin Invest 82:26-36, 1988
50. Lippincott-Shwartz JL, Bonifacio JS, Yuan LC, Klausner RD: Degradation from the endoplasmic reticulum: disposing of newly synthesised protein. Cell 54:209-220, 1988
51. Klausner RD, Sitia R: Protein degradation in the endoplasmic reticulum. Cell 62:611-614, 1990

52. Cheng SH, Gregory RJ, Marshall J, Paul S, Souza SW, White GA, O'Riodan CR: Defective intracellular transport and processing of CFT is the molecular basis of most cystic fibrosis. Cell 63:827-834, 1990
53. Karnik SS, Sakmar TP, Chen HB, Khorana HG: Cysteine residues 110 and 187 are essential for the formation of correct structure in bovine rhodopsin. Proc Nat Acad Sci USA 85:8459-8463, 1988
54. Karnik SS, Khorana HG: Assembly and functional rhodopsin requires a disulphide bond between cysteine residues 110 and 187. J Biol Chem 265:17520-17524, 1990
55. Doi T, Molday RS, Khorana HG: Role of the intradiscal domain in rhodopsin assembly and function. Proc Nat Acad Sci USA 87:4991-4995, 1990
56. Sung CH, Schneider BG, Agerwal N, Papermaster DS, Nathans J: Functional heterogeneity on mutant rhodopsins responsible for autosomal retinitis pigmentosa. Proc Nat Acad Sci USA 88:8840-8844, 1991
57. Connell G, Boscom R, McInnes R, Molday RS: Photoreceptor cell peripherin is the defective protein responsible for retinal degeneration slow (rds). Invest Ophthalmol Vis Sci (Suppl) 31:309, 1990
58. Travis G, Sutcliffe JG, Bok D: The retinal degeneration slow (rds) gene product is a photoreceptor disc membrane associated glycoprotein. Neuron 6:61-70, 1991
59. Travis G, Lloyd M, Bok D: Transgenic rescue of rod photoreceptors in rds mouse. Neuron 9:113-120, 1992
60. Hawkins RK, Jansen MG, Sanyal S: Development and degeneration of retina in rds mutant mice: photoreceptor abnormalities in the heterozygotes. Exp Eye Res 41:701-720, 1985
61. Moore T, Haig D: Genomic imprinting in mammalian development: a parental tug of war. Trends Genet 7:45-49, 1991
62. Willison K: Opposite imprinting of the mouse Igf2 and Igf2r genes. Trends Genet 7:107-109, 1991

UNUSUAL OCULAR COMPLICATIONS OF PREGNANCY

J. Donald M. Gass

Bascom Palmer Eye Institute, University of Miami School of Medicine, Miami, Florida, USA

Many physiologic alterations occur as part of normal pregnancy and they, along with pathological states peculiar to pregnancy, may be responsible for a variety of ocular disorders associated with loss of vision[1].

Idiopathic central serous chorioretinopathy

Patients during otherwise uncomplicated pregnancy may develop blurred vision, micropsia, and a positive scotoma in one or both eyes caused by serous detachment of the pigment epithelium and retina in the macular area[2,3]. This typically occurs during the last trimester of pregnancy. The detachment and the fluorescein angiographic findings are typical of that seen in young and middle-aged males with idiopathic central serous chorioretinopathy (ICSC). An unusual feature of the disorder in pregnant women is the presence of focal white subretinal exudate, probably fibrin, in the area of the pigment epithelium detachment or focal leak in over 90% of cases, compared to its incidence of only 10 to 15% of males with ICSC[3]. The exudate may be misinterpreted as focal retinitis, an ischemic retinal infarct, or subretinal neovascularization. Fluorescein angiography, which should not be necessary in most cases, usually shows intense fluorescein staining of the RPE detachment as well as the surrounding subretinal fluid. No treatment is necessary since the detachment resolves spontaneous soon after delivery or, in a few cases, beforehand. The cause of the high incidence of fibrinous exudation beneath the RPE and retina is unknown.

Valsalva hemorrhagic retinopathy

Either during pregnancy or during labor and delivery, the patient may experience sudden loss of vision caused by increased venous pressure associated with a Valsalva maneuver. Rupture of a superficial retinal capillary causes hemorrhagic detachment of the internal membrane, often in the macular area. The blood may dissect through the internal limiting membrane and cause a vitreous hemorrhage or may dissect externally to cause hemorrhagic retinal detachment. The prognosis for the spontaneous return of normal vision is good.

Macular detachment caused by benign choroidal tumors

During pregnancy alterations in hemodynamics may cause decompensation of the RPE overlying benign choroidal tumors including hemangiomas[4a,5] and osteomas[4b]. This usu-

Address for correspondence: J. Donald M. Gass, MD, Bascom Palmer Eye Institute, University of Miami School of Medicine, Miami, FL 33101, USA

Retina and Vitreous, pp. 309-310
Proceedings of the Symposium on Retina and Vitreous,
organized by the New Orleans Academy of Ophthalmology
New Orleans, LA, USA, March 12-15, 1992
edited by Rudolph M. Franklin

ally occurs during the second or third trimester and no treatment is required since the detachment typically resolves spontaneously soon after delivery. I have recently seen a woman who, during the third trimester, noted visual loss caused by a serous retinal detachment in the macula caused by a large partly pigmented tumor which was associated with an adjacent extensive zone of pigmentation of the pigment epithelium and bone-spicule migration of pigment into the overlying retina. This later suggested that in the distant past the tumor had caused a retinal detachment during its growth phase and that the detachment had spontaneously resolved. Ultrasonography revealed a highly reflective choroidal tumor atypical for a melanoma. The eye was enucleated and revealed a small spindle cell tumor compatible with a nevus. There were many dilated vascular spaces within the tumor. It is probable that vascular engorgement of this large benign tumor during pregnancy caused the serous macular detachment and that, had the patient been advised against enucleation, the retina would probably have re-attached spontaneously following delivery.

Post-partum Purtscher's-like retinopathy

During the first hours after either vaginal or Cesarian section delivery, the patient may experience rapid loss of vision in one or often both eyes associated with multiple large white ischemic inner retinal lesions and hemorrhages surrounding the optic disc in a pattern similar to that in Purtscher's retinopathy[4c,6]. Fluorescein angiography shows capillary non-perfusion corresponding with the areas of retinal whitening. A variety of prepartum complications including pancreatitis, toxemia, and oxytocin-induced labor have antedated this complication. The visual function often returns to near normal, but some evidence of optic atrophy may persist. The cause of this retinopathy is not known. Leukoembolization caused by abnormal aggregation of polymorphonuclear leukocytes stimulated by rapid elevation of complement C5A, has been postulated as the cause of Purtscher's retinopathy[4c,6,7]. This elevation has, however, not been demonstrated as yet in pregnant women with this disorder. Release of amniotic fluid or damaged placental tissue into the maternal circulation at the time of placental separation is a cause of activation of complement and has been associated with findings similar to Purtscher's retinopathy[8,9].

References

1. Sunness JS: The pregnant woman's eye. Surv Ophthalmol 32:219-238, 1988
2. Chumbley LC, Frank RN: Central serous retinopathy and pregnancy. Am J Ophthalmol 77:158, 1974
3. Gass, JDM: Central serous chorioretinopathy and white subretinal exudation during pregnancy. Arch Ophthalmol 109:677-681 1991
4. Gass JDM: Stereoscopic Atlas of Macular Diseases. Vol 2, pp (a)176, (b)178-179, (c)346-349, (d)558-559. St Louis: CV Mosby Co 1987
5. Pitta C, Bergen R, Littwin S: Spontaneous regression of a choroidal hemangioma following pregnancy. Ann Ophthalmol 11:772, 1979
6. Blodi BS, Johnson MW, Gass JDM, Fine SL, Joffe LM: Purtscher's-like retinopathy after childbirth. Ophthalmology 97:1654-1659, 1990
7. Jacob HS, Craddock PR, Hammerschmidt DE, Moldow CF: Complement-induced granulocytic aggregation: an unsuspected mechanism of disease. N Engl J Med 302:789, 1980
8. Chang M, Herbert WNP: Retinal arteriolar occlusions following amniotic fluid embolism. Ophthalmology 91:1634-1637, 1984
9. Hammerschmidt DE, Ogburn PL, Williams JE: Amniotic fluid activates complement: a role in amniotic fluid embolism syndrome? J Lab Clin Med 104:901-907, 1984

RETINOPATHY OF PREMATURITY

Sumit K. Nanda and Gary W. Abrams

Vitreoretinal Section, Eye Institute, Medical College of Wisconsin, Milwaukee, WI, USA

Introduction

Since Terry[1,2] first described an entity called "retrolental fibroplasia" in 1942, the management of this increasingly common retinal vascular disease of premature infants has been a challenge for the neonatologist and ophthalmologist alike. Within a decade after it was first described, retinopathy of prematurity (ROP) became the single largest cause of blindness in children in the United States; by the early 1950s, ROP cases exceeded all other causes of childhood blindness combined[3]. The incrimination of oxygen as the principal cause of ROP in the 1950s led to the practice of rigid curtailment of oxygen in the nursery and a reduction in the incidence of ROP followed. However, several reports subsequently reported that this strict restriction of oxygen had an adverse effect on premature infant morbidity and mortality rates. An increased incidence of deaths due to hyaline membrane disease and the idiopathic respiratory distress syndrome (RDS) were associated with this rigid oxygen restriction and the lack of arterial blood gas monitoring[4]. Consequently, in the late 1960s and 1970s there was a gradual trend towards the liberalization of oxygen use in neonatal intensive care units.

With recent advances in neonatology, more premature infants of low birth weight are surviving. Phelps[5] reported a greater than four-fold increase over earlier years in survival of infants weighing less than 1000 g. As ROP becomes an increasingly important clinical problem, there is renewed interest in its pathogenesis and therapy. In this treatise, we will describe the possible etiologies and pathogeneses, classification, and current medical and surgical therapies of ROP.

Incidence and risk factors

Prematurity, low birth weight, and supplemental oxygen are established risk factors for the development of ROP. In the Multicenter Trial of Cryotherapy for ROP[6], the incidence of ROP in 4099 infants weighing less than 1251 g was 65.8%; 81.6% of infants weighing less than 1000 g developed ROP to some degree. Earlier reports found an incidence of 52% in infants weighing between 501 and 1250 g[7,8]. In general, birth weight is inversely related to the incidence and severity of ROP[6,7,9-13]. Although the role of supplemental

Supported in part by Core Grant EY01931 from the National Eye Institute/NIH, Bethesda, MD

Dr. Nanda is a 1991-92 Heed Foundation Fellow

Address for correspondence: Gary W. Abrams, MD, Eye Institute, Medical College of Wisconsin, 8700 W. Wisconsin Avenue, Milwaukee, WI 53226, USA

Retina and Vitreous, pp. 311-322
Proceedings of the Symposium on Retina and Vitreous,
organized by the New Orleans Academy of Ophthalmology
New Orleans, LA, USA, March 12-15, 1992
edited by Rudolph M. Franklin

oxygen in increasing the incidence of ROP has been well documented clinically and experimentally[14-19], the occurrence of ROP does not appear to be related to arterial oxygen levels[7]. Moreover, the duration of supplemental oxygen therapy was unrelated to the incidence of ROP except in infants weighing more than 1500 g[12].

Vitamin E deficiency has been implicated as a possible risk factor for the development of ROP. However, results of studies evaluating the "antioxidant" properties of large doses of vitamin E in preventing ROP have been inconclusive[20-27]. Other possible risk factors associated with ROP include the following: cyanosis, apnea, prolonged parenteral nutrition, repeated blood transfusions, episodes of hypoxemia, hypercarbia, hypocarbia, mechanical ventilation, intraventricular hemorrhages, seizures, septicemia, anemia, patent ductus arteriosus, and xanthine administration[7,9-11,28-33]. Black infants appear to be less susceptible to ROP of all grades of severity than non-black infants[6].

Pathogenesis

The mode of retinal vascular development is key to understanding the possible pathogenesis of ROP. Michaelson[34] originally proposed that retinal capillaries arise by budding from pre-existent arteries and veins originating from the hyaloid vessels at the optic disc. Cogan and Kuwabara[35] suggested the budding of solid endothelial cords from the hyaloid vessels as the primary mechanism of retinal capillary formation. Ashton[36] suggested that the mesenchyme, the blood vessel precursor, grows from the optic disc through the nerve fiber layer to the retinal periphery. A fine meshwork of capillaries is presumably present on the posterior edge of the advancing mesenchyme. According to Ashton's theory, this fine meshwork of vessels then undergoes absorption and remodelling to develop into mature retinal vessels surrounded by the capillary meshwork.

Flynn *et al.*[31,37-39] offer the following hypothesis regarding the pathogenesis of ROP:

1. Injury to the endothelium occurs at the point where it differentiates from mesenchyme to form the primitive capillary meshwork. This phenomenon is analogous to that seen in Patz's kitten model in which a short duration of hyperoxia resulted in capillary damage to the most anterior and immature retinal vascular bed[40].
2. After injury to the vascular endothelium by some noxious agent(s), the few viable vascular channels unite to form a mesenchymal arteriovenous shunt. This shunt is located at the border between the avascular anterior retina and the vascularized posterior retina; it consists of a nest of primitive mesenchyme and maturing endothelial cells fed by mature arteries and veins. Flynn suggested that this structure represents the pathognomonic lesion of acute ROP[37]. When cells inside the shunt divide and differentiate into normal capillary endothelium, they form primitive endothelial tubes that project a "brush" border of capillaries into the avascular retina. This event allows regression of the disease. In progressive cases, however, the primitive cells inside the shunt proliferate and penetrate the internal limiting membrane (ILM) to grow on the retinal surface and into the vitreous cavity.

Foos describes a vanguard and rearguard of cells that contribute to the tissue changes of ROP[41,42]. The vanguard, or anterior component, contains spindle-shaped cells representing glia[35], while the rearguard consists of primitive endothelial cells. As the retina matures, the endothelial cells aggregate into cords and lumenize, becoming the primordial capillaries of the retina. The neovascularization of ROP presumably arises from these rearguard primitive endothelial cells. Foos noted that as the developing vessels reach their most anterior extent and mature, the spindle cells of the vanguard disappear.

Oxygen affects the immature kitten retinal vessels by inducing initial vasoconstriction and subsequent capillary closure[43]. Selective endothelial cell damage of immature vessels due to hyperoxia with sparing of the neural retina has been documented by electron microscopy[44]. After sustained hyperoxia is discontinued, a marked endothelial cell proliferation arises from the residual vascular complexes adjacent to the closed capillaries, leading to canalization and penetration through the ILM. An angiogenic factor has been implicated as the triggering mechanism for endothelial cell growth.

Most retinal detachments in ROP have a tractional as well as an exudative component[45]. Exudative detachments occur due to leaking new blood vessels; these detachments may resolve if the vessels spontaneously involute prior to the presence of significant traction (vitreous organization). However, if cellular migration and proliferation continues, predominantly tractional detachments occur. The effect of traction on the anterior avascular retina differs from that of the vascularized posterior retina[46]. The posterior retina is reinforced by larger vessels. Traction in this region readily causes detachment since these larger vessels are not stretchable. As traction is applied to the avascular anterior retina, however, the suction forces of the retinal pigment epithelium simultaneously keep the retina attached. The anterior retina stretches, and a peripheral trough develops with the most anterior retina attached and the more posterior retina detached.

Classification

The international classification of ROP adopted in 1984[47] categorizes the disease by location and severity. Anatomically, the retina is divided into three zones and the extent of the lesions is described by meridians (clock hours) involved. Zone I, the posterior pole or inner zone, is a circle centered on the disc that subtends an arc of 60 degrees. It extends from the disc to twice the distance from the disc to the center of the macula, in all directions from the disc. Zone II extends from the peripheral border of zone I to a circle tangen-

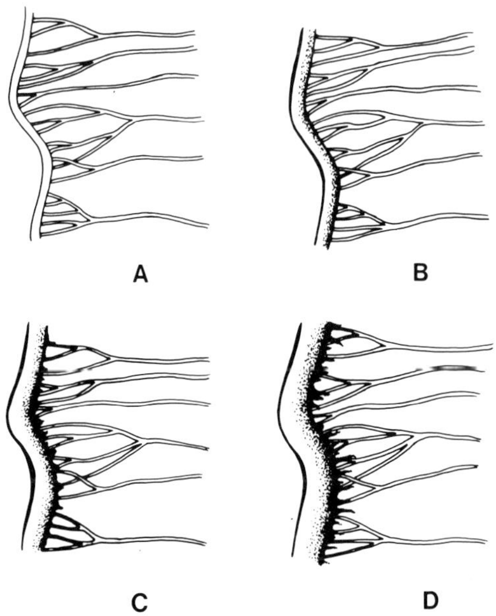

Fig. 1. Diagrams illustrating the patho-anatomy of ROP stages 1-3 based on the international classification. Vascular, more mature retina is depicted on the right and avascular retina is present on the left in the diagrams. *A.* Flat, white demarcation line of stage 1. *B.* Ridge extending anterior to the plane of the retina, characteristic of stage 2. *C.* Ridge associated with "mild" proliferation of extraretinal fibrovascular tissue (stage 3). *D.* "Moderate" proliferation of extraretinal fibrovascular tissue in more advanced stage 3. (Modified from: Patz A, Palmer EA: Retinopathy of prematurity. In: Ryan SJ (ed) Retina, Vol 2, Ch 84, pp 509-530. St. Louis: CV Mosby 1989. Permission granted.)

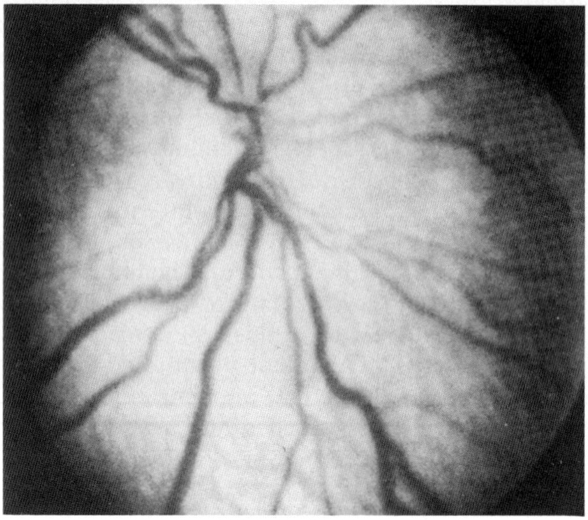

Fig. 2. Standard fundus photograph of threshold "plus" disease demonstrating increased retinal vascular dilation and tortuosity. (From: Cryotherapy for Retinopathy of Prematurity Cooperative Group: Multicenter trial of cryotherapy for retinopathy of prematurity. Preliminary results. Arch Ophthalmol 106:471-479, 1988. Copyright 1988, American Medical Association.)

tial to the nasal ora serrata and corresponds to the anatomic equator temporally. Zone III is the remaining temporal crescent of retina anterior to zone II. Zone III is the last region of the retina to become fully vascularized and is the most likely to be involved with ROP.

The severity of ROP is divided into five stages. Stage 1 is characterized by a demarcation line separating the anterior, avascular retina from the posterior, vascularized retina. The line is flat, white, and lies within the plane of the retina. In stage 2, this demarcation line develops height and width, occupies a volume, and extends anterior to the plane of the retina to form a ridge. Small tufts of new vessels may be present posterior to the ridge, but there is no fibrovascular growth from the surface of the ridge. In contrast, stage 3 is characterized by a ridge associated with extraretinal fibrovascular proliferation (Fig. 1).

Stage 4 is a partial retinal detachment and subclassified as 4A, with the macula attached, and 4B, with the macula detached. Extrafoveal retinal detachments (4A) are concave, traction-derived, and located in anterior zones II or III. They may be circumferential extending 360 degrees or segmental occupying only a portion of the circumference of the periphery. Partial retinal detachment involving the fovea is segmental and usually extends as a fold from the disc through zone I to zones II and III. Stage 5 implies a total retinal detachment which is funnel shaped. This funnel is subdivided into an anterior and posterior portion. When open both anteriorly and posteriorly, the detachment has a concave configuration and extends to the optic disc. Alternatively, the funnel may be narrow both anteriorly and posteriorly, and the detached retina is located just behind the lens. Less frequently, the funnel may be open anteriorly but narrow posteriorly. Least common is a funnel that is narrow anteriorly and open posteriorly.

"Plus" disease represents a more florid manifestation of ROP. It is characterized by increased dilation and tortuosity of retinal vessels, iris vascular engorgement, pupillary rigidity, and vitreous haze (Fig. 2). These clinical signs indicate progressive vascular incompetence and breakdown of the blood-retinal barrier.

Management

Non-surgical

The goals of managing infants with ROP are early detection of disease by careful screening and prevention of progression to retinal detachment (stages 4 and 5). We recommend screening all infants weighing 1250 g or less at four to six weeks of chronological age or 31-34 weeks of post-conceptional age (gestational age at birth plus chronological age)[6]. If ROP is absent during the initial screening, a repeat examination at biweekly intervals is advisable until vascularization proceeds to zone 3. If pre-threshold ROP (neovascularization with or without plus disease) is noted on initial examination, the infant should be re-examined at one to two week intervals until disease regression is documented. Infants with more severe disease should be examined more frequently than those with mild disease. Those near "threshold" (see following) should be re-examined within one week. If "threshold" ROP (Fig. 3) as defined by the Cryo-ROP trial (five or more contiguous or eight cumulative 30 degree sectors or clock hours of stage 3 ROP in zones 1 or 2 in the presence of plus disease) is present in one or both eyes, prompt treatment is recommended. The mean gestational age at birth of infants in the Cryo-ROP trial in whom disease reached threshold was 26.31 weeks; these data may serve to identify those infants who are at a higher risk of progression. Moreover, threshold was reached at a mean chronological age of 11.33 weeks, suggesting a postnatal time frame when close monitoring for progression is important.

Ablation of peripheral avascular retina is the mainstay of therapy of advanced ROP without retinal detachment. The recent three- and 12-month reports from the multicenter trial of cryotherapy for ROP demonstrated an anatomic and functional improvement in treated eyes[48-50]. Transscleral cryotherapy was applied circumferentially to the avascular retina anterior to and not including the ridge when threshold disease was identified (Figs. 4 and 5) At three months, there was an approximately 50% reduction in unfavorable events defined as the presence of a retinal fold involving the macula, a posterior retinal detachment, or a retrolental mass in the cryotherapy-treated group (31.1% of treated *versus* 51.4% of untreated eyes). Similar results were obtained at 12 months after randomization, when an unfavorable anatomic outcome was noted in 25.7% of treated eyes *versus* 47.4% of untreated eyes. Masked Teller Acuity Card assessment of grating acuity per-

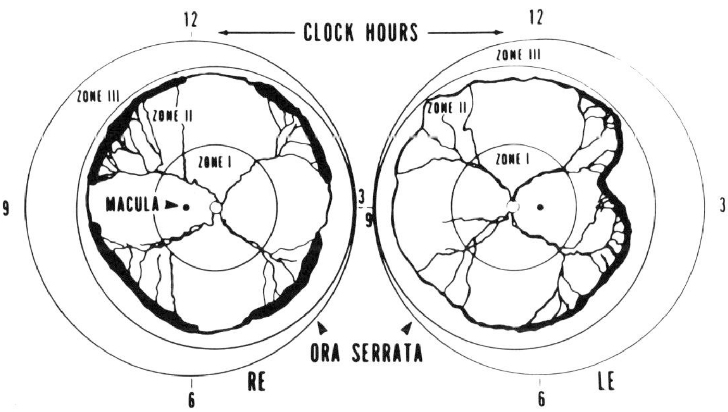

Fig. 3. Diagram of two representative eyes that have reached threshold ROP. Right eye (RE): at least eight cumulative 30-degree sectors (clock hours) of stage 3. Left eye (LE): at least five contiguous 30-degree sectors of stage 3. Thin line represents stage 1 or 2 ROP, and broader sketched line signifies stage 3 ROP. (From: Cryotherapy for Retinopathy of Prematurity Cooperative Group: Multicenter trial of cryotherapy for retinopathy of prematurity. Preliminary results. Arch Ophthalmol 106:471-479, 1988. Copyright 1988, American Medical Association.)

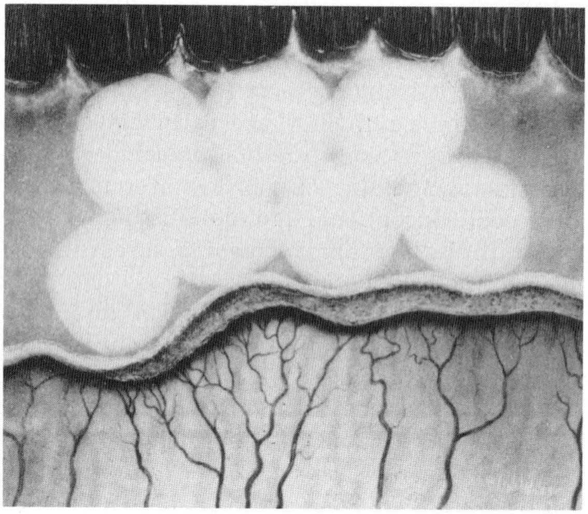

Fig. 4. Schematic illustration representing the avascular zone immediately following several applications of cryotherapy. The ideal spacing of freeze spots and relationship to ora serrata anteriorly and stage 3 ROP ridge posteriorly are shown. (From: Cryotherapy for Retinopathy of Prematurity Cooperative Group: Multicenter trial of cryotherapy for retinopathy of prematurity. Preliminary results. Arch Ophthalmol 106:471-479, 1988. Copyright 1988, American Medical Association.)

formed in the study group of 291 infants at 12 months revealed an unfavorable functional outcome in 35% of treated *versus* 56.3% of untreated eyes.

The rationale of cryotherapy is that treatment of avascular anterior retina causes regression of neovascularization. One hypothesis is that treatment obliterates the spindle cells in the avascular retina which secrete angiogenic factors; it may also injure the myofibroblasts which proliferate and contract to produce retinal distortion and detachment[51]. Another theory is that cryotherapy causes release of plasminogen activator inhibitors which may reduce neovascularization[52].

The most frequent ocular complication of cryotherapy reported in the multicenter trial[49] was retinal, preretinal, or vitreous hemorrhage, present in 22.3% of cases. Conjunc-

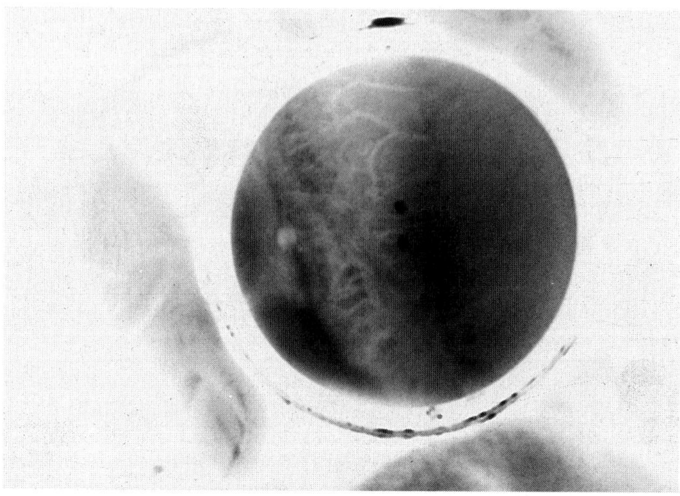

Fig. 5. Indirect ophthalmoscopic view of peripheral retina showing cryotherapy applications to avascular retina anterior to a ridge with extraretinal fibrovascular proliferation.

tival or subconjunctival hematomas were present in 11.7% of eyes and unintended conjunctival lacerations were noted in 5.3% of eyes. Transient closure of the central retinal artery was observed in one eye and inadvertent freezing to an area outside the target zone occurred in two eyes. Other complications consisted of a retinal break and dilation of the tunica vasculosa lentis in one case each. Long-term complications of cryotherapy are less well documented, but a recent report describes three patients who developed total rhegmatogenous retinal detachments one to four years following treatment[53]. In each case, a retinal tear was noted at the junction of the treated and untreated retina.

Systemic complications during administration of anesthesia and cryotherapy in the multicenter trial[49] consisted of bradycardia, arrhythmia, or apnea in 9.4% of cases; an additional 1.1% experienced cyanosis. Other complications including tachycardia, transient blood pressure changes, or hypoxemia were noted in 2.3% of infants; one infant (0.4%) had a seizure during therapy. In Brown *et al.*'s series[54] of 80 infants who underwent cryotherapy, four cases of respiratory arrest and one case of cardiorespiratory arrest were noted. They recommend the following measures to avert these systemic complications:
1. avoidance of excess subconjunctival anesthetic doses;
2. preoperative intravenous atropine administration to minimize the oculo-cardiac reflex;
3. preoperative systemic analgesia to minimize discomfort and exhaustion; and
4. close cardiorespiratory monitoring in a hospital setting.

The ability to administer laser photocoagulation to the peripheral avascular retina may minimize the above ocular and systemic complications of cryotherapy. Recent reports suggest that transpupillary argon laser photocoagulation is comparable to cryotherapy in preventing an unfavorable outcome in threshold ROP eyes[55-58]. Laser therapy may induce less full-thickness scleral and choroidal injury than cryotherapy. The extensive scarring of the retina, choroid, and sclera produced by cryoablation may predispose to late-onset rhegmatogenous retinal detachments[53]. As suggested by data from one series[58], laser therapy might reduce the incidence (22.3% in the Cryo-ROP trial) of hemorrhagic complications of cryotherapy. Furthermore, photocoagulation may reduce the amount of conjunctival scarring and eliminate the need for conjunctival incisions for posterior treatment. Laser treatment may obviate the need for general anesthesia which was required in 27.5% of cases in the Cryo-ROP trial; thus, we may be able to avoid the small but significant incidence (13.2%) of systemic complications associated with treatment in the Cryo-ROP study. A larger, prospective trial comparing these two treatment modalities (in terms of efficacy and complication rates) would be useful.

Indirect ophthalmoscopic diode laser photocoagulation may be a potentially useful modality in the treatment of "threshold" ROP. A preliminary study of seven infants with symmetric "threshold" ROP randomized to either cryotherapy or diode laser photocoagulation found disease regression in all treated eyes[59]. In our series of 15 "threshold" ROP eyes treated with indirect diode laser photocoagulation, complete regression was noted in all eyes at three months with no associated ocular or systemic complications[60].

The diode laser offers several advantages including compactness and portability. Transscleral delivery of the diode laser may be useful in some cases of ROP. While the small transscleral probe may be easier to use than a cryoprobe and allow more precise placement of burns because of the visible aiming beam, further study is needed before clinical use. Preliminary histopathologic studies of transscleral diode laser burns in the rabbit reveal inner scleral damage[61].

Surgical

Although the implementation of cryotherapy halves the risk of retinal detachment, 24.5% of infants in the Cryo-ROP trial still progressed beyond stage 3 despite therapy[50].

Two surgical techniques for retinal reattachment have been described: scleral buckling[62-65], and vitrectomy[66-74].

Although scleral buckling cannot release all circumferential and antero-posterior traction, it offers advantages over vitrectomy techniques in being less invasive and preserving the lens. Buckling need not be performed if the retinal detachment is confined to the periphery (stage 4A) and the disease is inactive, since spontaneous re-attachment may occur[75]. If the macula is detached (stage 4B), a circumferential flat 2 mm wide silicone band may be placed just posterior to the muscle insertions. If possible, the band should be localized to the area of the shunt. Although some authors advocate drainage of subretinal fluid, it is usually not necessary and the retina will re-attach in a short period of time. In addition, drainage can be risky in some eyes with posterior shunts in which the anterior retina remains attached. Despite the recent reports[64,65] of successful anatomic results for stages 4B and 5 (open funnel) retinal detachments treated by scleral buckling, functional outcome is still relatively poor. Greven and Tasman[64] reported a re-attachment rate of 100% in stage 4B and 48% in stage 5 eyes. Visual outcome better than 20/400 was achieved in 66% of Stage 4B eyes and 11% of stage 5 eyes. Noorily *et al.*[65] reported a 67% re-attachment rate for stage 4B eyes with a single scleral buckling operation, but only 20% of these infants achieved fix and follow acuities. The Advanced Retinopathy of Prematurity Study (AROPS) has been proposed to compare outcome between stage 4 and open funnel stage 5 eyes treated with a scleral buckle *versus* control eyes not treated with a scleral buckle.

Vitreous surgery is considered when preretinal and transvitreal proliferation prevent re-attachment of the retina with a scleral buckle and when vitreous opacities obscure the posterior retina. The surgical technique consists of lensectomy, vitrectomy with membrane peeling, and release of vitreoretinal traction. Both closed and "open sky" approaches are currently used. An advantage of closed vitrectomy over the open-sky approach is that it allows operating in a watertight globe with less anatomic distortion of the eye[46]. Open-sky vitrectomy may be necessary in eyes with opaque corneas[76]. In advanced cases, lensectomy is required since the lens is usually closely adherent to the fibrovascular tissue in the anterior vitreous. Moreover, since the infant eye has an incompletely developed pars plana, a relatively large crystalline lens, and an anteriorly pulled peripheral retina, a limbal or pars plicata entry is necessary to prevent iatrogenic retinal damage[46]. A recent report[77] describes lens-sparing vitreoretinal surgery utilizing a pars plicata approach and a dual-function endoillumination-vitreous infusion probe. The authors maintained phakia in infants by directing instruments away from the geometric center of the globe (in a line parallel to the visual axis) and by limiting surgical manipulation to the post-equatorial region.

Following lensectomy, using a two-handed technique, a central vertical slit is made in the retrolenticular membrane and extended using intraocular scissors. Trese[45] advocates use of healon during dissection but we and others infuse BSS plus during dissection. The retrolenticular tissue is then divided with forceps and scissors. After opening the center of the funnel, Trese describes a two-handed dissection of the posterior pole with careful dissection of tissue at the ridge and disc. Dissection and delamination of tissue at the ridge and in the anterior peripheral trough is then performed. Retinal breaks must be avoided, because residual traction will prevent retinal re-attachment if a retinal break is present. Usual techniques for treating retinal breaks are uniformly unsuccessful in eyes with ROP. External drainage of subretinal fluid may be performed if the retina is freely mobile and the base of the peripheral trough can be visualized. Tamponade with intraocular air or gas is sometimes used. Air injection with excessive pressure can tear the retina. If drainage of subretinal fluid appears risky, non-drainage may be an option since subretinal fluid usually resorbs spontaneously in several weeks. While drainage of subretinal fluid and injection of air or gas may speed retinal re-attachment, the risks must be weighed against the benefits. We usually do not drain subretinal fluid.

Anatomic success rates following vitrectomy range from 13-60%[73]. The prognosis for macular re-attachment following vitreous surgery is better for stage 4B compared to stage 5 eyes[72,78]. Macular re-attachment was accomplished in 64-83% of stage 4B eyes and only in 33-40% of stage 5 eyes. Moreover, 38% of stage 4B eyes achieved visual acuities of fixation and following or greater *versus* only 11% of stage 5 eyes[71]. Detachments with open or partially open funnels have a better prognosis for anatomic success[45,46,72]. In a recent study by Zilis *et al.* of 140 eyes, 63% of eyes with an open funnel both anteriorly and posteriorly were re-attached compared to 31% of eyes with a narrow funnel[72]. Reoperations only allowed re-attachment in 22% of cases and rarely improved visual outcome (4%)[72].

The appropriate timing of intervention is undetermined, but it is reasonable to await the resolution of active proliferation and "plus" disease. Anatomic success appears to be higher when surgery is performed after six months of age (61% *versus* 27%)[72].

Despite these encouraging results of anatomic outcome following surgery for stages 4B and 5 eyes, the visual prognosis is poor. Visual acuity data one year following surgery from 71 eyes which underwent vitrectomy for stage 5 ROP revealed only two eyes with pattern vision at the lowest measurable threshold[73,74]. None of the remaining eyes that underwent vitrectomy showed any evidence of pattern vision. Although better visual results were obtained in stage 4B and open funnel stage 5 eyes in the study by Zilis and co-workers[72], the results of surgery are still poor. Efforts must be directed towards arresting the disease prior to the development of retinal detachment.

References

1. Terry TL: Extreme prematurity and fibroblastic overgrowth of persistent vascular sheath behind each crystalline lens. 1. Preliminary report. Am J Ophthalmol 25:203-204, 1942
2. Terry TL: Fibroblastic overgrowth of persistent tunica vasculosa lentis in premature infants. 2. Report of cases-clinical aspects. Arch Ophthalmol 29:36-53, 1943
3. Patz A: The role of oxygen in retrolental fibroplasia. Trans Am Ophthalmol Soc 66:940-985, 1968
4. Avery ME, Oppenheimer EH: Recent increase in mortality from hyaline membrane disease. J Pediatr 57:553-559, 1960
5. Phelps DL: Retinopathy of prematurity: an estimate of vision loss in the United States-1979. Pediatrics 67:924-926, 1981
6. Palmer EA, Flynn JT et al: Incidence and early course of retinopathy of prematurity. Ophthalmology 98:1628-1640, 1991
7. Shohat M, Reisner SH, Krikler R et al: Retinopathy of prematurity: incidence and risk factors. Pediatrics 72:159-163, 1983
8. Reisner SH, Amir I, Shohat M et al: Retinopathy of prematurity: incidence and treatment. Arch Dis Child 60: 698-701, 1985
9. Bossi, Koenher F, Flury B, Zulali FM: Retinopathy of prematurity: a risk factor analysis with univariate and multivariate statistics. Helv Paediatr Acta 39:307-317, 1984
10. Gunn TR, Easdown J, Outerbridge EW, Aranda VJ: Risk factors in retrolental fibroplasia. Pediatrics 65:1096-1100, 1980
11. Hammer ME, Mullen PW, Ferguson JG et al: Logistic analysis of risk factors in acute retinopathy of prematurity. Am J Ophthalmol 102:1-6, 1986
12. Kinsey VE, Arnold HJ, Kalina RE et al: PaO2 levels and retrolental fibroplasia: a report of the cooperative study. Pediatrics 60:655-668, 1977
13. Patz A: Retrolental fibroplasia. Surv Ophthalmol 14:1-29, 1969
14. Lanman JT, Guy LP, Dancis J: Retrolental fibroplasia and oxygen therapy. JAMA 155:223-226, 1954
15. Patz A, Hoeck LE, De La Cruz E: Studies on the effect of high oxygen administration in retrolental fibroplasia. 1. Nursery observations. Am J Ophthalmol 35:1248-1253, 1952
16. Kinsey VE: Retrolental fibroplasia. Cooperative study of retrolental fibroplasia and the use of oxygen. Arch Ophthalmol 56:481-543, 1956
17. Ashton N, Ward B, Serpell G: Effect of oxygen on developing retinal vessels with particular reference to the problem of retrolental fibroplasia. Br J Ophthalmol 38:397-432, 1954

18. Ashton N, Ward B, Serpell G: Role of oxygen in the genesis of retrolental fibroplasia; a preliminary report. Br J Ophthalmol 37:513-520, 1953
19. Patz A, Eastham A, Higginbotham DH, Kleh T: Oxygen studies in retrolental fibroplasia. 2. The production of the microscopic changes of retrolental fibroplasia in experimental animals. Am J Ophthalmol 36:1511-1522, 1953
20. Johnson LH, Schaffer DB, Goldstein DE, Boggs TR: Influence of vitamin E treatment and adult blood transfusions on mean severity of retrolental fibroplasia (MS-RLF) in premature infants. Pediatr Res 11:535, 1977
21. Johnson L, Schaffer D, Boggs TR: The premature infant, vitamin E deficiency and retrolental fibroplasia. Am J Clin Nutr 27:1158-1171, 1974
22. Hittner HM, Godio LB, Rudolph AJ et al: Retrolental fibroplasia: efficacy of vitamin E in a double-blind clinical study of preterm infants. N Engl J Med 305:1365-1371, 1981
23. Phelps DL, Rosenbaum AL, Isenberg SJ, Leake RD, Dorey FJ: Tocopherol efficacy and safety for preventing retinopathy of prematurity: a randomized, controlled, double-masked trial. Pediatrics 79:489-500, 1987
24. Finer NN, Schindler RF, Peters KL, Grant GD: Vitamin E and retrolental fibroplasia: improved visual outcome with early vitamin E. Ophthalmology 90:428-435, 1983.
25. Puklin JE, Simon RM, Ehrenkranz RA: Influence on retrolental fibroplasia of intramuscular vitamin E administration during respiratory distress syndrome. Ophthalmology 89:96-103, 1982
26. Schaffer DB, Johnson L, Quinn GE, Weston M, Bowen FW: Vitamin E and retinopathy of prematurity: follow-up at one year. Ophthalmology 92:1005-1011, 1985
27. Institute of Medicine: Report of a study: Vitamin E and retinopathy of prematurity, pp 1-24. Washington DC: National Academy Press 1986
28. Aranda JV, Clark TE, Maniello R, Outerbridge EW: Blood transfusions (BT): possible potentiating risk factor in retrolental fibroplasia (RLF). Pediatr Res 9:362, 1975
29. Biglan AW, Brown DR, Reynolds JD, Milley JR: Risk factors associated with retrolental fibroplasia. Ophthalmology 91:1504-1511, 1984
30. Brown DR, Milley JR, Ripepi U, Biglan AW: Retinopathy of prematurity-risk factors in a five-year cohort of critically ill premature neonates. Am J Dis Child 141:154-160, 1987
31. Flynn JT: Retinopathy of prematurity. Pediatr Clin North Am 34:1487-1515, 1987
32. Majima A: Studies on retinopathy of prematurity. 1. Statistical analysis of factors related to occurrence and progression in active phase. Jpn J Ophthalmol 21:404-420, 1977
33. Procianoy RS, Garcia-Prats JA, Hittner HM, Adams JM, Rudolph AJ: An association between retinopathy of prematurity and intraventricular hemorrhage in very low birthweight infants. Acta Paediatr Scand 70:473-477, 1981
34. Michaelson IC: The mode of development of the vascular system of the retina with some observations on its significance for certain retinal diseases. Trans Ophthalmol Soc UK 68: 137-180, 1948
35. Cogan DG, Kuwabara T: Accessory cells in vessels of the perinatal human retina. Arch Ophthalmol 104:747-752, 1986.
36. Ashton N: Oxygen and the growth and development of retinal vessels: in vivo and in vitro studies. Am J Ophthalmol 62:412-435, 1966
37. Cantolino SJ, O'Grady GE, Herrera JA, Israel C, Justice J Jr, Flynn JT: Ophthalmoscopic monitoring of oxygen therapy in premature infants: fluorescein angiography in acute retrolental fibroplasia. Am J Ophthalmol 72:322-331, 1971
38. Flynn JT: Acute proliferative retrolental fibroplasia: evolution of the lesion. Graefe's Arch Klin Exp Ophthalmol 195: 101-111, 1975
39. Flynn JT, Bancalari E, Bachynski BN et al: Retinopathy of prematurity: a randomized, prospective trial of transcutaneous oxygen monitoring. Ophthalmology 94:630-638, 1987
40. Patz A: Oxygen studies in retrolental fibroplasia. 4. Clinical and experimental observations. Am J Ophthalmol 38:291, 1954
41. Foos RY: Acute retrolental fibroplasia. Graefe's Arch Clin Exp Ophthalmol 195:87-100, 1975
42. Foos RY: Retinopathy of prematurity-pathologic correlation of clinical stages. Retina 7:260-276, 1987
43. Patz A, Palmer EA: Retinopathy of prematurity. In: Ryan SJ (ed) Retina, Vol 2, Ch 84, pp 509-530. St Louis: CV Mosby 1989
44. Ashton N, Pedler C: Studies on developing retinal vessels. 9. Reaction of endothelial cells to oxygen. Br J Ophthalmol 46:257-276, 1962
45. Trese MT: Retinopathy of prematurity. In: Ryan SJ (ed), Vol 3, Ch 147, pp 551-563. St Louis: CV Mosby 1989

46. Machemer R, DeJuan E Jr: Retinopathy of prematurity: approaches to surgical therapy. Austral NZ J Ophthalmol 18:47-56, 1990
47. Committee for the Classification of Retinopathy of Prematurity: An international classification of retinopathy of prematurity. Arch Ophthalmol 102:1130-1134, 1984
48. Cryotherapy for Retinopathy of Prematurity Cooperative Group: Multicenter trial of cryotherapy for retinopathy of prematurity-preliminary results. Arch Ophthalmol 106:471-479, 1988
49. Cryotherapy for Retinopathy of Prematurity Cooperative Group: Multicenter trial of cryotherapy for retinopathy of prematurity: three month outcome. Arch Ophthalmol 108:195-204, 1990
50. Cryotherapy for Retinopathy of Prematurity Cooperative Group: Multicenter trial of cryotherapy for retinopathy of prematurity: one-year outcome: structure and function. Arch Ophthalmol 108:1408-1416, 1990
51. Kretzer FL, Mehta RS, Brown ES, Mintz-Hittner HA: The pathogenesis of retinopathy of prematurity as it relates to surgical treatment. Doc Ophthalmol 74:205-211, 1990
52. Trese M, Orgel I, Hartzer M, Williams GA, Chapman C: Intraocular plasminogen activator inhibitor-2 (PAI-2) levels in premature infant eyes. Invest Ophthalmol Vis Sci (Suppl) 33:1085, 1992
53. Greven CM, Tasman W: Rhegmatogenous retinal detachment following cryotherapy in retinopathy of prematurity. Arch Ophthalmol 107:1017-1018, 1989
54. Brown GC, Tasman WS, Naidoff M, Schaffer DB, Quinn G, Bhutani VK: Systemic complications associated with retinal cryoablation for retinopathy of prematurity. Ophthalmology 97:855-858, 1990
55. Landers MB III, Semple HC, Ruben JB, Serdahl C: Argon laser photocoagulation for advanced retinopathy of prematurity. Am J Ophthalmol 110:429-431, 1990
56. McNamara JA, Tasman W, Brown GC, Federman JL: Laser photocoagulation for stage 3+ retinopathy of prematurity. Ophthalmology 98:576-580, 1991
57. Iverson DA, Trese MT, Orgel IK, Williams GA: Laser photocoagulation for threshold retinopathy of prematurity. Arch Ophthalmol 109:1342-1343, 1991
58. Landers MB III, Toth CA, Semple NC, Morse LS: Treatment of retinopathy of prematurity with argon laser photocoagulation. Arch Ophthalmol 110:44-47, 1992
59. Hunter DG, Repka MX: Diode laser photocoagulation in retinopathy of prematurity (ROP): a randomized study. Invest Ophthalmol Vis Sci (Suppl) 33:1282, 1992
60. Wolf MD, Nanda SK, Arrindell EL, Mieler WF, Han DP, Abrams GW: Indirect diode laser photocoagulation for threshold retinopathy of prematurity. (in preparation)
61. Nanda SK, Arrindell EL, Han DP, Abrams GW: Transconjunctival diode laser retinal photocoagulation through silicone scleral exoplants: a histopathologic study. (in preparation)
62. Tasman W: Late complications of retrolental fibroplasia. Ophthalmology 86:1724-1739, 1979
63. McPherson A, Hittner AM, Lemos R: Scleral buckling in 2 1/2 to 11 month old premature infants with retinal detachment associated with acute retrolental fibroplasia. Ophthalmology 86:819-835, 1979
64. Greven C, Tasman W: Scleral buckling in stages 4B and 5 retinopathy of prematurity. Ophthalmology 97:817-820, 1990
65. Noorily SW, Small K, DeJuan E Jr, Machemer R: Scleral buckling surgery for stage 4B retinopathy of prematurity. Ophthalmology 99:263-268, 1992
66. Treister G, Machemer R: Results of vitrectomy for rare proliferative and hemorrhagic diseases. Am J Ophthalmol 84:394-412, 1977
67. Charles S: Vitreous surgery for retinopathy of prematurity. In: Syllabus: Retinopathy of Prematurity Conference. Washington, DC, 11:858-863, 1981
68. Schepens CL: Clinical and research aspects of subtotal open-sky vitrectomy. Am J Ophthalmol 91:143-171, 1981
69. Machemer R: Closed vitrectomy for severe retrolental fibroplasia in the infant. Ophthalmology 90:436-442, 1983
70. DeJuan E, Machemer R: Retinopathy of prematurity: surgical technique. Retina 7:63-69, 1987
71. Trese MT: Surgical therapy for stage V retinopathy of prematurity: a two-step approach. Graefe's Arch Ophthalmol 225:266-268, 1987
72. Zilis JD, DeJuan E, Machemer R: Advanced retinopathy of prematurity: the anatomic and visual results of vitreous surgery. Ophthalmology 97:821-826, 1990
73. Quinn GE, Dobson V, Barr CC et al: Visual acuity in infants after vitrectomy for severe retinopathy of prematurity. Ophthalmology 98:5-13, 1991
74. Kalina RE: Treatment of retinal detachment due to retinopathy of prematurity: a documented disappointment. Ophthalmology 98:3-4, 1991

75. Flynn JT, Bancalari E, Bachynski B et al: Retinopathy of prematurity: diagnosis, severity, and natural history. Ophthalmology 94:620-629, 1987
76. Tasman W, Borrone RN, Bolling J: Open-sky vitrectomy for total retinal detachment in retinopathy of prematurity. Ophthalmology 94:449-452, 1987
77. Maguire AM, Trese MT: Lens-sparing vitreoretinal surgery in infants. Arch Ophthalmol 110:284-286, 1992
78. Chong LP, DeJuan E, Machemer R: Vitrectomy for advanced stages of retinopathy of prematurity. Am J Ophthalmol 102:710-716, 1986

INDEX OF AUTHORS